Diabetes, Hematology/ Coagulation in Pregnancy

Editor

WINSTON A. CAMPBELL

CLINICS IN LABORATORY MEDICINE

www.labmed.theclinics.com

June 2013 • Volume 33 • Number 2

ELSEVIER

1600 John F. Kennedy Boulevard • Suite 1800 • Philadelphia, Pennsylvania, 19103-2899

http://www.theclinics.com

CLINICS IN LABORATORY MEDICINE Volume 33, Number 2
June 2013 ISSN 0272-2712, ISBN-13: 978-1-4557-7111-0

Editor: Patrick Manley

Reprints. For copies of 100 or more, of articles in this publication, please contact the Commercial Reprints Department, Elsevier Inc., 360 Park Avenue South, New York, New York 10010-1710. Tel. (212) 633-3813, Fax: (212) 462-1935, E-mail: reprints@elsevier.com.

Clinics in Laboratory Medicine (ISSN 0272-2712) is published quarterly by Elsevier Inc., 360 Park Avenue South, New York, NY 10010-1710. Months of issue are March, June, September, and December. Business and Editorial offices: 1600 John F. Kennedy Blvd., Suite 1800, Philadelphia, PA 19103-2899. Periodicals postage paid at NewYork, NY and additional mailing offices. Subscription prices are $240.00 per year (US individuals), $382.00 per year (US institutions), $129.00 per year (US students), $291.00 per year (Canadian individuals), $483.00 per year (Canadian institutions), $177.00 per year (Canadian students), $370.00 per year (foreign individuals), $483.00 per year (foreign institutions), $177.00 (foreign students). Foreign air speed delivery is included in all Clinics subscription prices. All prices are subject to change without notice. POSTMASTER: Send address changes to *Clinics in Laboratory Medicine*, Elsevier Health Sciences Division, Subscription Customer Service, 3251 Riverport Lane, Maryland Heights, MO 63043. **Customer Service: 1-800-654-2452 (US). From outside of the US and Canada, call 1-314-447-8871. Fax: 1-314-447-8029. E-mail: journalscustomerservice-usa@elsevier.com (for print support) or journalsonlinesupport-usa@elsevier. com (for online support).**

Clinics in Laboratory Medicine is covered in *EMBASE/Exerpta Medica, MEDLINE/PubMed (Index Medicus), Cinahl, Current Contents/Clinical Medicine, BIOSIS* and *ISI/BIOMED*.

Printed and bound by CPI Group (UK) Ltd, Croydon, CR0 4YY

Transferred to digital print 2012

Contributors

EDITOR

WINSTON A. CAMPBELL, MD
Professor, Obstetrics and Gynecology, Health Net Inc; Professor, Maternal-Fetal Medicine, Department of Obstetrics and Gynecology; Professor, Pediatrics; John Dempsey Hospital, University of Connecticut Health Center School of Medicine, Farmington, Connecticut

AUTHORS

NANCY DAY ADAMS, MD, FACP
Professor of Medicine, Chief of Nephrology, Training Program Director, Division of Nephrology, University of Connecticut Health Center, Farmington, Connecticut

TRACY M. ADAMS, DO
Maternal Fetal Medicine Fellow, Department of Obstetrics and Gynecology, Stony Brook-Winthrop University Hospitals; Clinical Assistant Instructor of Obstetrics and Gynecology, Stony Brook Medicine, Mineola, New York

M. BARAA ALLAF, MD
Maternal Fetal Medicine Fellow, Department of Obstetrics and Gynecology, Stony Brook-Winthrop University Hospitals; Clinical Assistant Instructor of Obstetrics and Gynecology, Stony Brook Medicine, Mineola, New York

BIREE ANDEMARIAM, MD
Assistant Professor of Medicine, Division of Hematology-Oncology, Lea Center for Hematologic Disorders; Director, Adult Sickle Cell Clinical and Research Center, University of Connecticut Health Center, Farmington, Connecticut

RAY BAHADO-SINGH, MD, MBA
Division of Maternal Fetal Medicine, Department of Obstetrics and Gynecology, Oakland University William Beaumont School of Medicine; Professor, Obstetrics and Gynecology, Oakland University William Beaumont Health System, Royal Oak, Michigan

PETER BENN, PhD, DSc
Professor, Department of Genetics and Developmental Biology, University of Connecticut Health Center School of Medicine, John Dempsey Hospital, Farmington, Connecticut

ADAM F. BORGIDA, MD
Associate Professor, Department of Maternal Fetal Medicine, Hartford Hospital, Hartford, Connecticut

SABRINA L. BROWNING, MD
Resident, Primary Care Internal Medicine, Yale University School of Medicine, New Haven, Connecticut

WINSTON A. CAMPBELL, MD
Professor, Obstetrics and Gynecology, Health Net Inc; Professor, Maternal-Fetal Medicine, Department of Obstetrics and Gynecology; Professor, Pediatrics; John Dempsey Hospital, University of Connecticut Health Center School of Medicine, Farmington, Connecticut

RICARD CERVERA, MD, PhD, FRCP
Department of Autoimmune Diseases, Hospital Clinic, Barcelona, Catalonia, Spain

KEITH A. EDDLEMAN, MD
Professor, Obstetrics, Gynecology and Reproductive Science; Professor, Genetics and Genomic Sciences; Director of Obstetrics, Icahn School of Medicine at Mount Sinai, New York, New York

GERARD ESPINOSA, MD, PhD
Department of Autoimmune Diseases, Hospital Clinic, Barcelona, Catalonia, Spain

YU MING VICTOR FANG, MD
Division of Maternal-Fetal Medicine, Department of Obstetrics and Gynecology, Hartford Hospital, Hartford, Connecticut

DEBORAH M. FELDMAN, MD
Division of Maternal-Fetal Medicine, Department of Obstetrics and Gynecology, Hartford Hospital, Hartford, Connecticut

KISTI P. FULLER, MD
Maternal Fetal Medicine Fellow, Department of Maternal-Fetal Medicine, John Dempsey Hospital, University of Connecticut, Farmington, Connecticut

JOSE A. GÓMEZ-PUERTA, MD, PhD
Department of Autoimmune Diseases, Hospital Clinic, Barcelona, Catalonia, Spain; Section of Clinical Sciences, Division of Rheumatology, Immunology and Allergy, Brigham and Women's Hospital, Boston, Massachusetts

PADMALATHA GURRAM, MD
Fellow, Maternal-Fetal Medicine, Department of Obstetrics and Gynecology, John Dempsey Hospital, University of Connecticut Health Center School of Medicine, Farmington, Connecticut

LALARUKH HAIDER, MBBS
Assistant Professor, Division of Nephrology, University of Connecticut Health Center, Farmington, Connecticut

KARI M. HOROWITZ, MD
Department of Maternal Fetal Medicine, University of Connecticut Health Center, Farmington, Connecticut

NAZLI HOSSAIN, MBBS, FCPS
Professor, Department of Obstetrics and Gynecology, Dow University of Health Sciences, Karachi, Pakistan

CHARLES J. INGARDIA, MD
Associate Professor, Department of Maternal Fetal Medicine, Hartford Hospital, Hartford, Connecticut

QUINETTA JOHNSON, MD
Resident, Department of Obstetrics and Gynecology, Oakwood Hospital and Medical Center, Dearborn, Michigan

THEODORE B. JONES, MD
Academic Chair, Department of Obstetrics and Gynecology, Oakwood Hospital and Medical Center, Dearborn, Michigan

MICHAEL D. LOCKSHIN, MD
Professor of Medicine and Obstetrics-Gynecology, The Barbara Volcker Center for Women and Rheumatic Disease, Hospital for Special Surgery, Weill Cornell Medical College, New York, New York

ANTHONY O. ODIBO, MD, MSCE
Department of Obstetrics and Gynecology, Washington University in Saint Louis, St Louis, Missouri

MICHAEL J. PAIDAS, MD
Professor, Baxter Clinical Fellowship Program, Yale Division of Maternal Fetal Medicine, Department of Obstetrics, Gynecology and Reproductive Sciences; Co-Director, National Hemophilia Foundation; Co-Director, Yale Women and Children's Center for Blood Disorders, Yale University School of Medicine, New Haven, Connecticut

SATYA POLAVARAPU, MD
Assistant Professor, Department of Maternal-Fetal Medicine, John Dempsey Hospital, University of Connecticut, Farmington, Connecticut

ANNE-MARIE PRABULOS, MD
Assistant Professor, Department of Maternal-Fetal Medicine, John Dempsey Hospital, University of Connecticut, Farmington, Connecticut

E. ALBERT REECE, MD, PhD, MBA
Vice President for Medical Affairs the John Z. and Akiko K. Bowers Distinguished Professor, and Dean of the School of Medicine, University of Maryland, Baltimore, Maryland

ZEYNEP ALPAY SAVASAN, MD
Assistant Professor, Division of Maternal Fetal Medicine, Department of Obstetrics and Gynecology, Oakland University William Beaumont School of Medicine, Royal Oak, Michigan

MOLLY J. STOUT, MD
Department of Obstetrics and Gynecology, Washington University in Saint Louis, St Louis, Missouri

NOEL K. STRONG, MD
Associate, Obstetrics, Gynecology and Reproductive Science, Icahn School of Medicine at Mount Sinai, New York, New York

GARRY TURNER, MD
Associate Professor, Department of Maternal-Fetal Medicine, John Dempsey Hospital, University of Connecticut, Farmington, Connecticut

ANTHONY M. VINTZILEOS, MD
Chairman, Department of Obstetrics and Gynecology, Winthrop University Hospitals; Professor of Obstetrics, Gynecology and Reproductive Medicine, School of Medicine, Stony Brook University, Mineola, New York

ZHIYONG ZHAO, PhD
Assistant Professor, Department of Obstetrics, Gynecology and Reproductive Sciences, University of Maryland School of Medicine, Baltimore, Maryland

Contents

fetal malformations and spontaneous abortion. Preconception counseling about risks of medications, control of comorbid conditions, stability of allograft function, and potential risks to mother, fetus, and allograft has to be done. Close and careful monitoring of mother, fetus, and allograft is important in ensuring a good outcome.

Maternal pregestational diabetes mellitus is a known risk factor for multiple nonchromosomal congenital anomalies, but there is no clear evidence that diabetes increases the risk for aneuploidy. However, diabetes affects maternal serum analyte concentrations that are used for aneuploidy screening and can alter the false-positive rates of the screening tests. Correction factors are used for women with pregestational diabetes for second-trimester serum analytes used in aneuploidy screening. There is considerable variation in the reported literature regarding the effect of diabetes on first-trimester serum analytes and how it might have an impact on aneuploidy screening.

Hemodynamic changes occur in pregnancy to prepare for expected blood loss at delivery. Physiologic anemia occurs in pregnancy because plasma volume increases more quickly than red cell mass. Anemia is most commonly classified as microcytic, normocytic, or macrocytic. Iron deficiency anemia accounts for 75% of all anemias in pregnancy. Oral iron supplementation is the recommended treatment of iron deficiency anemia in pregnancy. Parenteral iron and erythropoietin can also be used in severe or refractory cases. Outcomes and treatments for other forms of inherited and acquired anemias in pregnancy vary by disease, and include nutritional supplementation, corticosteroids, supportive transfusions, and splenectomy.

Life expectancy in sickle cell disease (SCD) has increased substantially and thus women with SCD are almost universally reaching child-bearing age. Studies on potential complications during pregnancy have generated mixed data; however, it is generally accepted that women with SCD are at higher risk for adverse pregnancy outcomes and maternal mortality. It is therefore critical that their care be provided by a team that includes a hematologist and a maternal-fetal medicine specialist. Despite the published risks, women with SCD are capable of successful pregnancy outcomes with proper education and well-coordinated multidisciplinary care. Further investigation is needed to standardize management.

Neonatal alloimmune thrombocytopenia (NAIT) is the most common cause of severe thrombocytopenia in the healthy newborn, occurring in 1 in 1000 live births. NAIT is analogous to rhesus alloimmunization in pathophysiology; however, it often presents unexpectedly in first pregnancies. Presentation of NAIT varies from mild thrombocytopenia to life-threatening intracranial hemorrhage. It has been observed to be more severe in subsequent affected pregnancies. It is important that the diagnosis of NAIT be considered in the work-up of all cases of neonatal thrombocytopenia to determine the risk to future pregnancies and corresponding management plans. This article discusses the pathogenesis and incidence of NAIT and the antenatal and postnatal management of this condition.

Thrombocytopenia is a common complication encountered in pregnancy, and can have a wide range of prognostic implications, from completely benign to life threatening. It is important for obstetricians to be aware of the various causes of thrombocytopenia in pregnancy, and to be able to diagnose and manage these patients. This article reviews the various causes of thrombocytopenia in pregnancy, highlights clinical and laboratory features of the most common and most severe causes, and provides an overview of management for these disorders.

This article reviews anticoagulant medications used for obstetric patients who have acute thrombosis or who require anticoagulant therapy for other indications. Medication options, dosing and monitoring, side effects, and complications are reviewed. Antepartum, intrapartum, and postpartum management of therapy is discussed, as well as breastfeeding options.

Pregnancy management with mechanical heart valves is best done collaboratively with experienced cardiologists and maternal fetal medicine specialists. All anticoagulation options are associated with risks and benefits. Pregnancy is one situation in which the benefit of warfarin use may outweigh the risks. In light of the absence of definitive research to suggest a superior regimen, the risks, benefits, and limitations of each strategy should be discussed with the patient and specific attention given to her individual clinical situation.

Knowledge of antiphospholipid antibodies and their impact on pregnancy continues to evolve. A variety of antiphospholipid antibodies have been identified, but not all of them seem to be pathologic for pregnancy outcome. Understanding of which patients are at high risk for adverse pregnancy outcome and the most effective treatment will require clinical trials based on risk stratification and long-term follow-up of infants.

CLINICS IN LABORATORY MEDICINE

Preface

Diabetes, Hematology/ Coagulation in Pregnancy

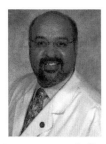

Winston A. Campbell, MD
Editor

As the editor of this issue of *Clinics in Laboratory Medicine*, I was asked to focus on the themes of Diabetes, Hematology/Coagulation in Pregnancy. While each topic in itself is important, I felt there was merit in providing a multifocus approach for this issue. Within the main topics, subtopics were selected that might present as a pregestational or gestational problem for the pregnant patient that could have significant impact on maternal care and pregnancy outcome.

The first theme focuses on diabetes. Any pregnancy has a 3% to 6% risk of being complicated by a birth defect. Diabetes is known to increase this risk in patients with poor preconception glucose control. Zhao and Reece present new concepts on mechanisms that may play a role in diabetes-associated birth defects. Gurram and colleagues continue with a theme on birth defects, but from the perspective of how diabetes may alter maternal serum analyte laboratory screening methods used to identify pregnancies at risk for chromosome abnormalities.

The remaining articles address basic and special prenatal management issues for pregnant diabetic patients. Fang and Feldman provide an update on the recent trend of using oral hypoglycemic agents along with the traditional approach of insulin and its newer analogues for optimal glucose control. Ischemic heart disease is a significant mortality risk for the pregnant diabetic patient. Jones and coworkers provide critical information on this risk and how patients should be evaluated and managed during pregnancy. Haider and Adams address how a long-term sequela of diabetes, renal failure, presents a very special set of management issues when organ transplant (renal) becomes a factor.

The hematology theme starts with a focus on anemia. This is very common in pregnancy, yet the practitioner may not consider all the causes that may be involved. Horowitz and colleagues provide the reader with a concise approach to evaluate this problem so that common and unusual causes will not be missed. As medical care of chronic illnesses improves, patients who are in their reproductive years might consider

Clin Lab Med 33 (2013) xiii–xiv
http://dx.doi.org/10.1016/j.cll.2013.03.026
labmed.theclinics.com

becoming pregnant. Andemariam and Browning provide an up-to-date approach on managing patients with sickle cell anemia. The principles of management for this specific hemoglobinopathy are likely applicable to other inherited hemoglobinopathies. Neonatal alloimmune thrombocytopenia is not a common condition, but it has severe consequences for the newborn infant. Strong and Eddleman provide an overview on pathophysiology and clinical presentation, as well as the current management algorithm based on clinical trials using risk-stratified management protocols. The final article by Adams and coworkers discusses maternal thrombocytopenia. Like anemia, this is a common complication during pregnancy and the practitioner may not always consider the various causes involved. This article provides a comprehensive approach to patient evaluation and management. It also points out overlap that thrombocytopenia might have with other medical conditions discussed in this issue.

Coagulation, the third and final theme, is the topic of five articles covering a range of basic information and specific management issues for conditions that continue to show an evolution in our management knowledge or are so uncommon that consensus opinion is the current cornerstone of management. Fuller and coworkers outline the current anticoagulation guidelines and provide a basis for patient management for the remaining articles. Caring for patients with prosthetic heart valves presents a difficult challenge due to concerns about medication side effects on the fetus. Stout and Odibo present current viewpoints on the compromise that has been reached to avoid fetal harm yet provide the best care for the mother. Thrombophilia presents unique challenges in obstetrics in regard to thromboembolic risk to the mother and concern about adverse pregnancy outcome. The article by Lockshin presents our evolving understanding of acquired thrombophilia and how management is becoming more focused on patient risk stratification. Hossain and Paidas address inherited thrombophilia and how the initial concerns that led to the broad use of anticoagulation to avoid adverse pregnancy outcome is being tempered. They show how recent randomized trial results are providing a more evidence-based management approach.

The last article addresses an unusual and very challenging problem to the practitioner. The article by Gomez-Puerta and colleagues on catastrophic antiphospholipid syndrome (CAPS) brings awareness to the practitioner of this unusual variant of acquired thrombophilia. An international CAPS registry has recorded about 400 patients with this condition. Even fewer have been pregnant. Thus there is still much that is being learned about this condition and best evaluation and management principles during pregnancy.

I want to thank all the authors for the significant effort they put forth for this issue of the *Clinics in Laboratory Medicine*. While the array of articles has its own focus, some share an overlap of information and management. I hope that readers find these articles beneficial in the daily care of their patients.

Winston A. Campbell, MD
University of Connecticut Health Center School of Medicine
John Dempsey Hospital
263 Farmington Avenue-CG 214
Farmington, CT 06030-4946, USA

E-mail address:
wcampbell@nso2.uchc.edu

New Concepts in Diabetic Embryopathy

Zhiyong Zhao, PhD[a],*, E. Albert Reece, MD, PhD, MBA[b]

KEYWORDS

- Diabetic embryopathy • Birth defects • Hyperglycemia • Apoptosis
- Cell proliferation • Metabolism • Intracellular stress • Intervention

KEY POINTS

- Diabetes mellitus in early pregnancy increases the risk of birth defects in infants.
- High glucose induces intracellular stress, increases programmed cell death (apoptosis), and decreases cell proliferation in the embryo.
- Reduction of the risk includes preconceptional and early gestational glycemic control.
- Interventions via dietary supplementation remain to be developed.
- Preconceptional counseling and planned pregnancy are encouraged for physicians and patients.

INTRODUCTION

Diabetes mellitus is a metabolic disease, primarily caused by high concentrations of glucose in the circulation.[1] Hyperglycemia interrupts normal cellular metabolism and signaling and causes organ dysfunction.[2,3] Nearly 2 centuries after diabetes was first recognized,[4] its association with congenital birth defects and fetal mortality in pregnancy was recognized and referred to as diabetic embryopathy.[4,5] Before the introduction of insulin, diabetes-associated fetal and maternal mortality were nearly 70% and 40%, respectively.[6,7] Since the administration of insulin to control glycemia in pregnant women, this mortality has decreased dramatically to nearly 12%.[8–15] In addition to the control of glycemia with insulin, aggressive perinatal care and neonatal management also contributed to the decline of maternal and fetal mortality.[10,16–19]

The present birth defect rate in diabetic pregnancies (about 10%) is still higher than that in the general population (3%) and seems to be on the increase.[7,12,13,15,20–25] The reasons for this increase in birth defect rates are complex. One reason is that there has been a rapid increase in diabetic patients in the population, which includes women of childbearing age.[26] It is estimated that approximately 8000 babies in the United States

[a] Department of Obstetrics, Gynecology and Reproductive Sciences, University of Maryland School of Medicine, 655 West Baltimore Street, BRB 11-041, Baltimore, MD 21201, USA;
[b] Department of Obstetrics, Gynecology and Reproductive Sciences, University of Maryland School of Medicine, 655 West Baltimore Street, BRB 14-029, Baltimore, MD 21201, USA
* Corresponding author.
E-mail address: zzhao@fpi.umaryland.edu

Clin Lab Med 33 (2013) 207–233
http://dx.doi.org/10.1016/j.cll.2013.03.017
0272-2712/13/$ – see front matter
labmed.theclinics.com

are born each year with maternal diabetes-associated congenital malformations. The incidence of these malformations also has risen to near-epidemic level in developing countries.

Tackling this issue involves battles on several fronts: diagnosing fetal anomalies must be improved; technologies that can recognize developmental malformations as early as the embryogenesis period are needed; and better prenatal and planned pregnancy consultations should be implemented to help reduce diabetes-associated birth defects. These remain ongoing challenges for perinatal care providers.

An important goal in eliminating birth defects is to develop therapeutic interventions that can protect embryos from hyperglycemic insult. This goal can be achieved only by understanding the cellular and molecular mechanisms underlying diabetic embryopathy. Basic research using animal models has contributed a considerable amount of information about the manifestations of fetal abnormalities, but more work is still needed.

Pregestational and Gestational Diabetes

Diabetes mellitus is a chronic disease manifested by hyperglycemia and its associated metabolic factors. This condition is usually diagnosed by measuring the levels of plasma glucose, expressed as mg/dL or mM, and glycosylated hemoglobin A (HbA_{1c}), indexed as percentage of total hemoglobin A.[27–29] Manifestation of diabetes can be the result of insulin deficiency (type 1) or insulin resistance (type 2).

- Type 1 diabetes, or insulin-dependent diabetes, is caused by autoimmune destruction of insulin-producing β-cells in the pancreas.[30,31]
- Type 2 diabetes, or non–insulin-dependent diabetes, is caused by failure in insulin signaling to regulate cellular glucose uptake.[32–34]

Diabetes mellitus, either type 1 or type 2, diagnosed in women before pregnancy is referred to as pregestational diabetes.[20,35–37] When hyperglycemia is detected after the onset of pregnancy, usually in the third trimester (24–28 weeks), the pregnant woman is considered to have gestational diabetes mellitus (GDM).[38–42] According to guidelines from the International Association of Diabetes in Pregnancy Study Group, women who have a fasting plasma glucose of 126 mg/dL or greater and HbA_{1c} of 6.5% or greater are diagnosed as having GDM.[43]

Congenital birth defects in infants of diabetic mothers have been found to be associated with pregestational diabetes that is uncontrolled in the first trimester of pregnancy.[44–48] Although a few cases have suggested a link between GDM and birth defects, this association remains unclear and lacks strong supporting evidence.[49,50] One possible reason for the controversy is that some women with early-onset type 2 diabetes are misdiagnosed as having GDM when first screened in the second trimester.[39,51] Nevertheless, it is well established that GDM can lead to many adverse fetal outcomes, including macrosomia, hypoglycemia, hypocalcemia, and hyperbilirubinemia.[51–53]

High Glucose as a Major Teratogenic Factor

Human studies have shown a strong link between maternal glycemic level, as indicated by the association of plasma glucose and HbA_{1c} levels[54,55] with the incidence of congenital malformations in offspring.[19,55–59] Other adverse metabolic factors produced in diabetes mellitus, such as ketone bodies, advanced glycation end products, and branched chain amino acids, may have synergetic effects with glucose on disrupting normal embryonic development.[60–64] The putative teratogenic effects of hyperglycemia are supported by studies that show a reduction in the incidence of birth

Table 1
Recommendations for preconception HbA$_{1c}$ targets

	United States	United Kingdom
DCCT (%)	<7.0	<6.1
IFCC (mmol/mol)	<53	<43

Abbreviations: DCCT, Diabetes Control and Complications Trials; IFCC, International Federation of Clinical Chemistry and Laboratory Medicine.

defects after clinical interventions targeted at achieving euglycemia.[10,65–67] Animal studies also have shown that isolated embryos in culture exposed to high concentrations of glucose develop malformations similar to those seen in human diabetic pregnancies.[60,68–70] These observations indicate that high glucose in either type 1 or type 2 diabetes is a major teratogenic factor that disturbs embryonic development.

The major effort to eliminate adverse outcome in pregnancies complicated by pregestational diabetes and GDM is to control glycemic levels.[20,71–73] Clinical management of diabetic pregnancy with insulin and oral hypoglycemic medications can achieve the euglycemic standards recommended by Diabetes Control and Complications Trials and International Federation of Clinical Chemistry and Laboratory Medicine (**Table 1**).[74–76] However, with respect to pregestational diabetes, optimal glycemic control before conception seems to be a challenge because:

- Most women with diabetes do not seek preconception care
- Most have unplanned pregnancies[77]
- Even in women who plan pregnancies and receive preconception counseling, euglycemia is difficult to achieve and maintain in nonclinical settings.

Therefore, alternative approaches to glucose control to prevent birth defects need to be developed and implemented.

MALFORMATIONS AND DIAGNOSIS

Maternal diabetes-associated fetal anomalies can be seen in any organ system but are most common and severe in the central nervous system (CNS), cardiovascular system (CVS), craniofacial region, and caudal structure (**Table 2**).[11,12,25,44,55,78,79]

Table 2
Developmental anomalies in major organ systems in diabetic embryopathy

CNS	Craniofacial System	CVS	Skeletal System
Anencephaly	Hemifacial microsomia	Conus arteriosus defects	Sacral agenesis
Encephalocele	Macrostomia	Transposition of great vessels	Sacral hypoplasia
Exencephaly	Cleft palate	Tetralogy of Fallot	Limb defects
Microcephaly	Cleft lip	Ventricular septal defects	Vertebral defects
Hydrocephaly	Microtia	Pulmonary valve defects	Caudal regression
Holoprosencephaly	Micrognathia	Patent ductus arteriosus	
Spina bifida	Craniosynostosis	Hypoplastic left heart syndrome	
	Anotia/microtia	Coarctation of the aorta	
	Eye defects	Right ventricular septal defects	
		Atrial septal defects	
		Heterotaxia	

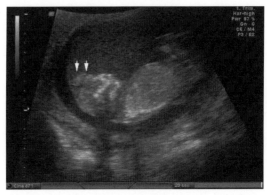

Fig. 1. Two-dimensional ultrasonic scanning of anencephaly in the first trimester. Arrows indicate missing forebrain. (*Modified from* Cameron M, Moran P. Prenatal screening and diagnosis of neural tube defects. Prenat Diagn 2009;29:403; with permission.)

CNS

The most common structural defects resulting from diabetic embryopathy occur in the brain region and spinal cord of the CNS.[12,25,80–83] Some of these defects can be recognized as early as in the first trimester using ultrasonography.

- Anencephaly is characterized as absence of the cerebral hemispheres, with the brain stem and portions of the midbrain intact. It is readily discernible in the first trimester (**Fig. 1**).[73,84,85] In the second trimester, it is more evident as poorly formed cranial bones and symmetric absence of the calvarium.[73,84,86]
- Holoprosencephaly, the complete or partial absence of the midline echo within the fetal brain, can be diagnosed as early as 14 weeks of gestation, although diagnosis at the 20-week anomaly scan is more common.[87–89]
- Excencephaly, the absence of the superior vault and convolution of the brain, can be diagnosed as early as 10 weeks of gestation (**Fig. 2**).[90]
- Ultrasonic diagnosis of CNS defects such as spina bifida usually occurs in conjunction with detection of the second trimester maternal blood biomarker α-fetoprotein.[78,91–94]

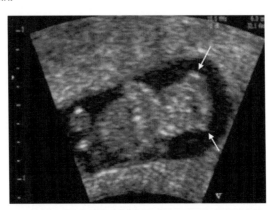

Fig. 2. Two-dimensional ultrasonic scanning of exencephaly in the first trimester. The contours of the brain are irregular (*arrows*). (*Modified from* Blaas HG, Eik-Nes SH. Sonoembryology and early prenatal diagnosis of neural anomalies. Prenat Diagn 2009;29:319; with permission.)

Craniofacial Structures

In newborns of diabetic mothers, the most common anomalies in the craniofacial regions are hemifacial microsomia and microtia.[79,95] Cleft palate and lip also occur in high frequency.[96–98] Hearing impairment in children has been found to be associated with diabetic pregnancy,[79,95,99] likely because of developmental defects in the inner and middle ear.[99]

Prenatal diagnosis of cleft lip and cleft palate relies on a combination of coronal and axial two-dimensional ultrasonographic scans.[100] Cleft lip can be easily recognized from coronal scan images; however, when cleft lip extends into the palate, the axial scan of the maxilla can provide the image of the defects.[101] Cases of lateral cleft lip/palate often present a so-called maxillary pseudomass visualized in two-dimensional sonographs.[102]

CVS

Fetal cardiac defects associated with maternal diabetes have been extensively characterized. Anomalies commonly are present in:

- Myocardium-derived structures
  - Atria
  - Ventricles
  - Interventricular septum
- Endocardium-derived structures
  - Conotruncal septum
  - Ventricular septum
  - Atrioventricular valves[44,47,103–105]

Sonographic imaging remains the standard method to diagnose fetal cardiac abnormalities. Technological advances in imaging, especially in high-frequency imaging and improvements in resolution, have aided perinatal care providers to recognize cardiac defects as early as 10 weeks of gestation.

Most heart anomalies, including double-outlet hearts, atrial septal defects, and ventricular septal defects, can be diagnosed using the 4-chamber view, a transverse projection through the fetal thorax above the level of the diaphragm (**Fig. 3**).[106] Measurement of the thickness of the ventricular walls in the sonographs can reveal myocardial hypoplasia. Because of the position of the canning plane, the 4-chamber view usually misses defects in the structures in the outflow tracts. A so-called base view, with scans superior to the 4-chamber view, can reveal abnormalities in the aorta and pulmonary artery. Complex defects such as tetralogy of Fallot, which involves ventricular septal defects and great vessel defects, may require a combination of 4-chambered and base views to be diagnosed.

Color Doppler provides an added advantage to practitioners, because it can detect minor defects in the heart by showing changes in blood flow pattern. The association of increased first trimester nuchal translucency with fetal cardiac defects has been observed; however, more studies are still needed to establish it as a diagnostic marker.[107,108]

Caudal Regression

Caudal regression syndrome, also known as caudal dysplasia, is characterized as the absence or hypoplasia of caudal trunk and limbs.[109,110] Caudal regression syndrome can be diagnosed by noting a shortened spine and abnormal lower limbs. This anomaly can be detected in the fetus as early as second trimester.

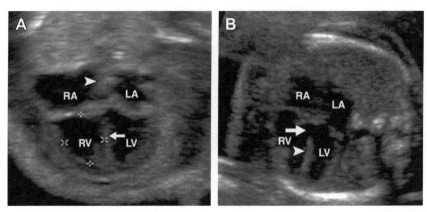

Fig. 3. Four-chamber view of fetal hearts. (*A*) Normal heart. Arrow indicates interventricular septum. Arrowhead indicates interatrial septum. (*B*) Heart with a ventricular septal defect (*arrow*) in the inlet portion of the interventricular septum (*arrowhead*). LA, left atrium; LV, left ventricle; RA, right atrium; RV, right ventricle. (*Modified from* Rajiah P, Mak C, Dubinksy TJ, et al. Ultrasound of fetal cardiac anomalies. AJR Am J Roentgenol 2011;197:W754, 756; with permission.)

MECHANISMS OF DIABETIC EMBRYOPATHY
Developmental Mechanisms

CNS

Diabetic embryopathy causes embryonic and fetal abnormalities as a result of a disturbance in normal organogenesis. In the CNS, most anomalies occur because of a failure of early neural tube formation, referred to as neural tube defects (NTDs).[111–113] The formation of the neural tube, or neurulation, occurs in human embryos from weeks 3 to 6 of gestation.[111] Neurulation begins with formation of the neural ectoderm, which develops into the neural folds. The neural folds grow dorsal-laterally and fuse at the dorsal midline along the body axis to form the neural tube.[114] In diabetic embryopathy, neurulation is perturbed in young embryos, leading to NTDs such as exencephaly or spina bifida.[60,70,115,116] Studies using diabetic rodents with poorly controlled hyperglycemia have recapitulated the same CNS defects observed in human fetuses (**Fig. 4**).[117–119]

CVS

The development of the heart is a complex process, involving multiple tissue types. The atria, ventricles, and interventricular septum are derived from the myocardium, whereas the membranous septa in the atrioventricular channel and the outflow tracts and associated valves are derived from the endocardium.[120–123]

The most common abnormality of the ventricles is hypoplastic heart syndrome.[44] It is associated with underdevelopment of the myocardium during early cardiogenesis.[118] Defects in endocardium-derived structures are often associated with endocardial cushions (**Fig. 5**),[118,124] bulbous structures that develop during early embryogenesis at the atrioventricular junction and the bulbous cortis (outflow tract) as a result of the production of the extracellular matrix.[125,126] During development of the endocardial cushions, endocardial (endothelial) cells differentiate into mesenchymal cells. This process is known as the endothelial-mesenchymal transformation.[125,127] These mesenchymal cells migrate into the extracellular matrix to fill the acellular space and promote the growth of the cardiac structures.[127] The endocardial cushions

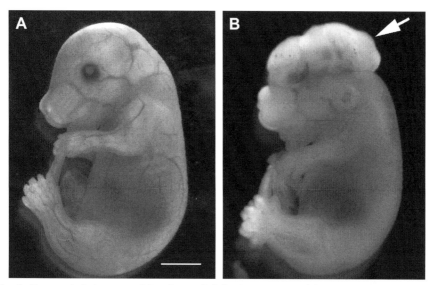

Fig. 4. Exencephaly in mouse E15.5 fetus of diabetic pregnancy. (*A*) Nondiabetic control. (*B*) Diabetes. Arrow indicates exencephaly. Scale bar = 3 mm.

develop toward each other and fuse to form a continuous septum.[122] After fusion, the endocardial tissues undergo dramatic remodeling to connect with the interventricular and primary atrial septum and form valves.[127,128]

In embryos of diabetic pregnancies, early development of the endocardial cushions is inhibited.[118] An impact of maternal hyperglycemia on later endocardial cushion remodeling also has been observed.[129] Further research is needed to determine the significance of these developmental processes in cardiac malformation in diabetic embryopathy.

Craniofacial

In the craniofacial region, abnormalities in facial structures may be associated with dysmorphogenesis of cartilages.[130,131] These cartilages, such as the Meckel cartilage in the mandibular arch, are not only involved in early morphogenesis of the facial processes but also give rise to many types of bony structures in the craniofacial regions, such as the auditory ossicles.[132,133]

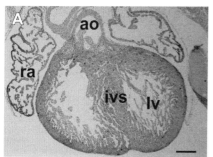
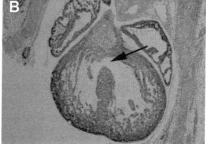

Fig. 5. A ventricular septal defect in mouse E15.5 fetus of diabetic pregnancy. (*A*) Heart of nondiabetic control. (*B*) Heart of diabetic group with a ventricular septal defect (*arrow*). ao, aorta; ivs, interventricular septum; lv, left ventricle; ra, right atrium. Scale bar = 200 μm.

Cellular mechanisms

The development of organ systems involves cell proliferation, death, migration, and differentiation. Excessive programmed cell death (apoptosis) has been observed in the dorsal region of the neural tube and is associated with NTDs in diabetic embryopathy.[68,119,134–139] In the developing heart, cell proliferation at the early stages and apoptosis at the late stages of cardiogenesis seem to be associated with cardiac malformations in the embryos of diabetic pregnancy.[118,129] In addition to cell proliferation, endocardial cell differentiation and migration also are suppressed by maternal hyperglycemia.[118,124]

Development of the cardiac outflow tract requires cell migration from the neural crest in the dorsal region of the neural tube. These neural crest cells contribute significantly to the septation of the outflow segment and the formation of the great vessels.[140,141] Malformations in the outflow segment may be caused by impaired neural crest cell migration, which can be caused by increased apoptosis.[142,143]

Craniofacial structure development also requires neural crest cells that migrate from the anterior neural tube during early embryogenesis.[144–146] Studies using animal models have shown that maternal diabetes perturbs neural crest cell migration in embryos.[130,147] Increased apoptosis in the mandibular arch has been observed in embryos of diabetic women, although it is uncertain whether those cells are of neural crest origin.[143] The impact of maternal diabetes on the differentiation of the neural crest origin craniofacial mesenchymal cells remains to be shown.

Molecular Mechanisms in Promoting Apoptosis in Diabetic Embryopathy

Endoplasmic reticulum stress

When exposed to high glucose, embryonic cells take up glucose via glucose transporters.[148,149] An influx of glucose disturbs intracellular metabolic homeostasis and organelle function. Dysfunction of the endoplasmic reticulum (ER) leads to aberrant protein folding and subsequent accumulation of unfolded and misfolded proteins in its lumen,[150–152] which cause ER stress.[153–156] Under stress conditions, the ER activates several molecular cascades, collectively known as the unfolded protein response (UPR), to increase expression of chaperone protein to resolve protein folding crisis, inhibit protein translation, suppress mitosis, and even trigger apoptosis (**Fig. 6**).[157–159] ER stress has been observed in the embryos from diabetic pregnancies.[124,160,161] The potential causative role of ER stress in embryonic malformation has been shown with experiments using a chemical chaperone to resolve protein folding crisis.[124]

Oxidative stress

High glucose also changes the morphology and function of mitochondria.[162] Changes in mitochondria interrupt the electron transport chain, leading to generation of reactive oxygen species (ROS).[163,164] High glucose also reduces the level of intracellular antioxidants, including glutathione (GSH) and thioredoxin.[165–168] The imbalance of ROS and antioxidative buffering results in oxidative stress, which perturbs intracellular signaling (**Fig. 7**).[169,170] Treating diabetic pregnant animals or embryos cultured in high glucose with antioxidants decreases embryonic malformation rates.[171–181] Moreover, embryos treated with antioxidants or overexpressing a transgene of superoxide dismutase resist maternal hyperglycemic insult.[182,183]

Nitrosative stress

Under hyperglycemic conditions, embryonic cells produce high levels of nitric oxide (NO). NO is a second messenger that regulates various intracellular signaling pathways[184,185] and also can react with ROS to produce more toxic radicals, called

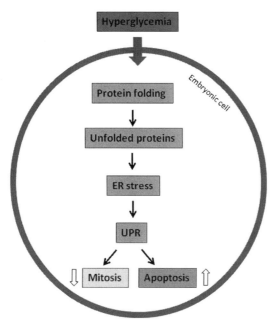

Fig. 6. ER stress in diabetic embryopathy.

reactive nitrogen species (RNS), than NO or ROS alone.[186,187] The high levels of RNS, such as peroxynitrite, generate a condition known as nitrosative stress (**Fig. 8**).

Synthesis of NO is catalyzed by NO synthase (NOS) enzymes. There are 3 main forms of NOS enzymes: neuronal (nNOS and NOS1); endothelial (eNOS and NOS3);

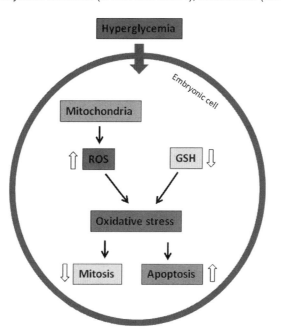

Fig. 7. Oxidative stress in diabetic embryopathy.

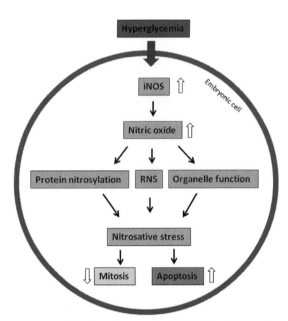

Fig. 8. Nitrosative stress in diabetic embryopathy. iNOS, inducible nitric oxide synthase.

and inducible (iNOS and NOS2).[188–190] Both nNOS and eNOS are constitutively expressed and do not vigorously respond to extracellular stimulation,[191,192] but iNOS actively responds to extracellular changes with marked upregulation in expression and activity.[193–195]

In embryos of diabetic animals, eNOS expression is decreased[196]; in contrast, iNOS expression is dramatically increased.[197,198] Experiments using an iNOS knockout model clearly show that a high level of NO is detrimental to the embryo (see **Fig. 8**).[117]

Stress response

Phospholipid peroxidation Cellular stress perturbs intracellular metabolic homeostasis. Phospholipid metabolism is initiated by phospholipases (PLs), including PLA, PLC, and PLD.[199,200] Cytosolic PL A2 (cPLA$_2$) cleaves arachidonic acid from the cell membrane.[201–203] In the cytoplasm, arachidonic acid undergoes 2 major pathways of metabolism: it can be converted into prostaglandin E$_2$ (PGE$_2$) by cyclooxygenase 2 (COX-2),[204,205] or it can be converted into PGE$_2$-like isoprostanes, such as 8-isoprostagladin F2 (8-iso-PGF$_2$), by non-COX-mediated peroxidation involving free radicals (**Fig. 9**).[206,207]

In embryos of diabetic animals or embryos exposed to high concentrations of glucose in vitro, the level of PGE$_2$ decreases dramatically.[208–212] On the other hand, the level of 8-iso-PGF$_2$ is dramatically increased in embryos under hyperglycemic conditions as well as in diabetic patients.[206,213] The reduction in PGE$_2$ in the embryo may be caused by a decrease in COX-2 activity and expression,[208,214,215] suggesting that a shift in arachidonic acid metabolism has occurred from producing PGE$_2$ to generating isoprostanes. These PGE$_2$-like isoprostanes have been shown to have damaging effects in animal models of diabetic pregnancy and embryos exposed to high glucose in culture,[213,216] whereas PGE$_2$ protects embryos from the damages caused by hyperglycemic conditions (see **Fig. 9**).[208,215,217]

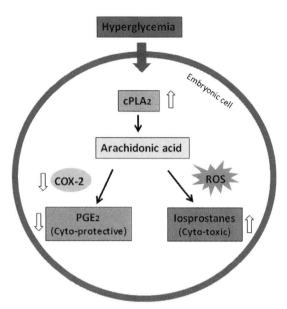

Fig. 9. Lipoperoxidation in diabetic embryopathy.

Protein kinase C family Under cellular stress conditions, several intracellular signaling systems are affected, including the ones regulated by members of the protein kinase C (PKC) family. The PKC family of serine/threonine protein kinases consists of 12 members, which can be divided into the following 3 groups, based on their activation mechanisms[218,219]: (1) PKCα, β$_1$, β$_2$, and γ require calcium and diacylglycerol (DAG) for activation; (2) PKCδ, ε, η, ν, and θ require only DAG; and (3) PKCμ, ξ, and ι/λ do not require calcium or DAG, but instead require distinct lipid cofactors (ie, ceramide and phosphatidylinositol-4-phosphate).[218]

In embryos of diabetic animals, each PKC isoform responds differently to hyperglycemia. For example, PKCα, β$_2$, and δ are phosphorylated and activated under hyperglycemic conditions.[138] Consequently, inhibiting PKCα, β$_2$, and δ with isoform-specific inhibitors reduces malformation rates in embryos cultured in a high concentration of glucose.[138,220] In addition, embryos from diabetic *pkcδ* knockout animal models show significantly lower malformation rate than embryos from diabetic mice having the gene.[161] These and other similar studies show that PKCs play critical roles in diabetic embryopathy.

Mitogen-activated protein kinase family The mitogen-activated protein kinase (MAPK) family also plays an important role in mediating the effects of maternal hyperglycemia on embryonic development. Members of the MAPK family, including extracellular signal-regulated kinases (ERKs) and c-jun N-terminal kinases (JNKs)/stress-activated protein kinases, can usually be inhibited or activated by oxidative stress. ERKs primarily regulate cell proliferation and survival, whereas JNKs act on proapoptotic pathways.[221–223] In embryos of diabetic animals, the levels of phosphorylated ERK1 and 2 are significantly reduced (see **Fig. 8**).[224,225] In contrast, JNKs are activated in embryos of diabetic animals.[224–227] Embryos treated with a JNK inhibitor and simultaneously incubated in a high concentration of glucose have a lower malformation rate compared with those without JNK inhibition.[228] More convincing evidence of the role of JNKs in diabetic embryopathy comes from the experiments using *jnk1* and *jnk2* knockout mice. Embryos homozygous for either *jnk1* or *jnk2* deletion show significantly lower malformation rates compared with a wild-type embryos from diabetic animals.[228,229]

Programmed Cell Death (Apoptosis)

Apoptosis is precisely regulated by several factors, including PKCs, JNKs, and members of the Bcl-2 and caspase families.[230] Although the mechanisms by which PKCs and JNKs promote apoptosis in diabetic embryopathy remain to be delineated, much is known about the roles that Bcl-2 and caspase family members play in programmed cell death.

In the Bcl-2 family, some members are proapoptotic, such as Bax, Bak, and Bid, whereas other members are antiapoptotic, such as Bcl-2 and Bcl-xL.[231] In the caspase family, some members play a role in executing apoptosis. These members, known as effector or executioner caspases, include caspase-3, caspase-6, and caspase-7.[232–234] Effector caspases can be activated by another group of caspases, known as initiator caspases, including caspase-8, caspase-9, and caspase-10.[232–234]

Bax and Bak form a pore in the outer membrane of mitochondria,[235,236] allowing cytochrome C to be release to cytoplasm to induce apoptosis.[237–239] During apoptosis, Bax and Bim expression levels increase in the cell.[235,236] Bax is activated by truncated Bid (tBid), which is produced when Bid is cleaved by serine/threonine proteases such as caspase-8.

In diabetic embryopathy, caspase-8 cleaves Bid into tBid, which stimulates the release of cytochrome C.[137] Cytochrome C binds to apoptosis protease-activating factor 1 (Apaf-1), and the resulting complex activates caspase-9 by forming an apoptosome. Activated caspase-9 then activates effector caspases, including caspase-3, caspase-6, and caspase-7, which turn on caspase-activated DNase and other factors, leading to DNA fragmentation and cell death (**Fig. 10**).[237,238]

In animal studies, suppression of apoptosis using caspase inhibitors can reduce embryonic malformations in the embryos cultured in high glucose.[137] The results imply potential interventional strategies to block apoptosis in embryos in diabetic pregnancies.

INTERVENTIONS AND CLINICAL CHALLENGES

Research conducted in animal models of diabetic pregnancy has revealed some of the major molecular changes and subsequent intracellular metabolic conditions that occur in embryos in response to hyperglycemia. This information has guided efforts to explore interventional approaches to reduce diabetes-induced embryonic malformations.[119,171,180,181,224,240–244]

Targeting Lipid Metabolism

One anomaly that occurs in diabetic embryopathy is aberrant phospholipid metabolism, especially lipoperoxidation. Dietary supplementation with arachidonic acid or myoinositol in diabetic pregnant animals has been shown to reduce embryonic malformations caused by lipoperoxidation.[180,181,241] Treatment of diabetic pregnancy animals with polyunsaturated fatty acids has also been shown to exert similar helpful effects on embryonic development.[224,245]

Antioxidative Strategies

Targeting oxidative stress to treat diabetic embryopathy, using lipoic acid, ergothioneine, vitamin C, and vitamin E, has been tested in diabetic pregnant animals and shown to decrease embryonic malformations.[171,178,180,181,240,246] *N*-acetylcysteine,

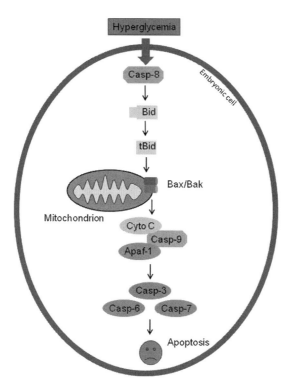

Fig. 10. Caspase-8-regulated apoptotic pathway in diabetic embryopathy. Casp, caspase; Cyto, cytochrome.

which has been used as an antioxidant in clinical practices to treat acetaminophen poisoning,[247,248] has been observed to reduce malformations in animal embryos in culture exposed to high glucose[249–251]; however, its effect in human diabetic pregnancy remains to be shown.

Folic acid, or water-soluble vitamin B9, has long been known to reduce NTDs in humans.[252,253] The effect of folic acid in reducing embryonic malformations associated with maternal diabetes has been explored in animal models. Treating cultured rodent embryos with folic acid can reduce neural tube dysmorphogenesis induced by high concentrations of glucose.[243] In in vivo experiments, diabetic pregnant rats injected with folic acid also show decreased NTDs in their embryos, compared with diabetic pregnant rats not given the supplement.[119,243,254]

Combination Approaches

The combination of antioxidants and phospholipids that target multiple molecular pathways could have more potent effects in reducing fetal abnormalities compared with monotherapy. Cocktails of vitamin E, arachidonic acid, and myoinositol have been explored in diabetic animal models and have been shown to decrease embryonic malformations.[180,181] The efficacy of antioxidants to prevent fetal defects in human diabetic pregnancy has not been examined. Antioxidant approaches tested to treat similar diseases, such as preeclampsia, have produced unsatisfactory results.[255–259] These results have tampered the enthusiasm in applying similar strategies to treat diabetic embryopathy, but exploration of other strategies is warranted.

Recently, alleviating nitrosative stress via iNOS inhibitors has been tested in diabetic embryopathy.[160] Oral treatment of diabetic pregnant animals with an iNOS inhibitor decreased embryonic malformation rates.[160] Additional studies are needed to test therapeutic agents or dietary supplements that inhibit iNOS to translate these basic research findings into clinical applications for human disease.

Clinical Challenges

Diabetic embryopathy involves complex molecular interactions. Extensive understanding of its mechanisms is essential for identifying therapeutic targets and developing effective interventions. Many challenges in developing these approaches lie ahead. First, interventions must be safe for the embryo and mother. The ideal approaches include dietary supplementation of nontoxic agents. Second, because developmental malformations occur early on in the first trimester of pregnancy, the dietary supplements must be easily accessible for women to take before conception or soon thereafter. Third, any therapeutic agents administered via oral treatments or dietary supplements must be able to pass the maternal-fetal barrier to exert potent effects on the developing embryo.

To overcome these challenges, it not only needs scientific research to decipher the molecular mechanisms underlying embryonic malformations and develop prevention strategies but also requires education of the public to raise awareness about the risk of birth defects in diabetic pregnancy. Preconception counseling and pregnancy planning have been shown to be correlated with reduction in adverse outcomes of pregnancies.[260–263] However, more cooperative efforts between perinatal care providers and patients are needed to achieve the goal of eliminating birth defects.

Concluding Remarks

Diabetic embryopathy is a global public health issue. Although pregestational screening for maternal diabetes, perinatal care, and postnatal management in developed countries is available to most pregnant women, the rate of birth defects in infants of diabetic mothers remains high. In developing countries, the rates of birth defects and even mortality are high because of unavailable and inadequate care for pregnant women. With the worldwide increase in obesity and type 2 diabetes, diagnosis and management of diabetic pregnancy is a big challenge for the medical community. The increasing public health burden of diabetes in women of childbearing age makes it important to develop interventional approaches to prevent embryonic malformations.

Further understanding of the mechanisms underlying diabetic embryopathy will provide crucial information for developing effective interventions. Clinical approaches must be safe to administer in early pregnancy and accessible to women before and soon after conception to be highly effective, because diabetes in early pregnancy often goes undetected and many women have unplanned pregnancies. Major cellular activities (ie, proliferation and apoptosis) and intracellular metabolic conditions (ie, nitrosative, ER, and oxidative stress) have been shown to be associated with diabetic embryopathy using animal models. Translating advances made in animal studies into clinical applications in humans will require collaborative efforts across the basic research, preclinical, and clinical communities.

REFERENCES

1. American Diabetes Association. Diagnosis and classification of diabetes mellitus. Diabetes Care 2012;35:S64–71.

2. Porte D Jr, Schwartz MW. Diabetes complications: why is glucose potentially toxic? Science 1996;272:699–700.

3. King GL. The role of hyperglycaemia and hyperinsulinaemia in causing vascular dysfunction in diabetes. Ann Med 1996;28:427–32.

4. Barnett DM, Krall LP. The history of diabetes. In: Kahn BB, King GL, Moses AC, et al, editors. Joslin's diabetes mellitus. Philadelphia: Lippincott Williams & Wilkins; 2005. p. 1–17.

5. LeCorche E. Du diabetic dans se rapports avec la vie uterine menstruation, et al grusesse. Annales de gynécologie 1885;24:257.

6. Duncan JM. On puerperal diabetes. Trans Obstet Soc London 1882;24:256.

7. Joslin EP. Treatment of diabetes mellitus. Philadelphia: Lea and Febiger; 1923.

8. Pedersen J. The pregnant diabetic and her newborn: problems and management. Baltimore (MD): Williams & Wilkins; 1977.

9. Olofsson P, Liedholm H, Sartor G, et al. Diabetes and pregnancy. A 21-year Swedish material. Acta Obstet Gynecol Scand Suppl 1984;122:3–62.

10. Kitzmiller JL, Gavin LA, Gin GD, et al. Preconception care of diabetes. Glycemic control prevents congenital anomalies. JAMA 1991;265:731–6.

11. Kucera J. Rate and type of congenital anomalies among offspring of diabetic women. J Reprod Med 1971;7:73–82.

12. Soler NG, Walsh CH, Malins JM. Congenital malformations in infants of diabetic mothers. Q J Med 1976;45:303–13.

13. Miodovnik M, Mimouni F, Dignan PS, et al. Major malformations in infants of IDDM women. Vasculopathy and early first-trimester poor glycemic control. Diabetes Care 1988;11:713–8.

14. Pedersen JF, Molsted-Pedersen L, Mortensen HB. Fetal growth delay and maternal hemoglobin A1c in early diabetic pregnancy. Obstet Gynecol 1984;64:351–2.

15. Rubin A, Murphy DP. Studies in human reproduction. III. The frequency of congenital malformations in the offspring of nondiabetic and diabetic individuals. J Pediatr 1958;53:579–85.

16. Damm P, Molsted-Pedersen L. Significant decrease in congenital malformations in newborn infants of an unselected population of diabetic women. Am J Obstet Gynecol 1989;161:1163–7.

17. Hanson U, Persson B, Thunell S. Relationship between haemoglobin A1C in early type 1 (insulin-dependent) diabetic pregnancy and the occurrence of spontaneous abortion and fetal malformation in Sweden. Diabetologia 1990;33:100–4.

18. Fuhrmann K, Reiher H, Semmler K, et al. Prevention of congenital malformations in infants of insulin-dependent diabetic mothers. Diabetes Care 1983;6:219–23.

19. Greene MF, Hare JW, Cloherty JP, et al. First-trimester hemoglobin A1 and risk for major malformation and spontaneous abortion in diabetic pregnancy. Teratology 1989;39:225–31.

20. Reece EA, Homko CJ. Assessment and management of pregnancies complicated by pregestational and gestational diabetes mellitus. J Assoc Acad Minor Phys 1994;5:87–97.

21. Kalter H, Warkany J. Medical progress. Congenital malformations: etiologic factors and their role in prevention (first of two parts). N Engl J Med 1983;308:424–31.

22. Tsang RC, Ballard J, Braun C. The infant of the diabetic mother: today and tomorrow. Clin Obstet Gynecol 1981;24:125–47.

23. Hadden DR. Diabetes in pregnancy 1985. Diabetologia 1986;29:1–9.

24. Ballard JL, Holroyde J, Tsang RC, et al. High malformation rates and decreased mortality in infants of diabetic mothers managed after the first trimester of pregnancy (1956-1978). Am J Obstet Gynecol 1984;148:1111–8.

25. Mills JL. Malformations in infants of diabetic mothers. Teratology 1982;25:385–94.
26. Harris MI, Flegal KM, Cowie CC, et al. Prevalence of diabetes, impaired fasting glucose, and impaired glucose tolerance in U.S. adults. The Third National Health and Nutrition Examination Survey, 1988-1994. Diabetes Care 1998;21:518–24.
27. Peacock I. Glycosylated haemoglobin: measurement and clinical use. J Clin Pathol 1984;37:841–51.
28. Lai LC. Global standardisation of HbA1c. Malays J Pathol 2008;30:67–71.
29. Consensus Committee. Consensus statement on the worldwide standardization of the hemoglobin A1C measurement: the American Diabetes Association, European Association for the Study of Diabetes, International Federation of Clinical Chemistry and Laboratory Medicine, and the International Diabetes Federation. Diabetes Care 2007;30:2399–400.
30. Eisenbarth GS. Type 1 diabetes mellitus. In: Kahn CR, Weir GC, King GL, et al, editors. Diabetes mellitus. Philadelphia: Lippincott Williams & Wilkins; 2005. p. 399–424.
31. Tisch R, McDevitt H. Insulin-dependent diabetes mellitus. Cell 1996;85:291–7.
32. Muoio DM, Newgard CB. Mechanisms of disease: molecular and metabolic mechanisms of insulin resistance and β-cell failure in type 2 diabetes. Nat Rev Mol Cell Biol 2008;9:193–205.
33. Meeuwisse-Pasterkamp SH, van der Klauw MM, Wolffenbuttel BH. Type 2 diabetes mellitus: prevention of macrovascular complications. Expert Rev Cardiovasc Ther 2008;6:323–41.
34. Hales CN, Barker DJ. Type 2 (non-insulin-dependent) diabetes mellitus: the thrifty phenotype hypothesis. Diabetologia 1992;35:595–601.
35. Meyer BA, Palmer SM. Pregestational diabetes. Semin Perinatol 1990;14:12–23.
36. Dunne FP. Pregestational diabetes mellitus and pregnancy. Trends Endocrinol Metab 1999;10:179–82.
37. Forsbach-Sanchez G, Tamez-Perez HE, Vazquez-Lara J. Diabetes and pregnancy. Arch Med Res 2005;36:291–9.
38. Ratner RE, Passaro MD. Gestational diabetes mellitus. In: LeRoith D, Taylor SI, Olefsky JM, editors. Diabetes mellitus: a fundamental and clinical text. Philadelphia: Lippincott Williams & Wilkins; 2004. p. 1291–300.
39. Reece EA, Leguizamon G, Wiznitzer A. Gestational diabetes: the need for a common ground. Lancet 2009;373:1789–97.
40. Ullrich I, Yeater R. Gestational diabetes. W V Med J 1995;91:148–51.
41. Persson B, Hanson U. Neonatal morbidities in gestational diabetes mellitus. Diabetes Care 1998;21(Suppl 2):B79–84.
42. Lucas MJ. Diabetes complicating pregnancy. Obstet Gynecol Clin North Am 2001;28:513–36.
43. International Association of Diabetes, Pregnancy Study Groups Consensus Panel, Metzger BE, Gabbe SG, Persson B, et al. International Association of Diabetes and Pregnancy study groups recommendations on the diagnosis and classification of hyperglycemia in pregnancy. Diabetes Care 2010;33:676–82.
44. Correa A, Gilboa SM, Besser LM, et al. Diabetes mellitus and birth defects. Am J Obstet Gynecol 2008;199:237.e1–9.
45. Reece EA. Diabetes-induced birth defects: what do we know? What can we do? Curr Diab Rep 2012;12:24–32.
46. Becerra JE, Khoury MJ, Cordero JF, et al. Diabetes mellitus during pregnancy and the risks for specific birth defects: a population-based case-control study. Pediatrics 1990;85:1–9.

47. Loffredo CA, Wilson PD, Ferencz C. Maternal diabetes: an independent risk factor for major cardiovascular malformations with increased mortality of affected infants. Teratology 2001;64:98–106.
48. Ramos-Arroyo MA, Rodriguez-Pinilla E, Cordero JF. Maternal diabetes: the risk for specific birth defects. Eur J Epidemiol 1992;8:503–8.
49. Farrell T, Neale L, Cundy T. Congenital anomalies in the offspring of women with type 1, type 2 and gestational diabetes. Diabet Med 2002;19:322–6.
50. Sheffield JS, Butler-Koster EL, Casey BM, et al. Maternal diabetes mellitus and infant malformations. Obstet Gynecol 2002;100:925–30.
51. Reece EA. The fetal and maternal consequences of gestational diabetes mellitus. J Matern Fetal Neonatal Med 2010;23:199–203.
52. Garcia Carrapato MR. The offspring of gestational diabetes. J Perinat Med 2003;31:5–11.
53. Jones CW. Gestational diabetes and its impact on the neonate. Neonatal Netw 2001;20:17–23.
54. Shields LE, Gan EA, Murphy HF, et al. The prognostic value of hemoglobin A1c in predicting fetal heart disease in diabetic pregnancies. Obstet Gynecol 1993; 81:954–7.
55. Miller E, Hare JW, Cloherty JP, et al. Elevated maternal hemoglobin A1c in early pregnancy and major congenital anomalies in infants of diabetic mothers. N Engl J Med 1981;304:1331–4.
56. Rose BI, Graff S, Spencer R, et al. Major congenital anomalies in infants and glycosylated hemoglobin levels in insulin-requiring diabetic mothers. J Perinatol 1988;8:309–11.
57. Lucas MJ, Leveno KJ, Williams ML, et al. Early pregnancy glycosylated hemoglobin, severity of diabetes, and fetal malformations. Am J Obstet Gynecol 1989;161:426–31.
58. Key TC, Giuffrida R, Moore TR. Predictive value of early pregnancy glycohemoglobin in the insulin- treated diabetic patient. Am J Obstet Gynecol 1987;156: 1096–100.
59. Ylinen K, Aula P, Stenman UH, et al. Risk of minor and major fetal malformations in diabetics with high haemoglobin A1c values in early pregnancy. Br Med J (Clin Res Ed) 1984;289:345–6.
60. Eriksson UJ, Borg LA, Cederberg J, et al. Pathogenesis of diabetes-induced congenital malformations. Ups J Med Sci 2000;105:53–84.
61. Horton WE Jr, Sadler TW. Effects of maternal diabetes on early embryogenesis. Alterations in morphogenesis produced by the ketone body, B-hydroxybutyrate. Diabetes 1983;32:610–6.
62. Hunter ES 3rd, Sadler TW, Wynn RE. A potential mechanism of DL-β-hydroxybutyrate-induced malformations in mouse embryos. Am J Physiol 1987;253:E72–80.
63. Hunter ES 3rd, Sadler TW. D-(-)-β-hydroxybutyrate-induced effects on mouse embryos in vitro. Teratology 1987;36:259–64.
64. Moore DC, Stanisstreet M, Clarke CA. Morphological and physiological effects of β-hydroxybutyrate on rat embryos grown in vitro at different stages. Teratology 1989;40:237–51.
65. Eriksson UJ, Cederberg J, Wentzel P. Congenital malformations in offspring of diabetic mothers–animal and human studies. Rev Endocr Metab Disord 2003; 4:79–93.
66. Persson B. Prevention of fetal malformation with antioxidants in diabetic pregnancy. Pediatr Res 2001;49:742–3.

67. Fuhrmann K, Reiher H, Semmler K, et al. The effect of intensified conventional insulin therapy before and during pregnancy on the malformation rate in offspring of diabetic mothers. Exp Clin Endocrinol 1984;83:173–7.
68. Gareskog M, Cederberg J, Eriksson UJ, et al. Maternal diabetes in vivo and high glucose concentration in vitro increases apoptosis in rat embryos. Reprod Toxicol 2007;23:63–74.
69. Akazawa S. Diabetic embryopathy: studies using a rat embryo culture system and an animal model. Congenit Anom (Kyoto) 2005;45:73–9.
70. Zhao Z, Reece EA. Experimental mechanisms of diabetic embryopathy and strategies for developing therapeutic interventions. J Soc Gynecol Investig 2005;12:549–57.
71. Lee-Parritz A. New technologies for the management of pregestational diabetes mellitus. Obstet Gynecol Surv 2012;67:167–75.
72. Ballas J, Moore TR, Ramos GA. Management of diabetes in pregnancy. Curr Diab Rep 2012;12:33–42.
73. Reece EA, Friedman AM, Copel JA, et al. Prenatal diagnosis and management of deviant fetal growth and congenital malformations. In: Reece EA, Coustan DR, editors. Diabetes mellitus in pregnancy. New York: Churchill Livingstone; 1995. p. 219–49.
74. Guideline Development Group. Management of diabetes from preconception to the postnatal period: summary of NICE guidance. BMJ 2008;336:714–7.
75. Ali S, Dornhorst A. Diabetes in pregnancy: health risks and management. Postgrad Med J 2011;87:417–27.
76. Kitzmiller JL, Block JM, Brown FM, et al. Managing preexisting diabetes for pregnancy: summary of evidence and consensus recommendations for care. Diabetes Care 2008;31:1060–79.
77. Holing EV, Beyer CS, Brown ZA, et al. Why don't women with diabetes plan their pregnancies? Diabetes Care 1998;21:889–95.
78. Reece EA, Hobbins JC. Diabetic embryopathy: pathogenesis, prenatal diagnosis and prevention. Obstet Gynecol Surv 1986;41:325–35.
79. Ewart-Toland A, Yankowitz J, Winder A, et al. Oculoauriculovertebral abnormalities in children of diabetic mothers. Am J Med Genet 2000;90:303–9.
80. Zacharias JF, Jenkins JH, Marion JP. The incidence of neural tube defects in the fetus and neonate of the insulin-dependent diabetic woman. Am J Obstet Gynecol 1984;150:797–8.
81. Barr M Jr, Hanson JW, Currey K, et al. Holoprosencephaly in infants of diabetic mothers. J Pediatr 1983;102:565–8.
82. Matsunaga E, Shiota K. Holoprosencephaly in human embryos: epidemiologic studies of 150 cases. Teratology 1977;16:261–72.
83. Rusnak SL, Driscoll SG. Congenital spinal anomalies in infants of diabetic mothers. Pediatrics 1965;35:989–95.
84. Aubry MC, Aubry JP, Dommergues M. Sonographic prenatal diagnosis of central nervous system abnormalities. Childs Nerv Syst 2003;19:391–402.
85. Cameron M, Moran P. Prenatal screening and diagnosis of neural tube defects. Prenat Diagn 2009;29:402–11.
86. Drugan A, Weissman A, Evans MI. Screening for neural tube defects. Clin Perinatol 2001;28:279–87, vii.
87. Turner CD, Silva S, Jeanty P. Prenatal diagnosis of alobar holoprosencephaly at 10 weeks of gestation. Ultrasound Obstet Gynecol 1999;13:360–2.
88. Peebles DM. Holoprosencephaly. Prenat Diagn 1998;18:477–80.

89. Wong HS, Tang MH, Yan KW, et al. Histological findings in a case of alobar holoprosencephaly diagnosed at 10 weeks of pregnancy. Prenat Diagn 1999;19:859–62.
90. Blaas HG, Eik-Nes SH. Sonoembryology and early prenatal diagnosis of neural anomalies. Prenat Diagn 2009;29:312–25.
91. Cuckle HS. Screening for neural tube defects. Ciba Found Symp 1994;181: 253–66 [discussion: 66–9].
92. Pergament E. α-fetoprotein and the prenatal diagnosis of neural tube defects. Obstet Gynecol Annu 1977;6:173–89.
93. Haddow JE, Knight GJ, Kloza EM. α-fetoprotein screening in pregnancy–a test whose time has come. Ariz Med 1982;39:436–9.
94. Haddow JE, Miller WA. Prenatal diagnosis of open neural tube defects. Methods Cell Biol 1982;26:67–94.
95. Wang R, Martinez-Frias ML, Graham JM Jr. Infants of diabetic mothers are at increased risk for the oculo-auriculo-vertebral sequence: a case-based and case-control approach. J Pediatr 2002;141:611–7.
96. Aberg A, Westbom L, Kallen B. Congenital malformations among infants whose mothers had gestational diabetes or preexisting diabetes. Early Hum Dev 2001; 61:85–95.
97. Garcia-Patterson A, Erdozain L, Ginovart G, et al. In human gestational diabetes mellitus congenital malformations are related to pre-pregnancy body mass index and to severity of diabetes. Diabetologia 2004;47:509–14.
98. Spilson SV, Kim HJ, Chung KC. Association between maternal diabetes mellitus and newborn oral cleft. Ann Plast Surg 2001;47:477–81.
99. Gratz ES, Pollack MA, Zimmerman RD. Congenital facial palsy and ipsilateral deafness: association with maternal diabetes mellitus. Int J Pediatr Otorhinolaryngol 1981;3:335–41.
100. Pilu G, Reece EA, Romero R, et al. Prenatal diagnosis of craniofacial malformations with ultrasonography. Am J Obstet Gynecol 1986;155:45–50.
101. Ghi T, Perolo A, Banzi C, et al. Two-dimensional ultrasound is accurate in the diagnosis of fetal craniofacial malformation. Ultrasound Obstet Gynecol 2002; 19:543–51.
102. Nyberg DA, Hegge FN, Kramer D, et al. Premaxillary protrusion: a sonographic clue to bilateral cleft lip and palate. J Ultrasound Med 1993;12:331–5.
103. Wren C, Birrell G, Hawthorne G. Cardiovascular malformations in infants of diabetic mothers. Heart 2003;89:1217–20.
104. Ferencz C, Rubin JD, McCarter RJ, et al. Maternal diabetes and cardiovascular malformations: predominance of double outlet right ventricle and truncus arteriosus. Teratology 1990;41:319–26.
105. Rowland TW, Hubbell JP Jr, Nadas AS. Congenital heart disease in infants of diabetic mothers. J Pediatr 1973;83:815–20.
106. Rajiah P, Mak C, Dubinksy TJ, et al. Ultrasound of fetal cardiac anomalies. AJR Am J Roentgenol 2011;197:W747–60.
107. Axt-Fliedner R, Gembruch U. Nuchal translucency and fetal cardiac malformations. Ultraschall Med 2010;31:144–50.
108. Clur SA, Ottenkamp J, Bilardo CM. The nuchal translucency and the fetal heart: a literature review. Prenat Diagn 2009;29:739–48.
109. Assemany SR, Muzzo S, Gardner LI. Syndrome of phocomelic diabetic embryopathy (caudal dysplasia). Am J Dis Child 1972;123:489–91.
110. Welch JP, Aterman K. The syndrome of caudal dysplasia: a review, including etiologic considerations and evidence of heterogeneity. Pediatr Pathol 1984;2: 313–27.

111. Sadler TW. Embryology of neural tube development. Am J Med Genet C Semin Med Genet 2005;135C:2–8.

112. Kaufman BA. Neural tube defects. Pediatr Clin North Am 2004;51:389–419.

113. Hollyday M. Neurogenesis in the vertebrate neural tube. Int J Dev Neurosci 2001;19:161–73.

114. Altmann CR, Brivanlou AH. Neural patterning in the vertebrate embryo. Int Rev Cytol 2001;203:447–82.

115. Loeken MR. Current perspectives on the causes of neural tube defects resulting from diabetic pregnancy. Am J Med Genet C Semin Med Genet 2005;135C: 77–87.

116. Chappell JH Jr, Wang XD, Loeken MR. Diabetes and apoptosis: neural crest cells and neural tube. Apoptosis 2009;14:1472–83.

117. Sugimura Y, Murase T, Oyama K, et al. Prevention of neural tube defects by loss of function of inducible nitric oxide synthase in fetuses of a mouse model of streptozotocin-induced diabetes. Diabetologia 2009;52:962–71.

118. Zhao Z. Cardiac malformations and alteration of TGFβ signaling system in diabetic embryopathy. Birth Defects Res B Dev Reprod Toxicol 2010;89: 97–105.

119. Oyama K, Sugimura Y, Murase T, et al. Folic acid prevents congenital malformations in the offspring of diabetic mice. Endocr J 2009;56:29–37.

120. Wessels A, Markman MW, Vermeulen JL, et al. The development of the atrioventricular junction in the human heart. Circ Res 1996;78:110–7.

121. Moorman A, Webb S, Brown NA, et al. Development of the heart: (1) formation of the cardiac chambers and arterial trunks. Heart 2003;89:806–14.

122. Anderson RH, Webb S, Brown NA, et al. Development of the heart: (2) septation of the atriums and ventricles. Heart 2003;89:949–58.

123. Anderson RH, Webb S, Brown NA, et al. Development of the heart: (3) formation of the ventricular outflow tracts, arterial valves, and intrapericardial arterial trunks. Heart 2003;89:1110–8.

124. Zhao Z. Endoplasmic reticulum stress in maternal diabetes-induced cardiac malformations during critical cardiogenesis period. Birth Defects Res B Dev Reprod Toxicol 2012;95:1–6.

125. Markwald R, Eisenberg C, Eisenberg L, et al. Epithelial-mesenchymal transformations in early avian heart development. Acta Anat 1996;156:173–86.

126. Mjaatvedt GH, Yamamura H, Wessels A, et al. Mechanisms of segmentation, septation, and remodeling of the tubular heart: endocardial cushion fate and cardiac looping. In: Harvey RP, Rosenthal N, editors. Heart development. New York: Academic Press; 1999. p. 159–77.

127. Person AD, Klewer SE, Runyan RB. Cell biology of cardiac cushion development. Int Rev Cytol 2005;243:287–335.

128. Zhao Z, Rivkees SA. Programmed cell death in the developing heart: regulation by BMP4 and FGF2. Dev Dyn 2000;217:388–400.

129. Kumar SD, Dheen ST, Tay SS. Maternal diabetes induces congenital heart defects in mice by altering the expression of genes involved in cardiovascular development. Cardiovasc Diabetol 2007;6:34.

130. Siman CM, Gittenberger-De Groot AC, Wisse B, et al. Malformations in offspring of diabetic rats: morphometric analysis of neural crest-derived organs and effects of maternal vitamin E treatment. Teratology 2000;61:355–67.

131. Tanigawa K, Kawaguchi M, Tanaka O, et al. Skeletal malformations in rat offspring. Long-term effect of maternal insulin-induced hypoglycemia during organogenesis. Diabetes 1991;40:1115–21.

132. Bowden RE. Development of the middle and external ear in man. Proc R Soc Med 1977;70:807–15.
133. Mallo M. Formation of the middle ear: recent progress on the developmental and molecular mechanisms. Dev Biol 2001;231:410–9.
134. Sun F, Kawasaki E, Akazawa S, et al. Apoptosis and its pathway in early post-implantation embryos of diabetic rats. Diabetes Res Clin Pract 2005;67:110–8.
135. Phelan SA, Ito M, Loeken MR. Neural tube defects in embryos of diabetic mice: role of the Pax-3 gene and apoptosis. Diabetes 1997;46:1189–97.
136. Fine EL, Horal M, Chang TI, et al. Evidence that elevated glucose causes altered gene expression, apoptosis, and neural tube defects in a mouse model of diabetic pregnancy. Diabetes 1999;48:2454–62.
137. Zhao Z, Yang P, Eckert RL, et al. Caspase-8: a key role in the pathogenesis of diabetic embryopathy. Birth Defects Res B Dev Reprod Toxicol 2009;86:72–7.
138. Zhao Z, Wu YK, Reece EA. Demonstration of the essential role of protein kinase C isoforms in hyperglycemia-induced embryonic malformations. Reprod Sci 2008; 15:349–56.
139. Singh CK, Kumar A, Hitchcock DB, et al. Resveratrol prevents embryonic oxidative stress and apoptosis associated with diabetic embryopathy and improves glucose and lipid profile of diabetic dam. Mol Nutr Food Res 2011;55:1186–96.
140. Brown CB, Baldwin HS. Neural crest contribution to the cardiovascular system. Adv Exp Med Biol 2006;589:134–54.
141. Stoller JZ, Epstein JA. Cardiac neural crest. Semin Cell Dev Biol 2005;16:704–15.
142. Morgan SC, Relaix F, Sandell LL, et al. Oxidative stress during diabetic pregnancy disrupts cardiac neural crest migration and causes outflow tract defects. Birth Defects Res A Clin Mol Teratol 2008;82:453–63.
143. Wentzel P, Gareskog M, Eriksson UJ. Decreased cardiac glutathione peroxidase levels and enhanced mandibular apoptosis in malformed embryos of diabetic rats. Diabetes 2008;57:3344–52.
144. Graham A, Begbie J, McGonnell I. Significance of the cranial neural crest. Dev Dyn 2004;229:5–13.
145. Chai Y, Maxson RE Jr. Recent advances in craniofacial morphogenesis. Dev Dyn 2006;235:2353–75.
146. Santagati F, Rijli FM. Cranial neural crest and the building of the vertebrate head. Nat Rev Neurosci 2003;4:806–18.
147. Cederberg J, Picard JJ, Eriksson UJ. Maternal diabetes in the rat impairs the formation of neural-crest derived cranial nerve ganglia in the offspring. Diabetologia 2003;46:1245–51.
148. Li R, Thorens B, Loeken MR. Expression of the gene encoding the high-K (m) glucose transporter 2 by the early postimplantation mouse embryo is essential for neural tube defects associated with diabetic embryopathy. Diabetologia 2007;50:682–9.
149. Matsumoto K, Akazawa S, Ishibashi M, et al. Abundant expression of GLUT1 and GLUT3 in rat embryo during the early organogenesis period. Biochem Biophys Res Commun 1995;209:95–102.
150. Stevens FJ, Argon Y. Protein folding in the ER. Semin Cell Dev Biol 1999;10:443–54.
151. Benyair R, Ron E, Lederkremer GZ. Protein quality control, retention, and degradation at the endoplasmic reticulum. Int Rev Cell Mol Biol 2011;292:197–280.
152. Groenendyk J, Sreenivasaiah PK, Kim do H, et al. Biology of endoplasmic reticulum stress in the heart. Circ Res 2010;107:1185–97.

153. Yoshida H. ER stress and diseases. FEBS J 2007;274:630–58.
154. Banhegyi G, Baumeister P, Benedetti A, et al. Endoplasmic reticulum stress. Ann N Y Acad Sci 2007;1113:58–71.
155. Fonseca SG, Burcin M, Gromada J, et al. Endoplasmic reticulum stress in β-cells and development of diabetes. Curr Opin Pharmacol 2009;9:763–70.
156. Lin JH, Walter P, Yen TS. Endoplasmic reticulum stress in disease pathogenesis. Annu Rev Pathol 2008;3:399–425.
157. Schroder M. Endoplasmic reticulum stress responses. Cell Mol Life Sci 2008;65: 862–94.
158. Malhotra JD, Kaufman RJ. The endoplasmic reticulum and the unfolded protein response. Semin Cell Dev Biol 2007;18:716–31.
159. Lai E, Teodoro T, Volchuk A. Endoplasmic reticulum stress: signaling the unfolded protein response. Physiology 2007;22:193–201.
160. Zhao Z, Eckert RL, Reece EA. Reduction in embryonic malformations and alleviation of endoplasmic reticulum stress by nitric oxide synthase inhibition in diabetic embryopathy. Reprod Sci 2012;19:823–31.
161. Cao Y, Zhao Z, Eckert RL, et al. The essential role of protein kinase Cδ in diabetes-induced neural tube defects. J Matern Fetal Neonatal Med 2012;25: 2020–4.
162. Yang X, Borg LA, Eriksson UJ. Altered mitochondrial morphology of rat embryos in diabetic pregnancy. Anat Rec 1995;241:255–67.
163. Genova ML, Pich MM, Biondi A, et al. Mitochondrial production of oxygen radical species and the role of coenzyme Q as an antioxidant. Exp Biol Med 2003;228:506–13.
164. Raha S, Robinson BH. Mitochondria, oxygen free radicals, and apoptosis. Am J Med Genet 2001;106:62–70.
165. Ishibashi M, Akazawa S, Sakamaki H, et al. Oxygen-induced embryopathy and the significance of glutathione-dependent antioxidant system in the rat embryo during early organogenesis. Free Radic Biol Med 1997;22:447–54.
166. Li R, Chase M, Jung SK, et al. Hypoxic stress in diabetic pregnancy contributes to impaired embryo gene expression and defective development by inducing oxidative stress. Am J Physiol Endocrinol Metab 2005;289(4): E591–9.
167. Menegola E, Broccia ML, Prati M, et al. Glutathione status in diabetes-induced embryopathies. Biol Neonate 1996;69:293–7.
168. Yan J, Hales BF. Depletion of glutathione induces 4-hydroxynonenal protein adducts and hydroxyurea teratogenicity in the organogenesis stage mouse embryo. J Pharmacol Exp Ther 2006;319:613–21.
169. Djordjevic VB. Free radicals in cell biology. Int Rev Cytol 2004;237:57–89.
170. Ueda S, Masutani H, Nakamura H, et al. Redox control of cell death. Antioxid Redox Signal 2002;4:405–14.
171. Sivan E, Reece EA, Wu YK, et al. Dietary vitamin E prophylaxis and diabetic embryopathy: morphologic and biochemical analysis. Am J Obstet Gynecol 1996; 175:793–9.
172. Viana M, Herrera E, Bonet B. Teratogenic effects of diabetes mellitus in the rat. Prevention by vitamin E. Diabetologia 1996;39:1041–6.
173. Siman CM, Eriksson UJ. Vitamin E decreases the occurrence of malformations in the offspring of diabetic rats. Diabetes 1997;46:1054–61.
174. Siman CM, Eriksson UJ. Vitamin C supplementation of the maternal diet reduces the rate of malformation in the offspring of diabetic rats. Diabetologia 1997;40: 1416–24.

175. Yang X, Borg LA, Siman CM, et al. Maternal antioxidant treatments prevent diabetes-induced alterations of mitochondrial morphology in rat embryos. Anat Rec 1998;251:303–15.
176. Viana M, Aruoma OI, Herrera E, et al. Oxidative damage in pregnant diabetic rats and their embryos. Free Radic Biol Med 2000;29:1115–21.
177. Zaken V, Kohen R, Ornoy A. Vitamins C and E improve rat embryonic anti-oxidant defense mechanism in diabetic culture medium. Teratology 2001;64: 33–44.
178. Guijarro MV, Indart A, Aruoma OI, et al. Effects of ergothioneine on diabetic embryopathy in pregnant rats. Food Chem Toxicol 2002;40:1751–5.
179. Gareskog M, Eriksson UJ, Wentzel P. Combined supplementation of folic acid and vitamin E diminishes diabetes-induced embryotoxicity in rats. Birth defects research part A. Birth Defects Res A Clin Mol Teratol 2006;76:483–90.
180. Reece EA, Wu YK, Zhao Z, et al. Dietary vitamin and lipid therapy rescues aberrant signaling and apoptosis and prevents hyperglycemia-induced diabetic embryopathy in rats. Am J Obstet Gynecol 2006;194:580–5.
181. Reece EA, Wu YK. Prevention of diabetic embryopathy in offspring of diabetic rats with use of a cocktail of deficient substrates and an antioxidant. Am J Obstet Gynecol 1997;176:790–7.
182. Li X, Weng H, Reece EA, et al. SOD1 overexpression in vivo blocks hyperglycemia-induced specific PKC isoforms: substrate activation and consequent lipid peroxidation in diabetic embryopathy. Am J Obstet Gynecol 2011; 205:84.e1–6.
183. Hagay ZJ, Weiss Y, Zusman I, et al. Prevention of diabetes-associated embryopathy by overexpression of the free radical scavenger copper zinc superoxide dismutase in transgenic mouse embryos. Am J Obstet Gynecol 1995;173: 1036–41.
184. Jawerbaum A, Gonzalez E. The role of alterations in arachidonic acid metabolism and nitric oxide homeostasis in rat models of diabetes during early pregnancy. Curr Pharm Des 2005;11:1327–42.
185. Jawerbaum A, Higa R, White V, et al. Peroxynitrites and impaired modulation of nitric oxide concentrations in embryos from diabetic rats during early organogenesis. Reproduction 2005;130:695–703.
186. Pacher P, Beckman JS, Liaudet L. Nitric oxide and peroxynitrite in health and disease. Physiol Rev 2007;87:315–424.
187. Szabo C, Ischiropoulos H, Radi R. Peroxynitrite: biochemistry, pathophysiology and development of therapeutics. Nat Rev Drug Discov 2007;6:662–80.
188. Knowles RG, Moncada S. Nitric oxide synthases in mammals. Biochem J 1994; 298(Pt 2):249–58.
189. Torreilles J. Nitric oxide: one of the more conserved and widespread signaling molecules. Front Biosci 2001;6:D1161–72.
190. Groves JT, Wang CC. Nitric oxide synthase: models and mechanisms. Curr Opin Chem Biol 2000;4:687–95.
191. Umar S, van der Laarse A. Nitric oxide and nitric oxide synthase isoforms in the normal, hypertrophic, and failing heart. Mol Cell Biochem 2010;333:191–201.
192. Zhou L, Zhu DY. Neuronal nitric oxide synthase: structure, subcellular localization, regulation, and clinical implications. Nitric Oxide 2009;20:223–30.
193. Hesslinger C, Strub A, Boer R, et al. Inhibition of inducible nitric oxide synthase in respiratory diseases. Biochem Soc Trans 2009;37:886–91.
194. Kleinert H, Schwarz PM, Forstermann U. Regulation of the expression of inducible nitric oxide synthase. Biol Chem 2003;384:1343–64.

195. Kroncke KD, Suschek CV, Kolb-Bachofen V. Implications of inducible nitric oxide synthase expression and enzyme activity. Antioxid Redox Signal 2000;2: 585–605.
196. Kumar SD, Yong SK, Dheen ST, et al. Cardiac malformations are associated with altered expression of vascular endothelial growth factor and endothelial nitric oxide synthase genes in embryos of diabetic mice. Exp Biol Med 2008;233: 1421–32.
197. Jawerbaum A, Gonzalez ET, Novaro V, et al. Increased prostaglandin E generation and enhanced nitric oxide synthase activity in the non-insulin-dependent diabetic embryo during organogenesis. Reprod Fertil Dev 1998; 10:191–6.
198. Yang P, Cao Y, Li H. Hyperglycemia induces inducible nitric oxide synthase gene expression and consequent nitrosative stress via c-Jun N-terminal kinase activation. Am J Obstet Gynecol 2010;203:185.e5–185.e11.
199. Waite M. Phospholipases, enzymes that share a substrate class. Adv Exp Med Biol 1990;279:1–22.
200. Kaiser E, Chiba P, Zaky K. Phospholipases in biology and medicine. Clin Biochem 1990;23:349–70.
201. Blobe GC, Khan WA, Hannun YA. Protein kinase C: cellular target of the second messenger arachidonic acid? Prostaglandins Leukot Essent Fatty Acids 1995; 52:129–35.
202. Bonventre JV. Phospholipase A2 and signal transduction. J Am Soc Nephrol 1992;3:128–50.
203. Clark JD, Schievella AR, Nalefski EA, et al. Cytosolic phospholipase A2. J Lipid Mediat Cell Signal 1995;12:83–117.
204. Liang X, Wu L, Wang Q, et al. Function of COX-2 and prostaglandins in neurological disease. J Mol Neurosci 2007;33:94–9.
205. Rouzer CA, Marnett LJ. Cyclooxygenases: structural and functional insights. J Lipid Res 2009;50(Suppl):S29–34.
206. Morrow JD, Hill KE, Burk RF, et al. A series of prostaglandin F2-like compounds are produced in vivo in humans by a non-cyclooxygenase, free radical-catalyzed mechanism. Proc Natl Acad Sci U S A 1990;87:9383–7.
207. Morrow JD. The isoprostanes: their quantification as an index of oxidant stress status in vivo. Drug Metab Rev 2000;32:377–85.
208. Wentzel P, Welsh N, Eriksson UJ. Developmental damage, increased lipid peroxidation, diminished cyclooxygenase-2 gene expression, and lowered prostaglandin E2 levels in rat embryos exposed to a diabetic environment. Diabetes 1999;48:813–20.
209. Wentzel P, Eriksson UJ. A diabetes-like environment increases malformation rate and diminishes prostaglandin E(2) in rat embryos: reversal by administration of vitamin E and folic acid. Birth Defects Res A Clin Mol Teratol 2005;73(7): 506–11.
210. Piddington R, Joyce J, Dhanasekaran P, et al. Diabetes mellitus affects prostaglandin E2 levels in mouse embryos during neurulation. Diabetologia 1996;39: 915–20.
211. Jawerbaum A, Gonzalez ET, Sinner D, et al. Diminished PGE2 content, enhanced PGE2 release and defects in 3H-PGE2 transport in embryos from overtly diabetic rats. Reprod Fertil Dev 2000;12:141–7.
212. Jawerbaum A, Sinner D, White V, et al. Modulation of PGE2 generation in the diabetic embryo: effect of nitric oxide and superoxide dismutase. Prostaglandins Leukot Essent Fatty Acids 2001;64:127–33.

213. Wentzel P, Eriksson UJ. 8-Iso-PGF(2α) administration generates dysmorphogenesis and increased lipid peroxidation in rat embryos in vitro. Teratology 2002;66:164–8.
214. El-Bassiouni EA, Helmy MH, Abou Rawash N, et al. Embryopathy in experimental diabetic gestation: assessment of PGE2 level, gene expression of cyclooxygenases and apoptosis. Br J Biomed Sci 2005;62:161–5.
215. Wentzel P, Eriksson UJ. Antioxidants diminish developmental damage induced by high glucose and cyclooxygenase inhibitors in rat embryos in vitro. Diabetes 1998;47:677–84.
216. Jawerbaum A, Rosello Catafau J, Gonzalez ET, et al. Glucose metabolism, triglyceride and glycogen levels, as well as eicosanoid production in isolated uterine strips and in embryos in a rat model of non-insulin-dependent diabetes mellitus during pregnancy. Prostaglandins 1994;47:81–96.
217. Goto MP, Goldman AS, Uhing MR. PGE2 prevents anomalies induced by hyperglycemia or diabetic serum in mouse embryos. Diabetes 1992;41:1644–50.
218. Dempsey EC, Newton AC, Mochly-Rosen D, et al. Protein kinase C isozymes and the regulation of diverse cell responses. Am J Physiol Lung Cell Mol Physiol 2000;279:L429–38.
219. Shirai Y, Saito N. Activation mechanisms of protein kinase C: maturation, catalytic activation, and targeting. J Biochem 2002;132:663–8.
220. Cao Y, Zhao Z, Eckert RL, et al. Protein kinase Cβ2 inhibition reduces hyperglycemia-induced neural tube defects through suppression of a caspase 8-triggered apoptotic pathway. Am J Obstet Gynecol 2011;204:226.e1–5.
221. Wada T, Penninger JM. Mitogen-activated protein kinases in apoptosis regulation. Oncogene 2004;23:2838–49.
222. Lin A, Dibling B. The true face of JNK activation in apoptosis. Aging Cell 2002;1:112–6.
223. Corson LB, Yamanaka Y, Lai KM, et al. Spatial and temporal patterns of ERK signaling during mouse embryogenesis. Development 2003;130:4527–37.
224. Reece EA, Wu YK, Wiznitzer A, et al. Dietary polyunsaturated fatty acid prevents malformations in offspring of diabetic rats. Am J Obstet Gynecol 1996;175:818–23.
225. Reece EA, Ma XD, Wu YK, et al. Aberrant patterns of cellular communication in diabetes-induced embryopathy. I. Membrane signalling. J Matern Fetal Neonatal Med 2002;11:249–53.
226. Yang P, Zhao Z, Reece EA. Activation of oxidative stress signaling that is implicated in apoptosis with a mouse model of diabetic embryopathy. Am J Obstet Gynecol 2008;198:130.e1–7.
227. Yang P, Zhao Z, Reece EA. Blockade of c-Jun N-terminal kinase activation abrogates hyperglycemia-induced yolk sac vasculopathy in vitro. Am J Obstet Gynecol 2008;198:321.e1–7.
228. Yang P, Zhao Z, Reece EA. Involvement of c-Jun N-terminal kinases activation in diabetic embryopathy. Biochem Biophys Res Commun 2007;357:749–54.
229. Li X, Xu C, Yang P. c-Jun NH2-terminal kinase 1/2 and endoplasmic reticulum stress as interdependent and reciprocal causation in diabetic embryopathy. Diabetes 2012;62(2):599–608.
230. Ola MS, Nawaz M, Ahsan H. Role of Bcl-2 family proteins and caspases in the regulation of apoptosis. Mol Cell Biochem 2011;351:41–58.
231. Cory S, Huang DC, Adams JM. The Bcl-2 family: roles in cell survival and oncogenesis. Oncogene 2003;22:8590–607.

232. Kumar S. Caspase function in programmed cell death. Cell Death Differ 2007; 14:32–43.

233. Taylor RC, Cullen SP, Martin SJ. Apoptosis: controlled demolition at the cellular level. Nat Rev Mol Cell Biol 2008;9:231–41.

234. Degterev A, Yuan J. Expansion and evolution of cell death programmes. Nat Rev Mol Cell Biol 2008;9:378–90.

235. Willis SN, Adams JM. Life in the balance: how BH3-only proteins induce apoptosis. Curr Opin Cell Biol 2005;17:617–25.

236. Antignani A, Youle RJ. How do Bax and Bak lead to permeabilization of the outer mitochondrial membrane? Curr Opin Cell Biol 2006;18:685–9.

237. Degterev A, Boyce M, Yuan J. A decade of caspases. Oncogene 2003;22: 8543–67.

238. Ferraro E, Corvaro M, Cecconi F. Physiological and pathological roles of Apaf1 and the apoptosome. J Cell Mol Med 2003;7:21–34.

239. Youle RJ, Strasser A. The BCL-2 protein family: opposing activities that mediate cell death. Nat Rev Mol Cell Biol 2008;9:47–59.

240. Wiznitzer A, Ayalon N, Hershkovitz R, et al. Lipoic acid prevention of neural tube defects in offspring of rats with streptozocin-induced diabetes. Am J Obstet Gynecol 1999;180:188–93.

241. Khandelwal M, Reece EA, Wu YK, et al. Dietary myo-inositol therapy in hyperglycemia-induced embryopathy. Teratology 1998;57:79–84.

242. Reece EA, Khandelwal M, Wu YK, et al. Dietary intake of myo-inositol and neural tube defects in offspring of diabetic rats. Am J Obstet Gynecol 1997; 176:536–9.

243. Wentzel P, Gareskog M, Eriksson UJ. Folic acid supplementation diminishes diabetes- and glucose-induced dysmorphogenesis in rat embryos in vivo and in vitro. Diabetes 2005;54:546–53.

244. Zabihi S, Eriksson UJ, Wentzel P. Folic acid supplementation affects ROS scavenging enzymes, enhances Vegf-A, and diminishes apoptotic state in yolk sacs of embryos of diabetic rats. Reprod Toxicol 2007;23:486–98.

245. Pinter E, Reece EA, Ogburn PL Jr, et al. Fatty acid content of yolk sac and embryo in hyperglycemia-induced embryopathy and effect of arachidonic acid supplementation. Am J Obstet Gynecol 1988;159:1484–90.

246. Packer L, Kraemer K, Rimbach G. Molecular aspects of lipoic acid in the prevention of diabetes complications. Nutrition 2001;17:888–95.

247. Zed PJ, Krenzelok EP. Treatment of acetaminophen overdose. Am J Health Syst Pharm 1999;56:1081–91.

248. Kanter MZ. Comparison of oral and i.v. acetylcysteine in the treatment of acetaminophen poisoning. Am J Health Syst Pharm 2006;63:1821–7.

249. Gareskog M, Wentzel P. N-Acetylcysteine and α-cyano-4-hydroxycinnamic acid alter protein kinase C (PKC)-δ and PKC-ζ and diminish dysmorphogenesis in rat embryos cultured with high glucose in vitro. J Endocrinol 2007;192:207–14.

250. Wentzel P, Ejdesjo A, Eriksson UJ. Maternal diabetes in vivo and high glucose in vitro diminish GAPDH activity in rat embryos. Diabetes 2003;52:1222–8.

251. Wentzel P, Wentzel CR, Gareskog MB, et al. Induction of embryonic dysmorphogenesis by high glucose concentration, disturbed inositol metabolism, and inhibited protein kinase C activity. Teratology 2001;63:193–201.

252. Honarbakhsh S, Schachter M. Vitamins and cardiovascular disease. Br J Nutr 2009;101:1113–31.

253. Van Patten CL, de Boer JG, Tomlinson Guns ES. Diet and dietary supplement intervention trials for the prevention of prostate cancer recurrence: a review of

the randomized controlled trial evidence. J Urol 2008;180:2314–21 [discussion: 721–2].

254. Higa R, Kurtz M, Mazzucco MB, et al. Folic acid and safflower oil supplementation interacts and protects embryos from maternal diabetes-induced damage. Mol Hum Reprod 2012;18:253–64.

255. Villar J, Purwar M, Merialdi M, et al. World Health Organisation multicentre randomised trial of supplementation with vitamins C and E among pregnant women at high risk for pre-eclampsia in populations of low nutritional status from developing countries. BJOG 2009;116:780–8.

256. Robinson I, de Serna DG, Gutierrez A, et al. Vitamin E in humans: an explanation of clinical trial failure. Endocr Pract 2006;12:576–82.

257. Polyzos NP, Mauri D, Tsappi M, et al. Combined vitamin C and E supplementation during pregnancy for preeclampsia prevention: a systematic review. Obstet Gynecol Surv 2007;62:202–6.

258. Briasoulis A, Tousoulis D, Antoniades C, et al. The oxidative stress menace to coronary vasculature: any place for antioxidants? Curr Pharm Des 2009;15:3078–90.

259. Steinhubl SR. Why have antioxidants failed in clinical trials? Am J Cardiol 2008;101:14D–9D.

260. Lipscombe LL, McLaughlin HM, Wu W, et al. Pregnancy planning in women with pregestational diabetes. J Matern Fetal Neonatal Med 2011;24:1095–101.

261. Gabbe SG, Graves CR. Management of diabetes mellitus complicating pregnancy. Obstet Gynecol 2003;102:857–68.

262. Janz NK, Herman WH, Becker MP, et al. Diabetes and pregnancy. Factors associated with seeking pre-conception care. Diabetes Care 1995;18:157–65.

263. Willhoite MB, Bennert HW Jr, Palomaki GE, et al. The impact of preconception counseling on pregnancy outcomes. The experience of the Maine Diabetes in Pregnancy Program. Diabetes Care 1993;16:450–5.

Use of Oral Hypoglycemic and Insulin Agents in Pregnant Patients

Deborah M. Feldman, MD, Yu Ming Victor Fang, MD*

KEYWORDS

- Insulin • Pregnancy • Glyburide • Metformin • Gestational diabetes
- Type 1 and type 2 diabetes

KEY POINTS

- Diabetes mellitus (DM) complicates 6% to 7% of all pregnancies in the United States, and 85% of the cases are caused by gestational diabetes.
- During pregnancy, women with type 1 DM require insulin because of their lack of insulin production, whereas women with type 2 DM are often transitioned from an oral hypoglycemic agent to insulin.
- The management of diabetes using insulin depends on a combination of short- and long-acting insulin.
- The goals of plasma glucose control during pregnancy are a fasting sugar of 60 to 95 mg/dL and 2-hour postmeal sugar of 120 mg/dL or less.
- Current studies indicate that the insulin analogue glargine (Lantus) is a safe and effective treatment of pregnant patients with diabetes.
- Oral hypoglycemic agents (glyburide, metformin) can be alternative medications to treat gestational DM. However, a larger percent of women using metformin (46.3%) compared with glyburide (4.0%) may need supplemental insulin for good control.

INTRODUCTION

Diabetes mellitus (DM) is a condition that results in elevated blood glucose levels. DM occurring outside of pregnancy has been classified as either type 1 or type 2.

- Type 1 DM results from the lack of production of insulin by the pancreas.
  - Accounts for 5% to 10% of patients diagnosed with diabetes in the general population[1]

Division of Maternal-Fetal Medicine, Department of Obstetrics and Gynecology, Hartford Hospital, 85 Jefferson Street, Hartford, CT 06102, USA
* Corresponding author.
E-mail address: yfang@harthosp.org

Clin Lab Med 33 (2013) 235–242
http://dx.doi.org/10.1016/j.cll.2013.03.015
0272-2712/13/$ – see front matter © 2013 Elsevier Inc. All rights reserved.

- Type 2 DM results from the body's resistance to the effects of insulin.
  - Accounts for 90% to 95% of all patients with diabetes and most women of reproductive age with diabetes

Gestational DM (GDM) is a complication of pregnancy characterized by carbohydrate intolerance diagnosed during pregnancy. As the rates of obesity and sedentary lifestyle increase among women in the United States, so do the rates of GDM, now affecting approximately 5% of all pregnancies. It has been estimated that DM complicates approximately 6% to 7% of all pregnancies in the United States, and 85% of those cases are caused by GDM.[2]

The treatment of diabetes in pregnancy starts with proper nutritional counseling and dietary intervention as well as a reasonable exercise program. Pregnant women with type 1 DM will require insulin therapy throughout their pregnancy because of their lack of insulin production. Women with type 2 DM are often transitioned from an oral hypoglycemic to insulin once their pregnancy is confirmed. Women diagnosed with GDM are initially treated with diet modification. Those patients with GDM who do not attain adequate glycemic control have traditionally been treated with insulin during pregnancy; however, over the past decade, based on results from various trials indicating the efficacy and safety of oral hypoglycemic medications (glyburide and metformin) are increasingly used for treatment of GDM.[3–9]

With proper treatment, the goals of plasma glucose levels in pregnancy are

- Fasting 60 to 95 mg/dL
- Two hours after meals 120 mg/dL or less

This review focuses on the use of insulin and oral hypoglycemic medications for the treatment of diabetes in pregnancy.

INSULIN

During the late nineteenth century, several scientists discovered the function of the pancreas: an organ that produced a substance that could regulate blood glucose as well as digestive enzymes. This substance was a peptide hormone and came to be known as insulin, the major signal regulating carbohydrate metabolism. It is produced by the B cell of the pancreas, secreted into the hepatic portal circulation, and acts by both (1) inhibiting hepatic gluconeogenesis and glycolysis and (2) stimulating glucose uptake in the liver, muscle, and fat.

During that era, diabetes in pregnancy was a known entity, which often led to rapid premature death because no treatment was available. It was Drs Frederick Banting and Charles Best who, in the early 1920s, extracted a substance from animal pancreas that eventually became well known as insulin. The treatment of humans with diabetes with this extract was a success, and the discovery led to the Nobel Prize in 1923. Although not a cure for diabetes, the commercial availability of insulin remains one of the most important discoveries in medicine.[10]

Before the use of insulin in pregnant women with diabetes, rates of perinatal morbidity and mortality were extraordinarily high.[11] Even until the mid 1940s, the perinatal mortality rate in the United States and Europe stood at 40%. Following subspecialty care for these patients, the perinatal morbidity and mortality sharply decreased over the next several decades.[12] This decline was in large part caused by the improvement in blood sugar control with the use of insulin. In addition, the widespread use of home glucose monitoring using portable monitors has allowed the management of gestational diabetes to shift from an inpatient to an outpatient setting.

TYPES OF INSULIN

The management of diabetes using insulin depends on a combination of short- and long-acting insulin. See **Table 1** for a summary of the various types of insulin and their characteristics. Rapid-acting insulin types include insulin lispro (Humalog) and insulin aspart (Novolog) and are used just before mealtime to help quickly reduce blood sugar. Their onset of action is on the order of a few minutes, and their biologic activity peaks within 1 to 3 hours. These types are usually used in combination with intermediate-acting insulin, NPH and Lente, and long-acting agents, such as Ultralente and insulin glargine (Lantus).

In addition to the agents mentioned earlier, there are several premixed combinations of insulin supplying a mixture of short- and long-acting agents in one injection, which are available either in bottle or insulin pen form. The combinations of insulin are available in various percentages depending on patient need. In general, they are given twice daily before mealtime.

TREATMENT OF DM IN PREGNANCY WITH INSULIN

Experience with insulin in pregnancy was historically confined to those patients with type 1 diabetes. Nowadays, it is common for pregnant patients with type 1 DM to control blood sugars with the assistance of a continuous subcutaneous insulin pump along with continuous blood sugar monitoring.[13]

As the incidence of type 2 DM and GDM has increased along with the average body mass index of pregnant women, the need for insulin to attain glycemic control in GDM has also increased. Since their introduction, insulin analogues are the preferred choice for the treatment of pregnant women with diabetes because of their superior pharmacologic profiles, leading to greater flexibility and convenience of dosing. But is there a benefit to treating patients with GDM, especially if only short-term? There have been several studies examining the efficacy of injectable insulin in GDM. Treating patients with GDM has been shown in various trials to reduce the risk of shoulder dystocia and macrosomia.[14] In addition, the Australian Carbohydrate Intolerance Study in Pregnant Women demonstrated a reduction in the rate of composite serious perinatal complications, including perinatal death, shoulder dystocia, nerve palsy, or birth trauma (adjusted relative risk [RR] 0.33; 95% confidence interval [CI] 0.14–0.75).[15]

Over the past few years, clinical experience with insulin analogues in pregnancy has increased. Relatively recent data support the use of longer-acting agents, such as insulin glargine, both in patients with pregestational and gestational diabetes. Before

Table 1
Various types of injectable insulin

Insulin Type	Generic	Brand Name	Onset	Peak	Duration (h)
Rapid acting	Lispro	Humalog	15–30 min	30–90 min	3–5
	Aspart	Novolog	10–20 min	40–50 min	3–5
	Glulisine	Apidra	20–30 min	30–90 min	1.0–2.5
Short acting	Regular (R)	Humulin novolin	30–60 min	2–5 h	5–8
	Insulin pump	Velosulin	30–60 min	2–3 h	2–3
Intermediate acting	—	NPH (N)	1–2 h	4–12 h	18–24
	—	Lente (L)	1.0–2.5 h	3–10 h	18–24
Long acting	—	Ultralente	30 min to 3 h	10–20 h	20–36
	Glargine	Lantus	1.0–1.5 h	No peak	20–24
	Detemir	Levemir	1–2 h	6–8 h	Up to 24

2009, there had been limited published experience with insulin glargine in pregnancy. Fang and colleagues[16] reported the results of 52 pregnant women receiving insulin glargine and compared them with a similar cohort of patients managed with NPH insulin. Both patients with pregestational and gestational diabetes were included in both groups. In this study, the investigators found no increased maternal or neonatal morbidity associated with the use of insulin glargine. Among patients with pregestational diabetes, there was a lower rate of macrosomia (relative risk [RR], 0.38; 95% confidence intervals [CI], 0.17–0.87), neonatal hypoglycemia (0% treated with glargine and 25% treated with NPH), and neonatal hyperbilirubinemia (RR, 0.27; 95% CI, 0.07–0.98) in the cohort taking insulin glargine when compared with NPH.

An observational study by Negrato and colleagues[17] in 2010 showed similar efficacy and safety of insulin glargine in pregnancy among both patients with pregestational and gestational diabetes, with decreased adverse outcomes when compared with patients with diabetes using NPH. The long-acting nature of insulin glargine accompanied by minimal peak activity makes it an ideal choice to maintain steady-state blood glucose control during pregnancy.[18] The hesitation in the widespread use of insulin analogues is likely caused by the limited data on safety in pregnancy. Although further research with larger numbers is warranted, the aforementioned studies suggest that insulin glargine is a safe and effective insulin analogue that may be considered in the treatment of pregnant patients with diabetes.

Although insulin has been the gold standard in the treatment of patients with diabetes in pregnancy, there are risks associated with its use:

- Allergic reactions
- Injection-site reactions
- Hypoglycemia

These risks, along with the issues of dissatisfaction among patients in having to take injections, noncompliance, and difficulty with monitoring and adjusting the insulin dosage, have made the use of oral hypoglycemics a more attractive option to pregnant patients.

ORAL HYPOGLYCEMIC MEDICATIONS

In the past, oral hypoglycemic agents were contraindicated in pregnancy because of concerns regarding fetal teratogenicity and the concern that these medications (primarily first-generation sulfonylurea agents) may cause fetal hyperinsulinemia resulting in increased rates of macrosomia (because insulin is a growth factor) and neonatal hypoglycemia.[19] Currently, women with pregestational diabetes (type 2 DM) who start pregnancy being treated with oral hypoglycemic medications are usually switched to insulin because of the lack of studies demonstrating the safety and efficacy of these medications in early pregnancy.[20]

Most pregnant women are screened for gestational diabetes during the second trimester (24–28 weeks). The pathophysiology of GDM is caused by insulin resistance and also the insufficient secretion of insulin by the pancreas.[21] Therefore, oral hypoglycemic agents that may improve insulin sensitivity or insulin secretion are logical treatment options for GDM.

Over the past decade, several studies have found that either glyburide (a second-generation sulfonylurea) or metformin (a biguanide) may be used as alternative therapeutic options for the treatment of GDM during pregnancy.[3–9] Because the treatment of GDM is initiated in the second trimester well after organogenesis, the concern for teratogenicity is minimal when used for the treatment of GDM. Compared with insulin, oral hypoglycemic medications

- Are less expensive
- Requires less patient education/skills to use
- Allows patients to avoid daily painful injections

Because glyburide and metformin are the 2 oral hypoglycemic medications that have been prospectively studied for the treatment of GDM, this review focuses on these 2 medications.

GLYBURIDE

Glyburide acts by enhancing the release of insulin from the pancreas. It is metabolized by the liver. Glyburide is the most well-studied oral hypoglycemic medication for the treatment of GDM and is the most common oral hypoglycemic medication used to treat GDM by obstetricians. The initial starting dosage of glyburide is 2.5 mg once or twice a day, with a maximum dosage of 20 mg/d.[22] It is available in 1.25-mg, 2.5-mg, and 5.0-mg tablets. Glyburide is associated with a much lower rate of hypoglycemia (1%–5%) as compared with insulin (71%).[22]

The placental transport of glyburide from mother to fetus studied using an ex vivo technique is much less (3.9%) when compared with first-generation sulfonylurea drugs, such as tolbutamide (21.5%) and chlorpropamide (11.0%).[23] These findings suggest that fetal exposure to maternally administered glyburide may be low or insignificant. Further evidence to support the minimal passage of glyburide across the placenta was seen in a randomized trial whereby glyburide was not detected in the cord serum of any infant whose mother had been treated with glyburide during pregnancy.[3]

In a randomized trial comparing glyburide with insulin in the treatment of GDM conducted by Langer and colleagues,[3] no significant differences were noted in the daily blood glucose concentrations and glycosylated hemoglobin values between women who were treated with glyburide versus insulin. There were also no significant differences between the two groups in the rates of macrosomia, large-for-gestational-age infants, lung complications, hypoglycemia, admission to the neonatal intensive care unit, and fetal anomalies.[3] About 4% of the women treated with glyburide did not obtain adequate glycemic control and had to be switched to insulin. A recent meta-analysis examining randomized trials comparing glyburide with insulin in the treatment of GDM found no substantial difference in maternal or neonatal outcomes.[5] Based on the results of these studies, glyburide may be considered an alternative medication for the treatment of GDM. Patients should be made aware that certain women may not achieve adequate glycemic control using glyburide and will, therefore, require insulin for treatment.

METFORMIN

Metformin acts primarily by suppressing glucose production by the liver. It also increases insulin sensitivity, enhances peripheral glucose uptake, and decreases the absorption of glucose from the gastrointestinal tract. The usual starting dosage is 500 to 850 mg/d, which can be increased to a maximum dosage of 2500 mg/d. It is available in 500-mg, 850-mg, and 1000-mg tablets. The most common adverse effects of metformin are the following:

- Common side effects
  - Gastrointestinal upset, including
    - Diarrhea
    - Cramps
    - Nausea

- Vomiting
- Increased flatulence
- Serious potential side effect
  - Lactic acidosis
    - Very rare
    - Most of these cases seem related to comorbid conditions (eg, impaired liver or kidney function)

Metformin is considered a first-line drug of choice for the treatment of type 2 diabetes. In ex vivo placental perfusion studies, metformin was noted to cross the placenta with a maternal-to-fetal transfer rate of 10% to 16%.[24,25] Therefore, an intriguing question is whether or not women with type 2 diabetes who are treated with metformin should continue taking this medication during the preconception period and throughout their pregnancy. There have been limited reports regarding the use of metformin in the treatment of type 2 diabetes from the preconception period through pregnancy. In studies published by Coetzee and Jackson,[26] 22 women treated with metformin were compared with 42 women who were treated with insulin. There were no differences in the perinatal mortality rate between the two groups. There were no cases of maternal hypoglycemia or lactic acidosis. Metformin use in the first trimester was not associated with an increased risk of congenital anomalies.[27]

The use of metformin in the first trimester of pregnancy during the time of organogenesis has also been examined in women with polycystic ovarian syndrome. These women were treated with metformin to improve fertility. In an observational trial of 72 women who conceived using 2.5 g/d of metformin, there were no cases of lactic acidosis, fetal anomalies, or maternal or neonatal hypoglycemia.[28] In a follow-up study, at 18 months, the infants whose mothers were exposed to metformin during the first trimester showed no differences in height, weight, or motor and social skills when compared with matched controls.[29]

In the largest randomized controlled trial comparing metformin with insulin in the treatment of GDM, Rowan and colleagues[4] randomized 733 women (363 received metformin and 370 received insulin) at between 20 and 33 weeks. They found that neonatal complications (neonatal hypoglycemia, rates of respiratory distress, need for phototherapy, birth trauma, 5-minute Apgar scores <7, and preterm birth <37 weeks) were not increased in the women treated with metformin as compared with insulin (RR, 1.00; 95% CI, 0.90–1.10). It is important to note that in this study, 46.3% of the women taking metformin required supplemental insulin at some point in their pregnancy to obtain adequate glycemic control. This study also found that women preferred metformin over insulin treatment.

Based on the limited number of studies regarding the long-term effects of in utero exposure, the use of metformin for the treatment of diabetes in pregnancy is limited and is often individualized depending on the patient's circumstances. Similar to glyburide, women who are treated with metformin in pregnancy should be aware that a certain number of women may not achieve adequate glycemic control with just the oral hypoglycemic medication and may need to be switched to insulin.

SUMMARY

Insulin remains the standard medication for the treatment of all types of patients with diabetes during pregnancy. The choice of the type of insulin to use should be individualized based on practitioner and patient preference. Glyburide and metformin may be considered as alternative medications in the treatment of GDM.

REFERENCES

1. Ballas J, Moore TR, Ramos GA. Management of diabetes in pregnancy. Curr Diab Rep 2012;12:33–42.
2. Wier LM, Witt E, Burgess J, et al. Healthcare cost and utilization project. Statistical brief #102. Hospitalizations related to diabetes in pregnancy, 2008. Rockville (MD): Agency for Health Care Policy and Research; 2010.
3. Langer O, Conway DL, Berkus MD, et al. A comparison of glyburide and insulin in women with gestational diabetes mellitus. N Engl J Med 2000;343:1134–8.
4. Rowan JA, Hague WM, Gao W, et al. Metformin versus insulin for treatment of gestational diabetes [published erratum appears in N Engl J Med 2008;359:106]. N Engl J Med 2008;358:2003–15.
5. Nicholson W, Bolen S, Witkop CT, et al. Benefits and risk of oral diabetes agents compared with insulin in women with gestational diabetes: a systematic review. Obstet Gynecol 2009;113:193–205.
6. Moore LE, Clokey D, Rappaport VJ, et al. Metformin compared with glyburide in gestational diabetes: a randomized trial. Obstet Gynecol 2010;115:55–9.
7. Moretti ME, Rezvani M, Koren G. Safety of glyburide for gestational diabetes: a meta-analysis of pregnancy outcomes. Ann Pharmacother 2008;42:483–90.
8. Nicholson W, Baptiste-Roberts K. Oral hypoglycaemic agents during pregnancy: the evidence for effectiveness and safety. Best Pract Res Clin Obstet Gynaecol 2011;25:51–63.
9. Lain KY, Garabedian MJ, Daftary A, et al. Neonatal adiposity following maternal treatment of gestational diabetes with glyburide compared with insulin. Am J Obstet Gynecol 2009;200:501.e1–6.
10. "The discovery of insulin, " Nobelprize.org. 2012. Available at: http://www.nobelprize.org/educational/medicine/insulin/discovery-insulin.html. Accessed January 12, 2013.
11. McElduff A, Moses RG. Insulin therapy in pregnancy. Endocrinol Metab Clin North Am 2012;41:161–73.
12. Henley WE. Diabetes and pregnancy. N Z Med J 1947;46:386–97.
13. Combs CA. Continuous glucose monitoring and insulin pump therapy for diabetes in pregnancy. J Matern Fetal Neonatal Med 2012;25:2025–7. http://dx.doi.org/10.3109/14767058.2012.670409.
14. Horvath K, Koch K, Jeitler K, et al. Effects of treatment in women with gestational diabetes mellitus; systematic review and meta-analysis. BMJ 2010;340:c1395.
15. Crowther CA, Hiller JE, Moss JR, et al, Australian Carbohydrate Intolerance Study in Pregnant Women (ACHOIS) Trial Group. Effect of treatment of gestational diabetes mellitus on pregnancy outcomes. N Engl J Med 2005;352:2477–86.
16. Fang YM, MacKeen D, Egan JF, et al. Insulin glargine compared with neutral protamine Hagedorn insulin in the treatment of pregnant diabetics. J Matern Fetal Neonatal Med 2009;22:249–53.
17. Negrato CA, Rafacho A, Negrato G, et al. Glargine vs. NPH insulin therapy in pregnancies complicated by diabetes: an observational study. Diabetes Res Clin Pract 2010;89:46–51.
18. Hirsch JB. Insulin analogues. N Engl J Med 2005;352:174–83.
19. Langer O. Oral hypoglycemic agents and the pregnant diabetic: "from bench to bedside". Semin Perinatol 2002;26:215–24.
20. ACOG Practice Bulletin #60 Pregestational Diabetes Mellitus. Obstet Gynecol 2005;105:675–85.

21. Maymone AC, Baillargeon JP, Ménard J, et al. Oral hypoglycemic agents for gestational diabetes mellitus? Expert Opin Drug Saf 2011;10:227–38.
22. Refuerzo JS. Oral hypoglycemic agents in pregnancy. Obstet Gynecol Clin North Am 2011;38:227–34.
23. Elliott BD, Schenker S, Langer O, et al. Comparative placental transport of oral hypoglycemic agents in humans: a model of human placental drug transfer. Am J Obstet Gynecol 1994;171:653–60.
24. Kovo M, Haroutiunian S, Feldman N, et al. Determination of metformin transfer across the human placenta using a dually perfused ex vivo placental cotyledon model. Eur J Obstet Gynecol Reprod Biol 2008;136:29–33.
25. Nanovskaya TN, Nekhayeva IA, Patrikeeva S, et al. Transfer of metformin across the dually perfused human placental lobule. Am J Obstet Gynecol 2006;195: 1081–5.
26. Coetzee EJ, Jackson WP. Pregnancy in established non-insulin-dependent diabetics. A five-and-a-half year study at Groote Schuur Hospital. S Afr Med J 1980;58:795–802.
27. Coetzee EJ, Jackson WP. Oral hypoglycaemics in the first trimester and fetal outcome. S Afr Med J 1984;65:635–7.
28. Glueck CJ, Wang P, Goldenberg N, et al. Pregnancy outcomes among women with polycystic ovary syndrome treated with metformin. Hum Reprod 2002;17: 2858–64.
29. Glueck CJ, Goldenberg N, Pranicoff J, et al. Height, weight, and motor–social development during the first 18 months of life in 126 infants born to 109 mothers with polycystic ovary syndrome who conceived on and continued metformin through pregnancy. Hum Reprod 2004;19:1323–30.

Management of Pregnant Patients with Diabetes with Ischemic Heart Disease

Theodore B. Jones, MD[a],*, Zeynep Alpay Savasan, MD[b],
Quinetta Johnson, MD[a], Ray Bahado-Singh, MD, MBA[b,c]

KEYWORDS

- Diabetes • Ischemic heart disease • Acute myocardial infarction • Angina
- Maternal mortality

KEY POINTS

- Multidisciplinary preconception counseling is imperative for diabetic women with ischemic heart disease (IHD) to improve outcomes for mother and infant.
- Untreated coronary artery disease has a high mortality and should be diagnosed before pregnancy, but 66% of diabetic women have unplanned pregnancies.
- Unstable angina is a contraindication to becoming pregnant.
- Women are more likely to have atypical clinical symptoms of IHD, which leads to delay in diagnosis and treatment.
- Diabetic women with IHD who have an acute myocardial infarction during pregnancy have a 62% mortality.
- A multidisciplinary team approach is key in the management of patients with diabetes with IHD during the pregnancy as well as postpartum.

MANAGEMENT OF PREGNANT PATIENTS WITH DIABETES WITH ISCHEMIC HEART DISEASE

As the number of diabetic women increases, the rate of complications secondary to pregestational diabetes increases. There are numerous microvascular disease processes that occur with diabetes. Proliferative diabetic retinopathy is a microvascular

[a] Department of Obstetrics and Gynecology, Oakwood Hospital and Medical Center, 18101 Oakwood Boulevard, PO Box 2500, Dearborn, MI 48124, USA; [b] Division of Maternal Fetal Medicine, Department of Obstetrics and Gynecology, Oakland University William Beaumont Health System, Oakland University William Beaumont School of Medicine, 3535 West 13 Mile Road, Royal Oak, MI 48073, USA; [c] Obstetrics & Gynecology, Oakland University William Beaumont Health System, Royal Oak, MI, USA
* Corresponding author. Division of Maternal Fetal Medicine, Department of Obstetrics and Gynecology, Wayne State University School of Medicine, Detroit, MI.
E-mail address: theodore.jones@oakwood.org

Clin Lab Med 33 (2013) 243–256
http://dx.doi.org/10.1016/j.cll.2013.03.020
0272-2712/13/$ – see front matter © 2013 Elsevier Inc. All rights reserved.

complication that is caused by the formation of new retinal blood vessels and can lead to blindness by retinal detachment and/or bleeding. Diabetic nephropathy is the most common cause of end-stage renal disease in the United States.[1] Cardiovascular complications that can occur in diabetic pregnancies include chronic hypertension, pregnancy-induced hypertension, and atherosclerotic heart disease.[1] This article considers one particular significant vascular complication: ischemic heart disease (IHD).

The maternal mortality of women with IHD has been reported to be as high as 66% to 75%.[2] It has been reported that pregnancy increases the risk of myocardial infarction (MI) by 3-fold to 4-fold.[3] The incidence of myocardial ischemia in pregnancy has been reported in numerous sources as 1 case per 10,000 deliveries. There have been several factors cited as contributors to the increased incidence of myocardial ischemia in pregnancy, including diabetes mellitus, hypertension, increasing rates of obesity, increasing maternal age, and smoking.[3]

CLASSIFICATION OF DIABETIC COMPLICATIONS

The classification of diabetes in pregnancy by obstetricians has relied on a classification system devised by Priscilla White in 1932 that focused on the onset and duration of disease and vascular complications. However, in recent years, this classification system has become a source of debate. In this article, the complication of interest would be given a designation of class H. However, as type 2 diabetes has become more prevalent compared with type 1 diabetes (for which the White classification system was mainly based), there has been discussion as to whether or not the classification system created by the American Diabetes Association (ADA) in 1997 (modified in 2007) should replace the White classification.[4] Although there may be occasional references to the White classification, this article adheres to the ADA's diagnostic and classification system.[1]

In distinction to myocardial ischemia in the older population, peripartum myocardial ischemia is not usually caused by atherosclerosis. There can be several causes of myocardial ischemia during the antepartum, peripartum, and postpartum periods, including coronary artery disease, coronary dissection, coronary thrombus, and coronary spasm. Acute coronary syndrome or myocardial ischemia during pregnancy poses a challenge because symptoms of myocardial ischemia can imitate complaints typical of normal pregnancy. Therefore, the diagnosis can be overlooked and missed. Diabetes further contributes to a blunted appreciation for ischemic pain that can result in silent ischemia and silent infarcts.[5]

It has been well recognized that adequate diabetic control decreases maternal and fetal mortality and morbidity. It is thought to be imperative that sufficient glycemic control and preconception care be ensured before pregnancy to facilitate favorable outcomes. Preconception counseling entails a multidisciplinary team that includes a diabetologist, a physician skilled in diabetes management, an obstetrician skilled in high-risk pregnancies, and diabetic educators.[6] Untreated coronary artery disease is associated with a high mortality and it is important to diagnose before pregnancy when possible. However, unplanned pregnancies occur in approximately two-thirds of women with diabetes, making preconception counseling unattainable in most cases.[6]

OVERVIEW OF IHD

IHD represents a unique challenge in women. It is the leading cause of death in women, with more than 421,000 IHD deaths reported in the United States in 2011.[7] Although there has been a decline in IHD-related mortality in women, this lags behind the improvement reported in men. Higher rates of sudden death before hospitalization occur in women.[8] The most likely explanations for the higher mortality are:

- Higher rates of comorbidities in affected women
  - Obesity
  - Diabetes
  - Hypertension
- More frequent hospitalizations
- Lower rates of overall well-being beyond cardiac concerns that are reported[9]

CHALLENGE IN DIAGNOSIS IN WOMEN

As noted earlier, risk factors seem to be more prevalent in women than men and, when they do occur, have greater impact on IHD. Such factors include elevated triglycerides, obesity, diabetes, and metabolic syndrome.[10] A significant contributory factor to worse outcomes in women seems to be an increased frequency of delay or failure to make the diagnosis. The atypical presentation of coronary artery disease in women results in delayed recognition by patients and physicians. A recent large meta-analysis of 26 studies found significant differences in symptoms in women compared with men.[11] These findings are consistent with the results of numerous prior studies and meta-analyses. Chest pain is widely recognized by both the general public and medical personnel to be a sign of ischemic heart disease. Significantly lower rates of chest pain were noted in a review of women compared with men (odds ratio 0.63, 95% confidence interval [CI] 0.59, 0.68) when data were pooled from multiple studies. There were similarly higher rates of nonspecific and, therefore, confounding symptoms in women. There were higher odds of presenting with:

- Fatigue: relative risk (RR) 1.19, 95% CI 1.06, 1.33
- Neck pain: RR 1.54, 95% CI 1.38, 1.73
- Nausea: RR 1.42, 95% CI 1.02, 1.46
- Syncope: RR 1.37, 95% CI 1.11, 1.70
- Right arm pain: RR 1.20, 95% CI 1.07, 1.33
- Dizziness: RR 1.22, 95% CI 1.01, 1.92
- Jaw pain: RR 1.39, 95% CI 1.01, 1.92[11]

The atypical nature of these symptoms contributes both to late recognition and presentation for care and late and missed diagnosis in women. Adjusting for age and other confounding variables, for the most part, did not have a significant impact on the effect of gender on the presenting symptoms in acute MI (AMI).

DISPARITIES IN CARE FOR WOMEN WITH IHD

Compounding the challenges in women's recognition of the significance of their symptoms and delayed and even missed diagnosis by physicians are concerns regarding gender differences in therapy for coronary artery disease between the sexes. As a consequence of the atypical presentation, there is a delay in the decision time, which represents the period between the development of symptoms and presentation for medical care. Women are said to experience reduced rates of diagnostic testing, delay in referral to specialists, and longer wait times in receiving care.[12] It is also thought that the treatment women receive tends to be less aggressive, with women frequently being treated with anxiolytics and antidepressants as a result of misdiagnosis for psychological and anxiety disorders.[13] Despite the equal incidence of coronary artery disease in men and women, only 30% of coronary artery bypass surgery is performed in women.[14] Reduced use in women has been partly ascribed to the smaller caliber of female coronary arteries, smaller body size, and increased comorbidities in women. Diagnosis and treatment of IHD is therefore a major challenge in contemporary health care and demands greater attention from health care policy makers, clinicians, researchers, as well as women themselves.

ACUTE MYOCARDIAL INFARCTION (AMI)

Coronary artery disease, particularly MI, is a rare but consequential event in pregnancy. A nationwide study based on the Nationwide Inpatient Sample (NIS) database for the years 2000 to 2002 reported a US prevalence of AMI of 6.2 (95% CI 3.0–9.4) per 100,000 deliveries.[15] There was a case fatality rate of as high as 37%. With the overall maternal mortality at 12 per 100,000, myocardial infraction accounts for a significant percentage of maternal mortality.

Risk factors significantly associated with AMI in pregnancy include increasing maternal age, with women older than 30 years of age showing significantly increased rates of AMI than those younger than that age threshold.[15] Preexisting medical disorders frequently increase the AMI risk: factors include chronic hypertension, thrombophilia, diabetes mellitus, as well as cigarette smoking. In thrombophilia and hypertension, the increase in risk based on the previously referenced NIS study was greater than 20-fold.[15]

Complication risks were also greater when an AMI occurred. The need for transfusion and the development of postpartum infection had a significantly increased association with AMI in pregnancy. In this large study group, traditionally quoted risk factors such as maternal race, preeclampsia, postpartum hemorrhage, and anemia did not persist as independent risk factors for AMI in pregnancy.[15] Other significant risk factors reported in pregnancy-related AMI include hyperlipidemia, family history of MI, and diabetes.

The overall rate of AMI is increased in pregnancy by 3-fold to 4-fold.[16] Apart from the known and suspected contributions to the increased risk discussed earlier, it seems that the physiologic changes of pregnancy might also enhance the risk of AMI. Coronary artery dissection is a rare cause of AMI in the nonpregnant population but occurred in between 16% and 27% of AMI in 2 case series reviewed by Roth and colleagues.[16] It has been suggested that the increased rate of dissection may be the result of the effect of progesterone on the vessel wall leading to loss and fragmentation of fibers in vessel walls[17] and decreased acid mucopolysaccharide. The profound hemodynamic changes in pregnancy increase the oxygen demand of the heart and could predispose to cardiac ischemic changes. During labor, the pain associated with uterine contractions could increase the work of the heart, further increasing the risk of AMI. In addition, during the postpartum period, increased venous return from reduced vena caval compression and expulsion of blood from the uterine circulation further exacerbates cardiac work and risk of ischemia.

RISK FOR IHD IN DIABETES

The frequency of diabetes based on surveys of individuals in the United States has increased to 9%.[18] The frequency of this disorder is known to be equal in men and women. In general, diabetes is known to be a significant risk factor for IHD. The pathogenesis of coronary artery disease in diabetes is multifactorial, with contributory factors being increased plaque formation with the risk of ulceration or thrombus formation. Hyperglycemia seems to promote endothelial dysfunction, hypercoagulability, and platelet dysfunction. In addition, hyperglycemia increases oxidative stress, which inhibits nitric oxide production. Nitric oxide is a potent vasolidator and regulates platelet activation factor.[19] Among women, the cooccurrence of both IHD and diabetes (ie, class H diabetes) in pregnancy is rare, with only a limited number of cases reported in the English literature. In a prior report, all 11 of 24 class H patients with diabetes with myocardial ischemia before pregnancy survived.[20] Of 13 with AMI in pregnancy, 5 (38.5%) survived. Although this finding seems to confirm a high risk of mortality when AMI occurs in pregnant patients with diabetes, advances in critical care may have reduced the mortality in contemporary practice.

In 2 separate series, Roth and Elkayam[16] reported that, among cases of AMI during pregnancy, 4% and 10.7% of such cases were diabetic. The frequency of diabetes reportedly varies with the timing of the AMI in pregnancy, with significantly higher rates in the antepartum versus postpartum ischemic event (19% vs 1.6%, $P<.001$). The national study by James and colleagues[15] confirmed that diabetes significantly increased the risk IHD in pregnancy by 3.6-fold. Most studies have not distinguished gestational and preexisting diabetes in terms of the increased AMI risk. However, the study by Ladner and colleagues[21] found that preexisting rather than gestational diabetes was the significant associated factor with IHD in pregnancy.

PRECONCEPTION COUNSELING OF WOMEN WITH IHD AND DIABETES

Counseling in the preconception period has become an important intervention for perinatal providers working with patients and their families considering beginning a pregnancy. In many cases, their understanding of the risks associated with pregnancy is informed primarily by their understanding of diabetes in general as well as a rationalized opinion that their current state of health is likely to be superior to tomorrow's. Although this conventional wisdom may be true in many cases, there may be justifiable concern about the current state of health and the advisability of pregnancy. Moreover, even if physician approval of a pregnancy is a possible recommendation, there is often a need for careful evaluation and health improvement before giving support for the conception.

Any discussion in this area must consider the limited information concerning the subject. Despite nearly 4 decades of recognition of increased risk for poor maternal and fetal outcomes for women with diabetes and vascular complications, information useful to the clinician remains difficult to assemble and evaluate. Much of the earlier information came from articles focused on case reports coupled with literature reviews. The complexity of these cases generally involved the management of other affected end organs as well, rendering definitive management inferences problematic.

It is important that the consultant have access to as much of the patient's medical documentation as is available to aid in understanding the magnitude of the patient's cardiac disease. Because multiple consultants are commonly a part of the patient's care, reconciling her records before final recommendations is required. An updated assessment of the patient's diabetic status and the state of her IHD is important. The New York Heart Association (NYHA) classification system is helpful in evaluating a patient's functional status. However, it has little specificity to the underlying cardiac abnormality. When a patient has an NYHA class I or II at the time of counseling, a reasonable assumption is that the rate of complications related to the cardiac disease is less than that of individuals with class III or IV disease.[22]

Additional useful information for counseling includes the maternal risk for complications, including death, associated with pregnancy. This risk ranges from minimal (<1%) to moderate (5%–15%) to major (>25%). IHD should be considered as a moderate risk for complications, consistent with the classification placing previous MI in this category. It is important to remember that the class of risk may change during a pregnancy, thereby leading to greater risk than was appreciated at the preconception counseling.[23]

Outcome information shared by investigators in the past must be sorted through carefully to maximize applicability to the patient. Much of the information related to IHD and diabetes mellitus in pregnancy is a result of reports in the literature about women with diabetes with either an MI during pregnancy or the management of a patient with an unplanned pregnancy with history of IHD. However, the counseling of such patients should exercise caution, because it seems that diabetic women with IHD in pregnancy face more risks than just the risks associated with their cardiac disease in isolation. There may be a precarious balance between the possibility of a successful pregnancy and the significant potential for fetal and maternal complications. Combined with the likelihood of a shorter life even without pregnancy, this finding creates many issues that must be discussed deliberately and with candor.

Counseling should use the following information:

- Evaluation of the patient should include diabetic control currently and in the recent past (review of glucose logs, hemoglobin A1C)
- Review of past history of evaluation, treatment, and care related to the patient's IHD
- If there has been no recent evaluation of cardiac function, consideration should be given to updating patient's assessment (electrocardiogram, echocardiogram, nuclear medicine cardiac imaging, cardiac catheterization)
- Assessment of diabetes-related noncardiac end organs for evidence of compromise

With this information, the counseling may proceed as follows:

- Recap findings from history review and any recent laboratory assessment. This information provides a starting point for the recommendations that follow. Any need for additional evaluation before final recommendation should be discussed as well.
- Emphasize that all women with diabetes and IHD considering pregnancy must acknowledge that there is a quantifiable risk for poor outcome associated with a pregnancy even in the best of circumstances.
- A review of complications associated with diabetes in pregnancy should include information about risk for potential worsening of function in their cardiac function as well as other target organs. Although such deterioration is usually transient, there are instances of permanent loss of function.
- Risk to the prospective mother who has experienced a recent MI or has unstable angina at the time of counseling is substantial. This risk is frequently thought to be an absolute contraindication to pregnancy until greater stability and elapse of time has occurred.[24] The physiologic changes associated with pregnancy may increase the risk for a repeat MI.
- Women who are currently on treatment of IHD are usually asked to discontinue medications that pose risk to the fetus. Discontinuation of these medications, such as angiotensin-converting enzyme inhibitors and statins, may lead to loss of stability of cardiac disease that had improved previously with interventions (eg, medications, stents).

It is important to be as balanced as possible about the chance of success when contrasted with the risk for poor outcome. It is common for patients and families to find encouragement in the seemingly minor aspects of the counseling. Although an argument can be made that it is unlikely that the patient's health will not improve substantially with additional time, there is often quantifiable risk at the start of the pregnancy that would make pregnancy unwise and, in some cases, a risk for premature death.

If a patient with a significantly guarded prognosis decides to proceed with a pregnancy against medical advice, clear documentation of the discussion should be followed by an outlined plan of care coordinated with other key specialists.

MANAGEMENT
First Trimester

Patients with pregestational diabetes with IHD should have preconceptional counseling and have their baseline evaluations before pregnancy. Detailed history and physical examination, electrocardiogram, echocardiogram, stress test, and, if indicated, coronary angiogram and nuclear studies should be performed before pregnancy in any woman if coronary artery disease is suspected. Every effort should be made to treat coronary insufficiency before conception (**Box 1**).

Pregnancy is usually discouraged in patients with coronary insufficiency because of a significantly increased risk of maternal mortality. However, a large proportion of these patients start obstetric care after they confirm their pregnancies. A detailed history and physical examination with baseline evaluations should be evaluated at the first prenatal visit (**Box 2**).

Electrocardiogram evaluation for IHD does not vary significantly in pregnancy.[24] Echocardiogram is valuable in defining cardiac wall motion abnormalities. Noninvasive stress testing with radiologic or electrocardiographic imaging techniques may be used in special circumstances. Angiographic evaluation can be used to better define the coronary disease and potentially correct the lesion. Abdominal shielding is used to limit fetal exposure. In women with angina, β-blockers, are the drug of choice because of their relative safety for the fetus. Low-dose aspirin can be used. Nitrates have also been used without adverse fetal effects.

Patients who have stable angina pectoris only experience chest pain at high levels of exertion. The treatment option for these patients is beta-adrenergic blocking agents. In this setting, the likelihood of major complications during pregnancy, labor, or delivery is low.

Unstable angina is diagnosed when there is confirmed angina at rest or with mild exertion. These unstable anginas typically, but not necessarily, follow a series of stable anginas and they are usually the warning signs for a major ischemic event such as AMI or fatal ventricular arrhythmia. Pregnancy under these circumstances is not advisable. Aggressive therapy including coronary angioplasty and percutaneous coronary

---

Box 1
Preconception care

Before conception:

- Detailed history and physical examination

- Electrocardiogram and echocardiogram

- Stress test and, if indicated, coronary angiogram and nuclear studies

- Pregnancy is usually discouraged, especially if AMI was recent or current condition is not stable

---

Box 2
Early antenatal care

First trimester:

- A detailed history and physical examination with baseline evaluations
  - ○ Electrocardiogram
  - ○ Echocardiogram
  - ○ Complete blood count with platelet count
  - ○ Prothrombin time and International Normalization Ratio, activated partial thrombin time
  - ○ Electrolytes, magnesium, blood urea nitrogen, creatinine
  - ○ Blood glucose, hemoglobin A1c
  - ○ 24-hour urine protein, creatinine clearance
  - ○ Ophthalmology examination
- Noninvasive stress testing in special circumstances
- Angiographic evaluation with abdominal shielding
- Diabetes should be controlled but not tight (to decrease the incidence of hypoglycemia)

---

intervention or coronary artery bypass is recommended. If the outcome is satisfactory and condition is stable, pregnancy can be considered.

If unstable angina develops during pregnancy, aggressive treatment should be initiated in an intensive care unit. Percutaneous coronary intervention with stenting or bypass surgery may be necessary (**Box 3**). A coronary bypass operation should be performed without cardiopulmonary bypass to decrease risk to the fetus.[1]

The treatment of an AMI during pregnancy includes starting IV morphine sulfate to control pain, oxygen by nasal cannula or mask, sublingual nitroglycerine, and chewable aspirin. The goal is to complete this treatment in less than 10 minutes to avoid permanent or extensive damage. A 12-lead electrocardiogram should be performed

---

Box 3
Acute MI care

Unstable angina:

- Coronary angioplasty and percutaneous coronary intervention or coronary artery bypass

AMI treatment:

- Intravenous (IV) morphine sulfate to control pain
- Oxygen by nasal cannula or mask
- Sublingual nitroglycerine
- Chewable aspirin
- IV heparin
- β-Blockers (unless acute heart failure is present)
- IV nitroglycerine
- Antiplatelet therapy (clopidogrel)
- Systemic thrombolytic therapy (tissue plasminogen activator) is controversial
- Percutaneous coronary intervention with extensive lead shielding

and repeated after 5 to 10 minutes if there is suspected MI despite an initial electro-cardiogram reading of no abnormalities. If there is any sign of ST elevation or new left bundle branch block, treatment of an AMI should be started and cardiologists should be consulted.

The recommended treatment is outlined in **Box 3**. The use of systemic thrombolytic therapy (tissue plasminogen activator) in pregnancy is controversial. There are some reports with successful outcomes.[25] However, there is a potential increased risk for both maternal and fetal hemorrhage with the use of thrombolytic agents. Therefore, percutaneous coronary intervention is the preferred procedure by many care givers.[26] Although there is radiation exposure risk to the fetus, extensive lead shielding can be used. The radial artery approach has been described and used successfully in preg-nancy.[27] This technique has a theoretical advantage in minimizing radiation to the fetus and prolonging maternal/fetal platelet inhibition.

An important consideration is that AMI is associated with excess catecholamine production, making optimal glycemic control more difficult to achieve in diabetic pa-tients. Moreover, excess catecholamine production may create a burden on the myocardial function and oxygenation.

After an AMI in a pregnancy, several important decisions have to be addressed. If the gestational age is less than 14 to 16 weeks, pregnancy termination should be considered, because there is a risk for potential reinfarction. Although Husaini and colleagues[28] claimed that an early gestational age for termination is safer for these patients, they reported no maternal deaths in 8 patients with first-trimester AMI who continued pregnancy without reinfarction. In these patients, the overall rate of reinfarc-tion was 6%. However, Silfen and colleagues[29] think that even an early abortion pre-sents serious risk and recommend continuing the pregnancy. In the study by Hankins and colleagues,[30] no maternal deaths occurred in women who delivered more than 2 weeks after infarction.

Unstable angina, heart failure, dysrhythmia, and reinfarction are some of the com-plications that may develop after an AMI. In these patients, pregnancy termination is usually advised because of the increased cardiac demand of pregnancy.[28] If preg-nancy is continued after the complications, medical therapy and limitation of maternal exertion with adequate bed rest should be encouraged to decrease the myocardial oxygen demand.[30] These patients have prolonged hospitalization and stay in cardiac rehabilitation units. Repeat echocardiogram to assess the recovery of cardiac function is helpful in determining maternal outcome.[31]

Diabetes should be controlled but hypoglycemia should be avoided to prevent cate-cholamine release and tachycardia, which increase myocardial demands.[30] Tight glucose control in patients with diabetes during pregnancy is the general practice. However, this type of management may lead to more frequent episodes of hypoglyce-mia. Therefore, some investigators recommend accepting higher glucose values to avoid hypoglycemia.[32]

Early ultrasound for the confirmation of pregnancy and correct dates is essential, particularly for the correct diagnosis of fetal growth restriction or small for gestational age as the pregnancy advances. First-trimester genetic screening should be offered to the patient, because early pregnancy associated placental protein A and human cho-rionic gonadotropin measurements with nuchal translucency have been used to pre-dict the poor outcome in high-risk population.

Second and Third Trimester

Detailed fetal anatomy and echocardiogram should be done to screen for fetal congenital defects (**Box 4**). Uterine artery Doppler measurements may be helpful in

---

Box 4
Late antenatal care

Second and third trimesters:

- Detailed fetal anatomy and fetal echocardiogram
- Uterine artery Doppler measurements
- Monitor closely for the signs and symptoms of coronary insufficiency
- Always remember the atypical presentation of MI in patients with autonomic neuropathy
- Start serial fetal growth evaluations and antenatal testing earlier

---

predicting preeclampsia or placenta-related maternal and fetal complications in this high-risk population.

These patients should be monitored closely for the signs and symptoms of coronary insufficiency. If there are any new symptoms the work-up and evaluation should be repeated. MI should be always in the differential even with vague symptoms. Particularly in diabetic patients, the autonomic neuropathy may predispose to infarction and result in atypical presenting symptoms, making diagnosis difficult and delaying treatment. The diagnostic approach and management for angina and AMI is the same as for nonpregnant patients.

The potential concomitant uteroplacental vascular abnormalities increase the risk of fetal growth restriction and fetal demise, therefore serial fetal growth evaluations and antenatal testing should start earlier in these patients.[30]

LABOR AND DELIVERY, AND POSTPARTUM

Delivery within 2 weeks of MI is associated with increased mortality so, if possible, attempts should be made to allow adequate convalescence before delivery (**Boxes 5** and **6**).

If the cervix is favorable, under controlled circumstances cautious induction after a period of hemodynamic stabilization is optimal. Labor in the lateral recumbent position, with oxygen administration and adequate pain relief, and preferably with epidural anesthesia and, in selected cases, hemodynamic monitoring with a pulmonary artery catheter, are important management considerations.

The route of delivery should be individualized and a maternal fetal medicine specialist should be consulted for the best management plan. In the past, recommendations for route of delivery have focused on an operative vaginal delivery (forceps, vacuum) to shorten the second stage of labor to decrease the Valsalva maneuver and cesarean section used for obstetric indications.[31] Continuous cardiac monitoring is routinely advised and the use of central line catheters should be individualized. Continuous epidural anesthesia is recommended to avoid pain-related stress and tachycardia along with the accompanying increased myocardial oxygen demand and increased risk of acute cardiac events.

The greatest risk is the delivery and postpartum period for these patients. Issues to be clarified with the maternal fetal medicine specialist include, but are not limited to, the following:

- Timing of delivery
- Use of central monitoring
- Type of anesthesia

Box 5
Labor and delivery care

Labor and delivery:

- After a recent MI, try to delay delivery until after 2 weeks of the event of MI
- If cervix is favorable, time induction for when the mother is hemodynamically stable
- Continuous cardiac monitoring
- Selected cases require hemodynamic monitoring with a pulmonary artery catheter
- Adequate pain relief, preferably with epidural anesthesia
- Cesarean section for obstetric indications
- Shortening of second stage of labor

- Route of delivery
- Type of anesthesia and the continuation of monitoring postpartum for complication detection

Time of infarction, maternal cardiac function and hemodynamic status, concomitant pregnancy-related maternal complications, fetal condition, and gestational age are important factors to be considered when timing the delivery. If both maternal and fetal conditions are stable, induction can be considered after confirmation of fetal lung maturity and that the cervix is favorable. The facility should be familiar with the central monitoring. Although not every patient needs central line and monitoring, patients with recent infarction (1–2 months), unstable angina, impaired cardiac function, or pulmonary edema should have central monitoring.[33]

In patients who have not had an MI in the 3 weeks before delivery, with or without evidence of ischemia, heart failure, or severe left ventricular dysfunction, simple electrocardiographic monitoring is sufficient during labor. If a large myocardial ischemia has occurred during pregnancy, arterial blood pressure, central venous pressure, and pulmonary arterial and pulmonary wedge pressure with cardiac output should be monitored invasively. Monitoring should continue until after delivery because the preload abruptly increases with the delivery.

The delivery route should be decided by obstetric indications. Cesarean section has not been shown to have benefit in the morbidity.[30] In contrast, one study noted that the incidence of maternal mortality was higher with cesarean delivery than with vaginal delivery, although there were multiple confounding factors.[30] Elective cesarean without labor can increase the cardiac output suddenly up to 50% of predelivery values compared with an appropriately managed labor.[33] In addition, cesarean delivery

---

Box 6
Postpartum care

Postpartum:

- Continuation of monitoring during postpartum
- Central catheters and epidural should stay for at least 24 hours after delivery
- Extended period of close postpartum follow-up evaluation
- Contraception options should be discussed

increases the blood loss and postpartum complications.[30] However, cesarean delivery with controlled analgesia may result in a less pronounced fluid shift. Timing the delivery, avoidance of long or unpredictable labor, and a possibility of rapid resolution of pulmonary edema are the proposed advantages of cesarean delivery.[33]

Epidural analgesia is effective in controlling pain in labor and is associated with decreased catecholamine excess and tachycardia and decreased cardiac stress. It may also decrease the afterload and preload and help to diminish the myocardial load.[33] During labor, oxygen supplementation, lateral recumbent position, and avoidance of tachycardia and hypertension are important. Cases with parenteral nitrate therapy during labor to decrease myocardial demand have been reported.[33] Some investigators recommend shortening of the second stage of labor to avoid the adverse effects of maternal pushing on cardiac function. However, there are limited data to support this approach.[1,31] Ergot alkoloids and prostaglandins should be avoided because they may cause coronary vasoconstriction.

After delivery, a series of important physiologic changes occur. There is a significant and immediate fluid shift and increase in the cardiac output by release of venocaval obstruction, autotransfusion of uteroplacental blood, and rapid mobilization of extravascular fluid. For these reasons, these patients must be closely monitored. Both central catheters and epidural analgesia should stay for at least 24 hours after delivery to help manage fluid shifts. An extended period of close postpartum follow-up evaluation is required because the cardiovascular hemodynamics do not return to the prepregnancy state even by 12 weeks postpartum.[33]

SUMMARY OF MANAGEMENT

It is essential to inform the patient with diabetes and IHD about the serious maternal risk of pregnancy. Preconception counseling with a maternal-fetal medicine (MFM) specialist should be strongly recommended by the patient's cardiologist, endocrinologist, or primary caregiver if the patient wishes to get pregnant. Risk and prognosis should be brought up by the MFM specialist and permanent sterilization should be considered, especially in severely affected patients.

If the patient is determined to become pregnant and is aware of the risks and accepts them, every effort should be made by the obstetrician, maternal-fetal medicine specialist, the endocrinologist, and the cardiologist to create a perinatal care plan that is collaborative and that fosters good communication. A thorough antenatal cardiac evaluation should be obtained and optimal glycemic control should be obtained while being mindful of the need to avoid hypoglycemia. Continuous surveillance of maternal and fetal status throughout the pregnancy and meticulous management of the delivery and postpartum period creates the best chance for success for the patient and her caregivers.

REFERENCES

1. Creasy RK, Resnik R, Iams JD, et al. Diabetes in pregnancy. Creasy & Resnik's maternal-fetal medicine. 6th edition. Pennsylvania: Saunders Elsevier; 2009. p. 953–93.
2. Davies GA, Herberet WN. Ischemic heart disease and cardiomyopathy in pregnancy. J Obstet Gynaecol Can 2007;29(7):575–9.
3. El-Deeb M, El-Menyar A, Gehani A, et al. Acute coronary syndrome in pregnant women. Expert Rev Cardiovasc Ther 2011;9(4):505–15.
4. Cormier CM, Martinez CA, Refuerzo JS, et al. White's classification of diabetes in pregnancy in the 21st century: is it still valid? Am J Perinatol 2010;27:349–52.

5. Boras J, Pavlic-Renar I, Car N, et al. Diabetes and coronary heart disease. Diabetol Croat 2002;31(4):199–208.

6. American Diabetes Association: preconception care of women with diabetes (position statement). Diabetes Care 2003;26:591.

7. Roger VL, Go AS, Lloyd-Jones DM, et al. Heart disease and stroke statistics – 2011 update: a report from the American Heart Association. Circulation 2011; 123:e18–209.

8. Ni H, Coady S, Rosanond W, et al. Trends from 1987 to 2004 in sudden death due to coronary heart disease: the Atherosclerosis Risk in Communities (ARIC) study. Am Heart J 2009;157:46–52.

9. Olson MB, Kelsey SF, Matthews K, et al. Symptoms, myocardial ischemia and quality of life in women: results from the NHLBI-sponsored WISE Study. Eur Heart J 2003;24:1506–14.

10. Guleltz M, Show LJ, Merz CN. Myocardial ischemia in women: lesson from the NHLBI WISE Study. Clin Cardiol 2012;35:14–8.

11. Coventry LL, Finn J, Bremner AP. Sex differences in symptom presentation in acute myocardial infarction: a systematic review and meta-analysis. Heart Lung 2011;40:477–91.

12. Rosenfeld A, Lindauer A, Darney B. Understanding treatment-seeking delay in women with acute myocardial infraction: descriptions of decision making patterns. Am J Crit Care 2005;14:285–93.

13. Cantus DS, Ruiz M. Ischemic heart disease in women. Rev Lat Am Enfermagem 2011;19:1464–9.

14. Lawton JS. Sex and gender differences in coronary artery disease. Semin Thorac Cardiovasc Surg 2011;23:126–30.

15. James AH, Jamison MG, Biswas MS, et al. Acute myocardial infarction in pregnancy: a United States population-based study. Circulation 2006;113:1564–71.

16. Roth A, Elkayam V. Acute myocardial infraction associated with pregnancy. J Am Coll Cardiol 2008;52:171–80.

17. Bonnet J, Aumailley M, Thomas D, et al. Spontaneous coronary artery dissection: case report and evidence for a defect in collagen metabolism. Eur Heart J 1986; 7:904–9.

18. Schiller JS, Lucas JW, Ward BW, et al. Summary health statistics for US adults National Health Interview Survey, 2010. Vital Health Stat 10 2012;(252):1–207.

19. D'Souza A, Hussain E, Howarth E, et al. Pathogenesis and pathophysiology of accelerated atherosclerosis in the diabetic heart. Molec Cell Biol Chem 2009; 331:89–116.

20. Bagg W, Henley PG, MacPherson P, et al. Pregnancy in women with diabetes and ischemic heart disease. Aust N Z J Obstet Gynaecol 1999;1:99–102.

21. Ladner HE, Danielsen B, Gilbert WM, et al. Acute myocardial infarction in pregnancy and the puerperium: a population-based study. Obstet Gynecol 2005;105:480–4.

22. Clark SL. Structural cardiac disease in pregnancy. In: Clark SL, Cotton DB, Phelan JP, editors. Critical care obstetrics. Madden (MA): Blackwell Science; 1997. p. 290–304.

23. Gast MJ, Rigg LA. Class H diabetes and pregnancy. Obstet Gynecol 1985;66:5S.

24. Veille JC, Kitzman DW, Bacevice AE. Effects of pregnancy on the electrocardiogram in healthy subjects during strenuous exercise. Am J Obstet Gynecol 1996; 175(5):1360–4.

25. Schumacher B, Belfort MA, Card RJ. Successful treatment of acute myocardial infarction during pregnancy with tissue plasminogen activator. Am J Obstet Gynecol 1997;176(3):716–9.

26. Sebastian C, Scherlag M, Kugelmass A, et al. Primary stent implantation for acute myocardial infarction during pregnancy: use of abciximab, ticlopidine, and aspirin. Cathet Cardiovasc Diagn 1998;45(3):275–9.

27. Sharma GL, Loubeyre C, Morice MC. Safety and feasibility of the radial approach for primary angioplasty in acute myocardial infarction during pregnancy. J Invasive Cardiol 2002;14(6):359–62.

28. Husaini MH. Myocardial infarction during pregnancy: report of two cases with a review of the literature. Postgrad Med J 1971;47(552):660–5.

29. Silfen SL, Wapner RJ, Gabbe SG. Maternal outcome in class H diabetes mellitus. Obstet Gynecol 1980;55(6):749–51.

30. Hankins GD, Wendel GD Jr, Leveno KJ, et al. Myocardial infarction during pregnancy: a review. Obstet Gynecol 1985;65(1):139–46.

31. Sheikh AU, Harper MA. Myocardial infarction during pregnancy: management and outcome of two pregnancies. Am J Obstet Gynecol 1993;169(2 Pt 1): 279–83 [discussion: 283–4].

32. Pombar X, Strassner HT, Fenner PC. Pregnancy in a woman with class H diabetes mellitus and previous coronary artery bypass graft: a case report and review of the literature. Obstet Gynecol 1995;85(5 Pt 2):825–9.

33. Gordon MC, Landon MB, Boyle J, et al. Coronary artery disease in insulin-dependent diabetes mellitus of pregnancy (class H): a review of the literature. Obstet Gynecol Surv 1996;51(7):437–44.

Pregnancy Management of Diabetic Renal Transplant Patients

Lalarukh Haider, MBBS, Nancy Day Adams, MD*

KEYWORDS

- Management of pregnancy • Diabetes mellitus • Kidney transplant recipient
- End stage renal disease

KEY POINTS

- End-stage renal disease (ESRD) leads to impaired fertility.
- Impaired fertility in ESRD can improve by 1 to 6 months after renal transplant; thus, pregnancy is a viable option for some diabetic kidney transplant recipients.
- Optimal management of diabetes mellitus before conception is imperative to minimize risks to mother and fetus.
- Optimal management of the transplanted kidney allograft is important before proceeding with pregnancy.
- Risks associated with pregnancy to the fetus, mother, and allograft must be discussed in detail before conception.

INTRODUCTION

Joseph E. Murray performed the first successful kidney transplant in 1954 between identical twins. No immunosuppression was required. Since then, the field of transplantation has grown by leaps and bounds. The number of immunosuppressive medications has also grown. Kidney transplantation accounts for the largest number of transplanted organs in the United States.[1]

Advanced kidney disease disrupts the hypothalamic-pituitary-gonadal axis. Thus, fertility is reduced in advanced kidney disease not requiring renal replacement therapy and in kidney disease requiring hemodialysis or peritoneal dialysis. Successful transplantation can restore fertility 1 to 6 months after transplant. Thus, pregnancy is now a realistic option for young female transplant recipients. The first child born to a renal transplant recipient turned 48 years old in 2006.[2] The transplant recipient had received a kidney from her identical twin.

Unfortunately, the vast majority of transplants are not among identical twins and thus require immunosuppression. The effects of immunosuppressive medications

Division of Nephrology, University of Connecticut Health Center, MC 1405, 263 Farmington Avenue, Farmington, CT 06030, USA
* Corresponding author.
E-mail address: adams@nso.uchc.edu

Clin Lab Med 33 (2013) 257–269
http://dx.doi.org/10.1016/j.cll.2013.03.014
0272-2712/13/$ – see front matter © 2013 Elsevier Inc. All rights reserved.

labmed.theclinics.com

on the fetus can be detrimental. There have been more than 14,000 pregnancies documented in case series, case reports, and registries among patients after transplants.[3] Not all post-transplant pregnancies and their outcomes are documented. Three main registries exist that have published data on maternal, paternal, fetal, and graft outcomes. The largest number of post-transplant pregnancies to date is reported by the National Transplantation Pregnancy Registry (NTPR) in the United States.[4] The NTPR was established in 1991 to study outcomes (maternal, fetal, and graft) of pregnancies in transplant recipients. It registers female transplant recipients who have had post-transplant pregnancies and male transplant recipients who have fathered offspring. This is a voluntary registry and there may be a bias not to report spontaneous or therapeutic abortions. Thus, the data may be skewed. A patient, transplant coordinator, or physician (after obtaining consent from the patient) can register a patient. The registration form is a 1-page questionnaire and is followed by telephone interviews, and data are obtained from physicians periodically. All pregnancy and postpregnancy outcomes are documented: live births, therapeutic abortions, spontaneous abortions, still births, ectopic pregnancies, structural malformations, and neonatal complications. Long-term effects to recipients, offspring, and grafts are also followed. The UK Transplant Registry collected information from the majority of the transplantation units from 1997 to 2002. European Renal Association - European Dialysis and Transplantation Association Registry collects information on outcomes from European countries. The pregnancies reported by all 3 registries capture a fraction of the post-transplant pregnancies.

SCOPE OF THE PROBLEM: END-STAGE RENAL DISEASE AND DIABETES MELLITUS

In 2010, approximately 79,000 patients ages 18 years and older were waiting for a kidney transplant (**Table 1**)[1] —26% of the patients (male and female) on the kidney

Table 1
Characteristics of adult patients (18 years and older) on the kidney transplant wait list on December 31, 2009[5]

	N	%
Age (y)		
18–44	20,893	26.3
45–64	43,999	55.4
65–74	12,838	16.2
75+	1631	2.1
Gender		
Male	46,446	58.5
Female	32,915	41.5
Primary cause of ESRD		
Diabetes (types 1 and 2)	24,104	30.4
Hypertension	20,326	25.6
Glomerulonephritis	11,663	14.7
Cystic kidney disease	6708	8.5
Others	16,560	20.9
Transplant history		
First transplant	66,802	84.2
Subsequent transplant	12,559	15.8

transplant wait list were in the child-bearing age group of 18 to 44 years (*Organ Procurement and Transplantation Network* and Scientific Registry of Transplant Recipients annual report, 2010)[5]; 41% of all wait list candidates were female. Diabetes mellitus (types 1 and 2) was the primary cause of ESRD in 30% of the wait list candidates.

In 2009, 15,964 patients ages 18 years and older in the United States underwent a kidney transplant.[5] Their characteristics are shown in **Table 2**; 41% were women and 42% (including men) of the transplant recipients were ages 18 to 49 years. This young share of transplanted patients is a much greater share than that of the wait-list population. Diabetes mellitus was the cause of ESRD in 25% of the transplant cases. The percentage of patients with diabetes mellitus is slightly higher on the wait list compared with the percentage transplanted.

Advanced renal failure leads to impaired reproductive function, specifically a suppressed/dysfunctional hypothalamic-pituitary-gonadal axis. Few pregnancies occur in patients on hemodialysis or peritoneal dialysis. Fertility is restored 1 to 6 months after a successful kidney transplant. This offers younger transplant recipients a chance to conceive. The first reported successful pregnancy in a kidney recipient occurred in March 1958. Since then, thousands of pregnancies have occurred in transplant recipients.

As of December 2011, 2054 pregnancies (with 2108 outcomes) in 1247 female recipients were documented by the NTPR. Of these, 1490 pregnancies with 1525 outcomes (due to multiple births) were in 922 kidney transplant recipients; 71% to 76% of pregnancies resulted in a live birth in kidney transplant recipients. This percentage of live births to kidney transplant recipients is lower than that of the general population. The incidence of birth defects in the live born is similar to that in the general population.

Table 2 Characteristics of adult (18 years and older) kidney transplant recipients on December 31, 2009 (OPTN and SRTR Annual Data Report 2010)		
	N	**%**
Age (y)		
18–34	2208	13.8
35–49	4541	28.4
50–64	6556	41.1
65+	2659	16.7
Gender		
Male	9642	60.4
Female	6322	39.6
Primary cause of ESRD		
Diabetes (types 1 and 2)	3921	24.6
Hypertension	3931	24.6
Glomerulonephritis	3060	19.2
Cystic kidney disease	2070	13
Others	2982	18.7
Transplant history		
First transplant	14,037	87.9
Subsequent transplant	1927	12.1

Pregnancies with in utero mycophenolate mofetil exposure, however, have a 23% incidence of birth defects.[4,6]

Pregnancy in transplant recipients is a high-risk pregnancy. Mother, fetus, and allograft are at risk of complications. Acute graft rejection, graft dysfunction, hypertension, and preeclampsia are seen in renal transplant mothers during pregnancy. Fetal complications, such as prematurity (delivery <37 weeks gestation) and growth retardation, are well known. One of the goals of the NTPR is to follow the offspring of solid organ transplant recipients. Exposure to immunosuppressive medications in utero may result in subtle immunologic defects, learning disabilities, and abnormalities of reproductive function in the offspring of transplanted recipients. These defects may not manifest in offspring until much later in life. Defects may be present despite normal development and renal function in infants. Long-term follow-up and continued surveillance of offspring are warranted and remain a goal of the NTPR.

PREPARATION FOR PREGNANCY FOR THE KIDNEY TRANSPLANT RECIPIENT

Counseling for pregnancy or prevention of pregnancy should ideally start at the time of the pretransplant evaluation with a potential transplant recipient and partner and should include[3]

- Updated vaccinations (hepatitis B, *Streptococcus pneumoniae*, and influenza)
- Discussion of risks of the pregnancy to mother, fetus, and graft
- Prematurity of the fetus and possible long-term complications (eg, cerebral palsy)
- Discussion of plan for contraception, because fertility may be restored in as little as 1 month after kidney transplant, ideally started either before (for transplant from live donors) or at the time of transplant
- Optimal timing of conceiving

The American Society of Transplantation recommendations for the timing of pregnancy are[3]

- No rejection in the past year
- Stable kidney function
- Serum creatinine level less than or equal to 1.5 mg/dL
- Minimal to no proteinuria: minimal level of proteinuria needs to be defined by controlled trials but generally accepted as less than 1000 mg/d
- No acute infections that may infect the fetus (eg, cytomegalovirus and hepatitis C virus)
- Maintenance immunosuppression at stable doses
- Normal appearance of allograft on ultrasound

If these criteria are fulfilled, recipients can proceed with pregnancy 1 year after transplant. The European Society for Organ Transplantation recommends, however, waiting until 2 years after transplant.[7]

MANAGEMENT OF THE PREGNANT KIDNEY TRANSPLANT PATIENT

The team caring for a pregnant diabetic kidney transplant recipient should include

- Transplant nephrologist and surgeon
- High-risk maternal-fetal medicine obstetrician
- Endocrinologist
- Pediatrician/neonatologist

Hypertension

Hypertension is common among kidney transplant recipients, likely reflecting underlying chronic kidney disease. Angiotensin-converting enzyme inhibitors (ACEIs) and angiotensin receptor blockers (ARBs) are used routinely in renal transplant recipients to control hypertension. Both these drugs are teratogenic and should be stopped before conception.

- Pregnant kidney transplant recipients should check blood pressure daily.[8]
- All kidney transplant recipients are considered to have chronic kidney disease even if serum creatinine is within the normal range. Serum creatinine level normally decreases during pregnancy because of increased plasma volume. Thus, serum creatinine level of 1 mg/dL may not represent a normal glomerular filtration rate.[9]
- The goal blood pressure is stricter than for nontransplant pregnant patients, at a goal blood pressure of less than 130/80.[8,9]
- ACEIs and ARBs should be discontinued before conception because they are teratogenic and cause fetal malformations.[8]
- Drugs routinely used to treat hypertension during pregnancy include α-methyldopa and labetalol. Calcium channel blockers and hydrochlorothiazide can be used as second-line agents.[8,9]
- Preeclampsia develops in 30% of pregnant kidney transplant recipients. Incidence of preeclampsia in the general population is 5% to 8%. Pregnant kidney transplant recipients must be monitored frequently (every 2–4 weeks) with quantification of urine protein excretion (if proteinuria is present) and serum creatinine evaluation. A high index of suspicion is necessary.[10]

Allograft Monitoring

- Graft function should be monitored during pregnancy at regular intervals. Optimal timing is not determined but serum creatinine should be checked monthly in the first and second trimesters and possibly every 2 weeks during the third trimester.[11]
- A high index of suspicion for allograft rejection is important. The signs and symptoms of allograft rejection are not specific. They may mimic preeclampsia or pyelonephritis. Clues to suspect allograft rejection are
  ○ Decreased urine output
  ○ Rapid increase in weight
  ○ Lower-extremity edema
  ○ Deteriorating blood pressure control
  ○ Increasing proteinuria
  ○ Increasing serum creatinine
  ○ Fever, chills, pain, or swelling over the allograft (pain over the allograft may be absent because the renal allograft is denervated)
  ○ Urinary tract infection
- If a rejection is suspected, an allograft biopsy should be performed early. Rejection should be treated, preferably with steroids. The safety of lymphocyte-depleting agents in pregnancy is not known.[11]

Patients should be evaluated every 2 weeks. A cesarean section is indicated for obstetric reasons only. The transplanted kidney in the false pelvis does not cause dystocia. The dose of steroids should be increased at the onset of labor to account for the stress of labor and prevent postpartum rejection. The mother and allograft need close monitoring in the postpartum period too.

Immunosuppression

Immunosuppressive medications should be adjusted and stabilized before conception.[12] The most common immunosuppression regimen used in the United States consists of tacrolimus, prednisone, and mycophenolate mofetil. Other agents that can be used are cyclosporine A, azathioprine, sirolimus, rituximab, and lymphocyte-depleting agents.[13,14] Food and Drug Administration (FDA) categories for the immunosuppressive medications are shown in **Table 3**.

Tacrolimus

- Tacrolimus is a calcineurin inhibitor.
- Tacrolimus may cause hypertension, nephrotoxicity, and diabetes mellitus in the mother.
- Tacrolimus levels must be followed every 2 to 4 weeks during pregnancy. Common tacrolimus dosage is 1 mg to 4 mg orally twice a day. Goal whole blood trough levels are 3 ng/mL to 7 ng/mL. The dosage may need to be increased by 20% to 40% to maintain adequate levels during pregnancy. Postpartum tacrolimus levels need to be followed closely as well because dosage needs to be decreased to prepregnancy levels.
- Tacrolimus is excreted in breast milk; avoid breastfeeding.
- Tacrolimus may be better than cyclosporine in pregnant patients because risk of preeclampsia is thought to be less.

Table 3	
FDA categories for immunosuppressive medications	
Medication	**FDA category**
Azathioprine	C
Cyclosporine	C
Methylprednisolone	C
Mycophenolate mofetil	D
Prednisone	B
Sirolimus	C
Tacrolimus (FK506)	C
Thymoglobulin/OKT3	C
FDA categories for teratogenicity potential of medications	
FDA Category	
A	Controlled studies have not demonstrated a risk to the fetus in the first trimester and no evidence of risk in later trimesters.
B	Animal reproduction studies have shown no risk to fetus with no controlled studies in pregnant women OR animal control studies show an adverse effect on fetus but controlled studies in women failed to show this effect.
C	Animal studies have shown an adverse risk to fetus and there are no controlled studies in women OR studies in animals and women are not available.
D	There is evidence to show human fetal risk BUT benefit for use by a pregnant woman may be justified despite risk.
X	Contraindicated in pregnant women; studies demonstrate fetal risk in humans and/or animals and risk of drug outweighs any possible benefit.

Prednisone/corticosteroids

- Inhibit all stages of T-cell activation and blocks production of interleukin-1 and interleukin-6
- Used for induction, maintenance, and treatment of acute rejection
- May cause hypertension, diabetes mellitus, osteoporosis, weight gain, peptic ulcer disease, and premature rupture of membranes in the mother
- May cause fetal growth retardation, low birth weight, adrenal insufficiency and thymic hypoplasia
- Compatible with breastfeeding
- Common dosage in stable kidney transplant recipients 5 mg to 15 mg per oral daily, sometimes split as twice a day, with two-thirds of the dose in the morning and one-third in the evening

Mycophenolate mofetil

- Impairs B-cell and T-cell proliferation[4,6]
- May cause nausea, vomiting, and myelosuppression in the mother
- Increased risk of first-trimester pregnancy loss and congenital malformations, especially of the external ear and other facial abnormalities; malformations of the distal limbs, heart, esophagus, and kidneys described
- Breastfeeding not recommended
- Should be stopped 6 weeks before conception
- Common dosage 2000 mg to 3000 mg per oral divided twice a day; higher dose used more often in recipients of African descent; trough levels not routinely followed

Azathioprine

- Antimetabolite that inhibits DNA and RNA synthesis[15]
- Metabolized to the active form 6-mercaptopurine, which crosses the placental barrier
- May cause leukopenia, thrombocytopenia, nausea, vomiting, or hepatitis in the mother
- May cause growth retardation in the fetus
- Excreted in breast milk; avoid breastfeeding
- Common maintenance dose for azathioprine 1.5 mg/kg to 2.5 mg/kg body weight; usually 100 mg to 150 mg per oral divided twice a day

Cyclosporine

- May cause nephrotoxicity, hyperkalemia, hyperlipidemia, glucose intolerance, or malignancy in the mother[16]
- May cause growth retardation, low birth weight, premature birth in fetus
- May cause preeclampsia
- Levels need to be monitored every 2 to 4 weeks; common maintenance dose for cyclosporine 2 mg/kg to 5 mg/kg body weight, usually 150 mg to 300 mg per oral divided twice a day; goal trough cyclosporine whole blood or plasma levels 50 ng/mL to 150 ng/mL; dosage may need to be increased by 25% because metabolism may increase during pregnancy; cyclosporine levels need to be closely monitored in the postpartum period because dosage needs to be decreased.
- Excreted in breast milk; avoid breastfeeding
- Shown to induce permanent nephron deficit in young rabbits exposed to cyclosporine in utero

Sirolimus

- T-cell proliferation inhibitor
- Approved by FDA in 1999
- Relatively sparse data in humans
- Caused delayed ossification and low fetal weight in animal studies
- NTPR reports 15 kidney transplant recipients with 17 pregnancies: 13 live births, 3 spontaneous abortions, and 1 therapeutic abortion[4]; 2 pregnancies had exposure to mycophenolate mofetil as well; structural defects occurred in 2 of the live born: cleft lip, cleft palate, microtia, and tetralogy of Fallot.
- Common maintenance dose for sirolimus 2 mg to 4 mg per oral daily; goal whole blood sirolimus trough levels 3 ng/mL to 7 ng/mL

Monoclonal and polyclonal antibodies

- OKT3 (IgG monoclonal antibody anti-CD3), thymoglobulin, and antithymocyte globulin are examples of lymphocyte-depleting antibodies.
- These are used for induction during initial transplant and to treat acute rejection. They are not used as maintenance immunosuppression.
- Effect on the developing fetus is unknown and, therefore, should be avoided in rejection during pregnancy. High-dose steroids are the mainstay of treatment of rejection during pregnancy.

DIABETES MELLITUS: PREEXISTING VERSUS NEW-ONSET DIABETES AFTER TRANSPLANT

In 2003, international consensus guidelines defined new-onset diabetes after transplantation (NODAT).[17] NODAT can be diagnosed at any time after transplant (in patients not previously diagnosed with diabetes mellitus) using the following criteria:

- Symptoms of diabetes and a random glucose of greater than or equal to 200 mg/dL
- Fasting blood glucose (FBG) greater than or equal to 126 mg/dL on 2 separate occasions
- Two-hour plasma glucose greater than or equal to 200 mg/dL during an oral glucose tolerance test using 75 g of anhydrous glucose dissolved in water

The incidence of NODAT is highest 3 months after transplant. The cumulative incidence of 1-year post-transplant is 10% to 30%.

Common risk factors for developing NODAT are

- Increased age (greater than 40 years old)
- Obesity (body mass index greater than 30)
- African American or Hispanic race
- Family history of diabetes mellitus
- Hepatitis C virus infection
- Glucocorticoid therapy
- Calcineurin inhibitors (tacrolimus has a higher incidence of NODAT compared with cyclosporine)
- Sirolimus
- Preoperative impaired glucose tolerance or postoperative hyperglycemia

Implications of NODAT

- Increased cardiovascular mortality
- Increased risk of infection

- Decreased allograft survival (diabetic nephropathy in the allograft and increased risk of rejection)

Management of NODAT

- Pretransplant
  - Screen for impaired fasting glucose and high-risk characteristics (as listed previously).
  - Educate patients about risk of developing NODAT.
- Post-transplant
  - Check FBG weekly for 4 weeks, at 3 months, at 6 months, and then annually.
  - Hemoglobin A_{1C} (HbA$_{1C}$) can be checked if FBG is difficult to obtain. Wait 3 months post-transplant, however, to check the first HbA$_{1C}$. The threshold to diagnose diabetes mellitus is HbA$_{1C}$ greater than 6.5%.[7,18]
  - Consider modifying immunosuppression.
    - Minimize dose of steroids. Steroids should not be discontinued because this may precipitate graft rejection.
    - Reduce tacrolimus dose.

DIABETES MELLITUS AND PREGNANCY

The key issues that need to be followed in pregnant diabetic patients are

- Achieving and maintaining adequate glycemic control ideally before conception through the postpartum period
- Screening, monitoring, and treating maternal and fetal complications

As with kidney transplant recipients, counseling for pregnancy or prevention of pregnancy should start when diabetes is diagnosed. Preconception counseling should address maternal risks, fetal risks, and possibility of disease progression and complications. The possible teratogenic nature of medications should be clearly discussed.

Preparation for Pregnancy in the Diabetic Patient

Before pursuing pregnancy, baseline maternal medical status needs to be determined and subsequent issues addressed.

Glycemic control (HbA$_{1C}$)

In the general population, major congenital malformation occurs in 1% to 2% of the population.[18,19] In diabetic women with poor glycemic control in the periconception period, the risk of birth defects is 4 to 8 times greater than in the general population. The risk of spontaneous abortion is high if glycemic control is poor during pregnancy. The rate of major congenital malformation is 22.4%, with HbA$_{1C}$ greater than 8.5% in the periconceptional period.[19] This rate improves drastically to 3.4%, with improvement of HbA$_{1C}$ to less than 8.5%.[19] With good glycemic control, the risk of fetal malformation and spontaneous abortion approaches that of the general population. Current concepts of diabetic embryopathy by Zhao and Reece are discussed elsewhere in this issue. The risk of preeclampsia is also high with poor glycemic control. Optimization of glycemic control is important before conception. The American Diabetes Association (ADA) target goal for HBA$_{1C}$ in the nonpregnant adult population is less than 7%. The preconception/pregnancy HbA$_{1C}$ goal is more intensive, less than 6%. Oral hypoglycemic agents and insulin can be used before conception to optimize glycemic control. Medications that are safe during pregnancy are reviewed and discussed by Fang and Feldman in more detail elsewhere in this issue.

Presence of nephropathy

An American Congress of Obstetricians and Gynecologists (ACOG) practice bulletin reports increased risk of progression to ESRD if serum creatinine level is greater than 1.5 mg/dL and proteinuria is greater than 3 g/d.[20] The risk of preeclampsia is 15% for type 1 diabetes mellitus patients (risk in general population is 7%) and increases with nephropathy. At baseline, measurement of serum creatinine, glomerular filtration rate, and presence/quantification of proteinuria (either with a 24-hour urine collection or with a first-void urine specimen for albumin-to-creatinine ratio [if urine dipstick for protein is negative] or protein-to-creatinine ratio) is imperative. The earliest sign of diabetic nephropathy is the presence of microalbuminuria. Microalbuminuria is present when the first-void urine or random spot urine specimen albumin-to-creatinine ratio is between 30 μg and 299 μg albumin/mg of creatinine. Microalbuminuria can also be performed on a 24-hour urine collection (30–299 mg of albumin/24 h). Overt nephropathy has greater than 300 mg of protein excretion per 24-hour period. The higher the degree of overt nephropathy, the greater the incidence of complications associated with diabetes mellitus, such as progression of chronic kidney disease. ACEIs and/or ARBs are widely used to minimize proteinuria in diabetics. These are teratogenic and should be discontinued before conception.

Thyroid function status

Among patients with type 1 diabetes mellitus, 40% have coexisting autoimmune thyroid disorders.[18] Thus, if an existing thyroid disorder is unknown, serum TSH and free T_4 level should be assessed as part of the initial preconception work-up.

Blood pressure control

Patients with chronic kidney disease often have hypertension as a comorbid condition.[18] New-onset hypertension during pregnancy is defined as development of blood pressure greater than or equal to 140/90 on 2 occasions more than 6 hours apart with or without proteinuria. After 20 weeks of gestation, new-onset hypertension should raise concern about preeclampsia. If new-onset hypertension resolves in the postpartum period (by 12 weeks postpartum), then patients are considered to truly have had gestational hypertension. Hypertension is associated with a higher incidence of preeclampsia even in the absence of proteinuria. Blood pressure goals during pregnancy are more liberal than in the nonpregnant state. Treatment is recommended if blood pressure is greater than 150/100 to 160/100 in the absence of end-organ damage. In the setting of underlying diabetes mellitus and chronic kidney disease (such as a kidney transplant recipient), however, a more stringent blood pressure control (ie, less than 130/80) is desirable. Therefore, antihypertensive therapy is initiated or titrated up when the blood pressure is greater than 130/80. Aggressive blood pressure control can lead to a small-for-gestational-age child. As discussed previously, medications, such as ACEIs and ARBs, must be discontinued because of their teratogenic nature. α-Methyldopa and labetalol are the usual first-line agents.

Management of the Pregnant Diabetic Patient

Glycemic control

The ADA recommends a goal HbA_{1C} of less than 6% for pregnant diabetic patients.[18] Hemoglobin A1C should be repeated monthly starting at the prenatal visit. Pregnancy causes decreased insulin sensitivity thought to be due to the hormones associated with pregnancy. Insulin requirements fluctuate during pregnancy. There may be an initial decrease in the insulin dose during the first 10 weeks of gestation, followed by a substantial increase (up to 50%) in the insulin dosage until 35 to 37 weeks of gestation.

Insulin management is tailored to individual patients. A 4-times daily insulin regimen allows for better glycemic control. A twice-a-day insulin regimen may be associated with periods of hypoglycemia and hyperglycemia. A 4-times daily regimen also requires intensive self-monitoring of blood glucose (SMBG). The ADA recommends checking SMBG before and 1 hour after each meal, at bedtime, and occasionally between 2:00 AM and 4:00 AM (to detect nocturnal hypoglycemia).

The ADA recommendations for the goal of the SMBG levels are

- 1-Hour to 2-hour postprandial SMBG concentration of 100 mg/dL to 129 mg/dL
- Preprandial, bedtime, and overnight SMBG concentration of 60 mg/dL to 99 mg/dL
- Continuous infusion insulin pumps (CIIPs) are usually not initiated during pregnancy. If good glycemic control is maintained with a CIIP prepregnancy, however, the CIIP is continued during pregnancy but requires considerable titration of the dose of insulin.

Lack of awareness of hypoglycemia is common in type 1 diabetes mellitus. During pregnancy, tight glycemic control and increasing insulin requirements may make hypoglycemic events more common. Patient and family awareness of this is important.

Diabetic ketoacidosis (DKA) is less common than hypoglycemia during pregnancy. Presence of DKA should always elicit a search for the underlying cause. Maternal death due to DKA is uncommon. Fetal demise has been reported, however, in up to 35% of cases of DKA.

Hypoglycemic medications

An ADA consensus statement recommends insulin for optimal glycemic control for pregnant women with types 1 and 2 diabetes mellitus. The ACOG also recommends insulin as the preferred hypoglycemic agent.[20] ACOG also states oral hypoglycemic agents may be used for pregnant women with type 2 diabetes mellitus. Their use should be limited, however, and individualized pending stronger data showing safety of oral hypoglycemic agents in pregnancy.

Neutral protamine Hagedorn (NPH) insulin is an FDA category B drug. It can be given 2 to 3 times a day to help maintain normoglycemia. There are several studies published over the past few decades to show safety of NPH. In 2012, insulin detemir was changed from a category C to a category B drug based on one study that showed noninferiority compared with NPH.[21] Insulin glargine is an FDA category C drug. It has been shown to have a strong affinity to the insulinlike growth factor receptor in osteosarcoma cell lines. A recent retrospective study of 102 pregnancies of type 1 diabetic mothers who used insulin glargine showed no increase in congenital malformations. Both aspart and lispro insulin are category B drugs.

Diabetic retinopathy

Diabetic retinopathy may progress during pregnancy, and particularly when rapid correction occurs in pregnant diabetic patients with poor glycemic control may accelerate it. The ADA recommends an ophthalmology evaluation during the first trimester with close follow-up throughout pregnancy and the postpartum period. Ideally, the presence of diabetic retinopathy should be assessed in the preconception period.

SUMMARY

Optimal care for pregnant diabetic renal transplant recipients hinges on adequate monitoring and control of diabetes mellitus, allograft function, and comorbid conditions. These factors must be addressed before conception. The potential risks to mother, allograft, and fetus should be addressed.

No specific guidelines exist on the management of pregnant diabetic kidney transplant recipients. Recommendations on pregnant diabetic patients and pregnant renal transplant patients exist. These are based on expert opinion, observational data, case series, and so forth. Unfortunately, large and robust randomized control trials to guide management of these complex patients are lacking. Care of diabetic renal transplant patients requires teamwork, optimization of the various medical issues before conception, education of transplant recipients, and collection of strong data to help guide decision making in the future.

Pregnant diabetic kidney transplant patients have high-risk pregnancy. With adequate preconception planning, a dedicated team of physicians addressing the underlying comorbid conditions, and close and careful follow-up before, during, and after pregnancy, however, outcomes have improved in the past several years. In general, maternal and child outcomes are gratifying in patients who as young adults may have been concerned about reduced fertility, chronic kidney disease, and the specter of dialysis.

REFERENCES

1. Available at: http://www.usrds.org. 2012 USRDS data report. Accessed December 1, 2012.
2. McKay DB, Josephson MA. Pregnancy in recipients of solid organs—effects on mother and child. N Engl J Med 2006;354:1281–93.
3. McKay DB, Josephson MA, Armenti VT, et al. Reproduction and transplantation: report on the AST Consensus Conference on Reproductive Issues and Transplantation. Am J Transplant 2005;5:1592–9.
4. Annual Report: National Transplantation Pregnancy Registry. 2011. Available at: http://www.tju.edu/ntpr. Accessed December 1, 2012.
5. Organ Procurement and Transplantation Network and Scientific Registry of Transplant Recipients (OPTN and SRTR) Annual Data Report 2010. Available at: http://www.srtr.org/annual_reports/2010/. Accessed December 1, 2012.
6. KDIGO Transplant work group. KDIGO clinical practice guideline for the care of kidney transplant recipients. Chapter 25: sexual function and fertility. Am J Transplant 2009;9(Suppl 3):S106–9.
7. EBPG Expert Group on Renal Transplantation. European best practice guidelines for renal transplantation. Section IV: Long-term management of the transplant recipient. IV.10. Pregnancy in renal transplant recipients. Nephrol Dial Transplant 2002;17(Suppl 4):50–5.
8. Concepcion BP, Schaefer HM. Caring for the pregnant kidney transplant recipient. Clin Transplant 2011;25:821–9.
9. Maynard SE, Thadani R. Pregnancy and the kidney. J Am Soc Nephrol 2009;20: 14–22.
10. Levidiotis V, Chang S, McDonald S. Pregnancy and maternal outcomes among kidney transplant recipients. J Am Soc Nephrol 2009;20:2433–40.
11. McKay DB, Josephson MA. Pregnancy after kidney transplantation. Clin J Am Soc Nephrol 2008;3:S117–25.
12. Josephson MA, McKay DB. Pregnancy in the renal transplant recipient. Obstet Gynecol Clin North Am 2010;37:211–22.

13. Armenti VT. Immunosuppression and teratology: evolving guidelines. J Am Soc Nephrol 2004;15:2759–60.
14. Mukherjee S, Shapiro R. Transplantation and Pregnancy. Available at: http://www.emedicine.medscape.com/article/429932-overview. Accessed December 1, 2012.
15. Fischer T, Neumayer HH, Fischer R, et al. Effect of pregnancy on long-term kidney function in renal transplant recipients treated with cyclosporine and with Azathiprine. Am J Transplant 2005;5:2732–9.
16. Tendron A, Decramer S, Justrabo E, et al. Cyclosporin A administration during pregnancy induces a permanent nephron deficit in young rabbits. J Am Soc Nephrol 2003;14:3188–96.
17. Davidson J, Wilkinson A, Dantal J, et al. New-onset diabetes after transplantation: 2003 International consensus guidelines. Proceedings of an international expert panel meeting. Barcelona, Spain, 19 February 2003. Transplantation 2003;75: SS3.
18. American Diabetes Association. Standards of medical care in diabetes—2012. Diabetes Care 2012;35(Suppl 1):S11–63.
19. Moore TR. Diabetes Mellitus and Pregnancy. Medscape Reference. Available at: http://www.emedicine.medscape.com/article/127547-overview. Accessed January 5, 2013.
20. ACOG Committee on Practice Bulletins. ACOG Practice Bulletin. Clinical Management Guidelines for Obstetricians-Gynecologists. Pregestational Diabetes Mellitus. Obstet Gynecol 2005;105:675.
21. Mathiesen ER, Hod M, Ivanisevic M, et al. Maternal efficacy and safety outcomes in a randomized controlled trial comparing insulin detemir with NPH insulin in 310 pregnant women with type I diabetes mellitus. Diabetes Care 2012;35(10): 2012–7.

Impact of Diabetes on Aneuploidy Screening

Padmalatha Gurram, MD[a],*, Peter Benn, PhD, DSc[b],
Winston A. Campbell, MD[a]

KEYWORDS

- Pregestational diabetes • Aneuploidy • Second trimester screening
- First trimester screening • Maternal serum alpha-fetoprotein (MSAFP)
- Human Chorionic gonadotropin (hCG) • Unconjugated estriol (uE3) • Inhibin-A
- Pregnancy associated plasma protein-A

KEY POINTS

- Currently, aneuploidy screening is offered to all pregnant women regardless of age and relies on use of maternal serum analytes to adjust patients' a priori age-related risk.
- Pregestational diabetes does not increase the risk for fetal Down syndrome; however, it affects the levels of maternal serum analytes used in the screening tests. In the first trimester, pregnancy-associated plasma protein A (PAPP-A) and β human chorionic gonadotropin (β-hCG) are decreased. In the second trimester, MSAFP and unconjugated estriol (uE3) are decreased but β-hCG and inhibin A (inhA) are not affected.
- An adjustment to MSAFP to nondiabetic levels is performed in most screening centers. Further studies are required to assess if 10% upward adjustment is sufficient.
- Adjustment of PAPP-A to nondiabetic levels should be considered in the calculation and interpretation of the first-trimester screening tests, at least for women with type 2 diabetes mellitus. The amount of adjustment required and the effect of these adjustments on performance of the screening tests need further clarification.
- Given the increasing incidence of type 2 diabetes mellitus, it is important to determine the precise effect type 2 diabetes mellitus and oral hypoglycemic agents (OHGs) may have on the screening test results.

INTRODUCTION

Prenatal diagnosis for aneuploidy (primarily Down syndrome) has been evolving since the introduction of amniocentesis and fetal karyotyping in 1966.[1] Prenatal diagnosis by amniocentesis was initially focused on women considered at highest risk for

[a] Maternal-Fetal Medicine, Department of Obstetrics and Gynecology, University of Connecticut Health Center School of Medicine, John Dempsey Hospital, 263 Farmington Avenue, Room CG 214, Farmington, CT 06030, USA; [b] Department of Genetics and Developmental Biology, University of Connecticut Health Center School of Medicine, John Dempsey Hospital, 263 Farmington Avenue, L1049, Farmington, CT 06030-3808, USA
* Corresponding author.
E-mail address: PGurram@resident.uchc.edu

Clin Lab Med 33 (2013) 271–280
http://dx.doi.org/10.1016/j.cll.2013.03.022
0272-2712/13/$ – see front matter © 2013 Elsevier Inc. All rights reserved.

labmed.theclinics.com

Down syndrome (≥35 years old at delivery). The limitations of this maternal age screen was that only a small portion of the pregnant population (≥35 years at delivery) would be eligible for testing and less than 30% of cases of Down syndrome would be detected. Amniocentesis is an invasive diagnostic test with a potential risk of miscarriage (0.3%[1]–1.0%[2]) as a complication of the procedure. In the mid-1980s to 1990s, several maternal serum markers (analytes) measured during the second trimester of pregnancy (15–22 weeks) were reported as helpful in identifying pregnancies at a higher than expected risk for Down syndrome.[3–8]

The combination of the 4 serum analytes (maternal serum alpha fetoprotein [MSAFP]), hCG, uE3, and inhA) is known as the second-trimester quad screen. This screening test has a detection rate for fetal Down syndrome of 67% to 71% for a 5% false-positive rate.[9] At the same time that maternal serum analyte markers were evaluated to detect pregnancies complicated by Down syndrome, ultrasound markers were reported to identify at-risk pregnancies.[10,11] A combination of sonographic features of fetuses with Down syndrome (genetic sonogram) by itself has a reported detection rate for Down syndrome of 72% (range 63%–80%).[12]

In the 1990s there was a shift to developing prenatal screening for aneuploidy in the first trimester of pregnancy (10–14 weeks' gestation). Nicolaides and colleagues[13] and Snijders and colleagues[14] reported that the ultrasound measurement of nuchal translucency (NT) behind the fetal neck allows detection of 80% of Down syndrome affected pregnancies. In a retrospective analysis of 3 datasets assessing ultrasound (NT measurement) and maternal serum analytes (free β-hCG and PAPP-A), Wald and Hackshaw[15] reported that a combination of ultrasound and these serum analytes could allow the detection of Down syndrome to 80%. Several large prospective studies assessing combined first-trimester screening (ultrasound and maternal serum analytes) with or without integrating second-trimester maternal serum analyte screening (quad screen) can increase detection of Down syndrome to 90% or more with a 5% false-positive rate.[16–18]

The evolution of screening for prenatal diagnosis has allowed more flexibility and options for clinical management. Ultrasound screening using the genetic sonogram alone has aneuploidy (Down syndrome) detection rates approaching that of maternal serum analyte screening. The genetic sonogram was only evaluated, however, in women who were identified as at high risk for aneuploidy (maternal age or serum analyte adjusted risk). In contrast, first-semester or second-trimester maternal serum analyte–based screening can be offered to all women and those found at high risk may desire additional evaluation. This additional evaluation could be an invasive procedure (amniocentesis or chorionic villi sampling), recently introduced noninvasive testing based on the analysis of cell-free fetal DNA in maternal plasma, or a genetic sonogram. Invasive testing involving amniocentesis or chorionic villi sampling is reserved for those pregnancies found a high-risk after the application of the sequential screening tests.

As experience is gained with maternal serum analyte screening, there have been observations that certain factors might alter the serum analyte levels and this, in turn, could have an impact on the aneuploidy risk adjustment. Diabetes is one such condition that can alter maternal serum analyte concentrations. This article reviews the effect of diabetes on the second-trimester and first-trimester screening analytes and how the adjustments to the various analyte values might improve the performance of screening tests.

DIABETES IN PREGNANCY: EPIDEMIOLOGY AND CLASSIFICATION

Diabetes mellitus in pregnant women can be classified as pregestational (type 1 or type 2, diagnosed before the pregnancy) or gestational (diagnosed during the pregnancy). In a retrospective study, the prevalence of maternal diabetes at delivery in the United States was 4.2% of all live births.[19] Gestational diabetes accounted for 84.7%, followed by type 1 diabetes mellitus (7%), type 2 diabetes mellitus (4.7%), and unspecified diabetes (3.6%). The study reported an increasing incidence for all types of diabetes, especially type 2 diabetes mellitus in young women.

During pregnancy, there is no clear distinction between type 1 diabetes mellitus and type 2 diabetes mellitus and the management is similar in both groups. Prior to pregnancy, women with type 1 diabetes mellitus typically receive insulin for blood sugar control. Women with type 2 diabetes mellitus can be managed with insulin OHG or with diet. Women with type 2 diabetes mellitus receiving OHGs before pregnancy are usually switched to insulin at the beginning of pregnancy because the data regarding safety and efficacy of OHG medications are limited.[20]

The risk of birth defects is increased 4-fold to 8-fold among women with pregestational diabetes compared with 1% to 2% risk of general population.[21] There is no clear evidence, however, for an increased risk for aneuploidy in women with pregestational diabetes.[22] Narchi and Kulaylat[23] reported that Down syndrome is more common in infants born to mothers with gestational diabetes. A study by Martínez-Frías and colleagues[24] in 2004 showed that after correction for maternal age there seemed to be no relationship between Down syndrome incidence and any type of diabetes. No increase incidence of autosomal trisomy was seen in diabetic women in a study by Moore and colleagues.[25] Moore and colleagues,[25] however, did report an increase in numeric sex chromosome defects, especially Klinefelter syndrome and triple X defects, among the offspring of women with gestational diabetes. They suggested that women with gestational diabetes might have underlying risk factors, such as autoantibodies that induce nondisjunction, leading to chromosomal anomalies.

There is no increased risk of birth defects in women who develop gestational diabetes after the first trimester. Nondisjunction leading to nonmosaic trisomy 21 occurs before or shortly after fertilization and, therefore, gestational diabetes is not a causal factor for aneuploidy.

SCREENING FOR ANEUPLOIDY

In the absence of prenatal screening, diagnosis, and intervention, Down syndrome would occur in approximately 1 in 500 newborns and is the most common nonlethal trisomy. Trisomy 18 would occur in 1 in 4200 newborns and approximately 72% of fetuses die between 12 weeks and term.[26–29] Prenatal screening for aneuploidy has been largely focused on detection of trisomy 21 and trisomy 18. Most cases of trisomy are the result of meiotic nondisjunction and the risk increases with maternal age.

Serum analytes are measured as standardized units of mass and are converted to multiples of median (MoM) to allow serum analyte levels changing with gestational age. Log transformations are applied to the MoM values and these log (MoM) values show approximately gaussian distributions. For any particular woman, likelihood ratios are determined from the relative heights of the affected and unaffected gaussian distributions. An individual specific aneuploidy risk is calculated by multiplying a priori risk aneuploidy based on maternal age and previous aneuploidy history by the likelihood ratios, with adjustment for the correlations that exist between the analytes.

FACTORS AFFECTING THE SCREENING TESTS

A variety of factors are known to affect the performance of the aneuploidy screening tests. These include maternal weight, race/ethnicity, parity, multifetal gestation, smoking, in vitro fertilization pregnancies, and diabetes mellitus.[30,31]

Most screening laboratories adjust for maternal race, weight, and multiple gestations in the interpretation of the results of the test. Serum alpha fetoprotein (AFP), PAPP-A, and β-hCG, are increased and inhA levels are decreased in African American women. As maternal weight increases, concentrations of serum markers decrease, at least in part due to larger blood volume. In twin gestations, serum marker concentrations are approximately doubled compared with singleton pregnancies.

Some of the second-trimester analyte levels are reduced in patients with type 1 diabetes mellitus and most of the centers correct for AFP. Data in the literature vary regarding the first-trimester markers and pregestational diabetes.

SECOND-TRIMESTER SERUM SCREENING

Second-trimester aneuploidy screening is usually performed between 15 and 21 weeks. Maternal serum screening analytes used in the second trimester include AFP, uE3, β-hCG), and inhA measurements (quad screen). The quad screen has detection rates of approximately 67% to 71% using a fixed false-positive rate of 5% for Down syndrome. Women with Down syndrome pregnancies have low MSAFP (median 0.73 MoM), elevated β-hCG (2.02 MoM), low uE3 (0.73 MoM), and elevated inhA (1.85 MoM) levels.[9]

SECOND-TRIMESTER ANEUPLOIDY SCREENING: IMPACT OF TYPE 1 DIABETES MELLITUS ON SERUM ANALYTES
MSAFP and Type 1 Diabetes Mellitus

In 1979, Wald and colleagues[32] reported that maternal serum AFP in diabetic pregnancies is significantly lower than that of nondiabetic controls. This could falsely increase the risk of Down syndrome screen results. Since then, a correction factor has been applied to women with type 1 diabetes mellitus in most laboratories. Based on a series of 366 diabetic women, the median AFP MoM reported in diabetic pregnancies was 0.88 (95% CI, 0.84–0.93).[33]

In the past decade, several studies re-examined the use of a correction factor for MSAFP in diabetic women.[33–37] Traditionally, a 20% upward adjustment is made to MSAFP by many laboratories for women with type 1 diabetes mellitus. Recent studies suggest a 20% adjustment may result in overcorrection and 10% upward adjustment may be more appropriate.[34]

Due to the increase in prevalence of obesity, some investigators suggested that maternal weight correction alone might be sufficient to account for the difference in diabetic women,[35–37] whereas other studies suggested that MSAFP levels were lower despite adjustment for weight in diabetic patients.[34]

There was no distinction between patients with type 1 diabetes mellitus and patients with type 2 diabetes mellitus in earlier studies that observed lower levels of MSAFP. More recent studies that examined women with type 1 diabetes mellitus and type 2 diabetes mellitus separately reported lower levels of MSAFP in both groups and suggested adjustment for both type 1 diabetes mellitus and type 2 diabetes mellitus.[34]

AFP and OHGs

There are few data as to whether patients with type 2 diabetes mellitus treated with OHGs or controlled with diet require the same adjustment. A recent report suggests that OHGs may not require the adjustments to nondiabetic levels.[38] The number of patients in that study, however, were small and the investigators also reported that type 1 diabetes mellitus patients had weight-adjusted MSAFP values similar to nondiabetic controls.

AFP and Glycemic Control

The association between MSAFP levels and glycosylated hemoglobin (hemoglobin A_{1C} [HbA_{1C}]) has been controversial.[38–41] Some studies suggested that a lower MSAFP level is due to poor glycemic control and reported an inverse correlation between MSAFP and HbA_{1C}.[38–41] It has been suggested that adjustments should be made only to women with poor glycemic control.[40] This correlation was not seen in another study, however.[41] A difficulty with applying a glycemic control adjustment is that the degree of glycemic control may not always be known at the time of the aneuploidy screen.

Unconjugated Estriol and Type 1 Diabetes Mellitus

The median MoM value reported for 366 diabetic pregnancies was 0.95 (95% CI, 0.91–0.99) for uE3.[33] The estriol levels, therefore, seem reduced by 5% in diabetic pregnancies and some studies recommend adjustment to estriol in type 1 diabetes mellitus pregnancies,[33] whereas others do not.[42]

β-hCG and Type 1 Diabetes Mellitus

The median MoM values for total β-hCG in 178 diabetic pregnancies was reported as 0.90 but this value was not statistically significantly different from women without diabetes (95% CI, 0. 80–1.01).[33] Similarly, for 188 women with diabetes mellitus, the free β-hCG median MoM was 0.98 (95% CI, 0.88–1.08), also not significantly different from nondiabetic women.

Inhibin A and Type 1 Diabetes Mellitus

The median MoM value for inhA, 0.99 (95% CI, 0.89–1.10), in 150 women was not significantly different from nondiabetic women.[33]

FIRST-TRIMESTER ANEUPLOIDY SERUM SCREENING

First-trimester screening for aneuploidy includes combining maternal serum PAPP-A and β-hCG, either free or total, levels along with ultrasound measurement of fetal NT (fluid-filled space behind the fetal neck) between 11 + 0 to 13 + 6 weeks of gestation. The combined test has detection rates of approximately 80% to 87% using a fixed false-positive rate of 5% for Down syndrome.[9]

The serum levels of PAPP-A are decreased in fetuses with Down syndrome, and a mean PAPP-A of 0.40 MoM to 0.65 MoM was reported in fetuses with Down syndrome. The free β-hCG levels were elevated, with a mean value of 1.66 MoM to 2.30 MoM. NT measurement is greater than 95th percentile in more than 70% of pregnancies affected with Down syndrome. The serum levels of PAPP-A (0.14 MoM) and free β-hCG (0.44 MoM) are decreased and NT measurement increased in trisomy 18 compared with unaffected pregnancies.[22]

FIRST-TRIMESTER ANEUPLOIDY SCREENING: IMPACT OF TYPE 1 DIABETES MELLITUS ON SERUM ANALYTES
PAPP-A and Type 1 Diabetes Mellitus

Early studies by Spencer and colleagues[43] suggested that there were no significant differences between the type 1 diabetes mellitus and non–type 1 diabetes mellitus patients in median maternal weight corrected PAPP-A (type 1 diabetes mellitus 1.02 MoM; 95% CI, 0.83 to 1.05 MoM; non–type 1 diabetes mellitus 1.01 MoM). A recent study by the same investigators, however, involving a much larger number of pregnancies showed that PAPP-A levels are lower in patients with type 1 diabetes mellitus (type 1 diabetes mellitus 0.88 MoM, non–type 1 diabetes mellitus 1.03 MoM; $P<.0001$). This study showed no significant difference in the measured fetal NT or free β-hCG. It concluded that in the calculation of risks for chromosomal defects, it is necessary to make adjustments to PAPP-A in women with PGDM.[44]

In most of the studies that investigated the first-trimester screening, there was no distinction between type 1 diabetes mellitus and type 2 diabetes mellitus. A study by Savvidou and colleagues[45] that investigated type 1 diabetes mellitus and type 2 diabetes mellitus pregnancies separately showed that PAPP-A was reduced by 25% in type 2 diabetes mellitus and there was a 9% (nonsignificant) reduction in type 1 diabetes mellitus at 11 to 13 weeks of gestation. This study concluded that adjustments for PAPP-A should be considered for women with type 2 diabetes mellitus.

A more recent study by Ball and colleagues[46] also showed there was no significant change in PAPP-A in type 1 diabetes mellitus, but in women with type 2 diabetes mellitus, serum PAPP-A was decreased by 23%. Madisen and colleagues[47] studied only type 1 diabetes mellitus and showed a 15% decrease in PAPP-A at 9 to 11 weeks' gestation (0.86 MoM in diabetic pregnancies and 1.01 MoM in nondiabetic pregnancies, $P<.0001$). The authors' recent findings show there is a significant 12% reduction in PAPP-A in pregestational diabetics versus nondiabetic pregnant patients.[48] The observed variation in the literature,[43–51] from 5% to 20% reduction of PAPP-A MoM for women with unspecified types of diabetes, could, therefore, be due to the difference in the types of diabetes included in each of the studies.

PAPP-A and OHGs

It is not unusual for women with type 2 diabetes mellitus receiving OHGs to be switched to insulin during pregnancy. There are few limited data in the literature regarding the first-trimester screening and type-2 diabetics receiving oral hypoglycemic agents.

PAPP-A and Glycemic Control

PAPP-A is zinc-binding matrix metalloproteinase and regulates insulin growth factor–binding protein. In nonpregnant diabetic women, lower levels of PAPP-A were observed and the levels were inversely related to HbA_{1C}, suggesting that expression of PAPP-A is related to glycemic control.[52]

It is possible that pregestational diabetics with normal HbA_{1C} might have normal PAPP-A levels and only poorly controlled diabetics might need correction. If pregestational diabetic women with normal HbA_{1C} are corrected for PAPP-A, Down syndrome rates may be underestimated. Madsen and colleagues[47] reported a weak correlation between serum PAPP-A and HbA_{1C}. Other studies, however, did not show any correlation between PAPP-A and HbA_{1C}.[48,51]

β-hCG and Type 1 Diabetes Mellitus

There is considerable variation in the literature regarding the effect of type 1 diabetes mellitus on β-hCG, with some studies reporting no difference whereas others show up to a 26% reduction in free β-hCG.[43–47,49] In the majority of studies where reductions were reported, they were not statistically significant. Ong and colleagues,[50] however, reported a statistically significant reduction in β-hCG in pregestational diabetic women. The mean free β-hCG reported in a study on pregestational diabetes was 0.93 MoM.[45]

There are few data in the literature regarding the impact of pregestational diabetes on total β-hCG. The authors' recent findings show, however, a statistically significant reduction (18%) in total β-hCG in women with pregestational type 1 diabetes mellitus versus nondiabetic pregnant patients.[48]

Nuchal Translucency and Type 1 Diabetes Mellitus

Published literature is consistent in regards to NT measurement in women pregestational diabetic pregnancies. The studies did not find any significant difference in NT measurement among the women with pregestational diabetes compared with nondiabetic women.[43–45,48]

EFFECT OF ADJUSTMENTS TO MATERNAL SERUM MARKERS ON DETECTION RATES AND FALSE POSITIVE RATES

In women with diabetes, the decreased levels of PAPP-A result in an increase in false-positive screening tests unless the difference is adjusted to nondiabetic levels. Studies by Savvidou and colleagues[45] showed that the false-positive rates of first-trimester screening doubled in women with type 2 diabetes. Ball and colleagues[46] also pointed out that failure to adjust for women with diabetes would result in an increase in the false-positive rates. They noted that the relative increase in the false-positive rates in patients with type 2 diabetes mellitus was inversely related to gestational age (90% at 9 weeks and 21% at 13 weeks). Because the prevalence of diabetes is low, however, the net effect on an overall screening program is small.

DIABETES AND CELL-FREE FETAL DNA

Noninvasive prenatal screening for aneuploidy by measuring fetal cell-free DNA in maternal plasma has been incorporated into the screening programs recently. Studies reported a Down syndrome detection rate of 98.6% with a false-positive rate of 0.2%[53] in high-risk pregnancies. A minimal fetal fraction of 4% is required in the maternal circulation for the detection of trisomy, and very low levels of the cell-free DNA can result in failure of the test.[54]

There are few data on the maternal and fetal factors that affect the fetal fraction of the maternal plasma cell-free DNA. A study by Ashoor and colleagues[54] showed that fetal fraction of cell-free DNA increases with PAPP-A and β-hCG and decreases with maternal obesity. Maternal race, smoking, plasma storage time, fetal crown-rump length, NT thickness, and gender did not have any effect on fetal cell-free DNA. There are no studies to date on the effect of pregestational diabetes on cell fetal cell-free DNA and aneuploidy screening. In nonpregnant patients, however, cell-free DNA measured by PCR was found higher in patients with type 2 diabetes mellitus compared with controls.[55]

REFERENCES

1. NICHD National Registry for Amniocentesis Study Group. Midtrimester amniocentesis for prenatal diagnosis: safety and accuracy. JAMA 1976;236: 1471–6.
2. Tabor A, Madsen M, Obel EB, et al. Randomized controlled trial of genetic amniocentesis in 4606 low-risk women. Lancet 1986;1:1287–93.
3. Merkatz IR, Nitowsky HM, Macri JN, et al. An association between low maternal serum alpha-fetoprotein and fetal chromosomal abnormalities. Am J Obstet Gynecol 1984;148:886–94.
4. Cuckle HS, Wald NJ, Lindenbaum RH. Maternal serum alpha-fetoprotein measurement: a screening test for Down's syndrome. Lancet 1984;323:926–9.

5. Bogart MH, Pandian MR, Jones OW. Abnormal maternal serum chorionic gonadotropin levels in pregnancies with fetal chromosome abnormalities. Prenat Diagn 1987;7(9):623–30.
6. Canick JA, Knight GJ, Palomaki GE, et al. Low second trimester serum unconjugated oestriol in pregnancies with Down's syndrome. Br J Obstet Gynaecol 1988;95(4):330–3.
7. Cuckle H. Established markers in second trimester serum. Early Hum Dev 1996; 47(Suppl):S27–9.
8. Wald NJ, Densem J, George L, et al. Prenatal screening for Down's syndrome using inhibin-A as a serum marker. Prenat Diagn 1996;16:143–53.
9. Cuckle H, Benn P, Wright D. Down syndrome screening in the first and/or second trimester: model predicted performance using meta-analysis parameters. Semin Perinatol 2005;29(4):252–7.
10. Benacerraf BR, Neuberg B, Bromley B, et al. Sonographic scoring index for prenatal detection of chromosomal abnormalities. J Ultrasound Med 1992;9: 449–58.
11. Vintzileos AM, Campbell WA, Rodis JF, et al. The use of second trimester genetic sonogram in guiding clinical management of patients at increased risk for fetal trisomy 21. Obstet Gynecol 1996;87:948–52.
12. Hobbins JC, Lezotte DC, Persutte WH, et al. An 8-center study to evaluate the utility of midterm genetic sonograms among high-risk pregnancies. J Ultrasound Med 2003;22:33–8.
13. Nicolaides KH, Azar G, Byrne D, et al. Fetal nuchal translucency; ultrasound screening for chromosomal defects in first trimester of pregnancy. BMJ 1992; 304:867–9.
14. Snijders RL, Noble P, Sebire N, et al. UK multicenter project on assessment of risk of trisomy 21 by maternal age and fetal nuchal-translucency thickness at 10-14 weeks of gestation. Lancet 1998;352:343–6.
15. Wald NJ, Hackshaw AK. Combining ultrasound and biochemistry in first-trimester screening for Downs syndrome. Prenat Diagn 1997;17:821–9.
16. Wapner R, Thom E, Simpson JL, et al. First-trimester screening for trisomies 21 and 18. First-trimester maternal serum biochemistry and fetal nuchal translucency screening (BUN) study group. N Engl J Med 2003;349:1405–13.
17. Wald NJ, Rodeck C, Hackshaw AK, et al. First and second trimester antenatal screening for Downs syndrome: the results of the Serum, Urine and Ultrasound Screening Study (SURUSS). Health Technol Assess 2003;7:1–77.
18. Malone FD, Canick JA, Ball RH, et al. First-trimester or second-trimester screening or both, for down's syndrome [faster]. N Engl J Med 2005;353: 2001–11.
19. Albrecht SS, Kuklina EV, Bansil P. Diabetes trends among delivery hospitalizations in the U.S., 1994–2004. Diabetes Care 2010;33:768–73.
20. Pregestational Diabetes Mellitus. Committee on Practice Bulletins. Obstet Gynecol 2005;105:675–85.
21. Creasy R, Resnik R, Iams J. Creasy and Resniks Maternal–Fetal Medicine Principles and Practice 6th edition, 2009.
22. Bell R, Glinianaia SV, Tennant PW, et al. Periconception hyperglycaemia and nephropathy are associated with risk of congenital anomaly in women with preexisting diabetes: a population-based cohort study. Diabetologia 2012;55(4): 936–47.
23. Narchi H, Kulaylat N. High incidence of Down's syndrome in infants of diabetic mothers. Arch Dis Child 1997;77(3):242–4.

24. Martínez-Frías ML, Rodríguez-Pinilla E, Bermejo E. Epidemiological evidence that maternal diabetes does not appear to increase the risk for Down syndrome. Am J Med Genet 2002;112(4):335–7.

25. Moore LL, Bradlee ML, Singer MR, et al. Chromosomal Anomalies among the Offspring of women with gestational diabetes. Am J Epidemiol 2002;155(8): 719–24.

26. Morris J, Mutton DE, Alberman E. Revised estimates of the maternal age specific live birth prevalence of Down's syndrome. J Med Screen 2002;9:2–6.

27. Morris J, Alberman E. Trends in Down's syndrome live births and antenatal diagnoses in England and Wales from 1989 to 2008: analysis of data from the National Down Syndrome Cytogenetic Register. BMJ 2009;339:b3794.

28. Morris JK, Savva GM. The risk of fetal loss following a prenatal diagnosis of trisomy 13 or trisomy 18. Am J Med Genet A 2008;146:827–32.

29. Savva G, Walker K, Morris J. The maternal age-specific live birth prevalence of trisomies 13 and 18 compared to trisomy 21 (Down syndrome). Prenat Diagn 2010;30:57–64.

30. Kagan K, Wright DK, Nicolaides K, et al. First-trimester screening for trisomy 21 by free beta-human chorionic gonadotropin and pregnancy-associated plasma protein-A: impact of maternal and pregnancy characteristics. Ultrasound Obstet Gynecol 2008;31:493–502.

31. Lambert-Messerlian G, Palomaki GE, Canick JA. Adjustment of serum markers in first trimester screening. J Med Screen 2009;16(2):102.

32. Wald NJ, Cuckle H, Boreham J, et al. Maternal serum alpha-fetoprotein and diabetes mellitus. Br J Obstet Gynaecol 1979;86(2):101.

33. Huttley W, Rudnicka A, Wald J. Second trimester prenatal serum markers for Down syndrome in women with Insulin. Prenat Diagn 2004;24:804–7.

34. Thornburg LL, Knight KM, Peterson CJ, et al. Maternal serum alpha-fetoprotein values in type 1 and type 2 diabetic patients. Am J Obstet Gynecol 2008;199(2): 135.

35. Sancken U, Bartels I. Biochemical screening for chromosomal disorders and neural tube defects (NTD): is adjustment of maternal alpha-fetoprotein (AFP) still appropriate in insulin-dependent diabetes mellitus (IDDM)? Prenat Diagn 2001; 21:383–6.

36. Sprawka N, Lambert-Messerlian G, Palomaki GE. Adjustment of maternal serum alpha-fetoprotein levels in women with pregestational diabetes. Prenat Diagn 2011;31(3):282–5.

37. Evans MI, Harrison HH, O'Brien JE, et al. Correction for insulin-dependent diabetes in maternal serum alpha-fetoprotein testing has outlived its usefulness. Am J Obstet Gynecol 2002;187(4):1084.

38. Baumgarten A, Robinson J. Prospective study of an inverse relationship between maternal glycosylated hemoglobin and serum alpha-fetoprotein concentrations in pregnant women with diabetes. Am J Obstet Gynecol 1988; 159(1):77.

39. Martin AO, Dempsey LM, Minogue J. Maternal serum alpha-fetoprotein levels in pregnancies complicated by diabetes: implications for screening programs. Am J Obstet Gynecol 1990;163(4 Pt 1):1209.

40. Baumgarten A, Reece EA, Davis N, et al. A reassessment of maternal serum alpha-fetoprotein in diabetic pregnancy. Eur J Obstet Gynecol Reprod Biol 1988;28(4):289.

41. Tharakan T, Baxi L, Kramer D. Alpha-fetoprotein in diabetic pregnancy. J Reprod Med 1993;38(12):952–4.

42. Evans MI, O'Brien JE, Dvorin E, et al. Similarity of insulin-dependent diabetics' and non-insulin-dependent diabetics' levels of beta-hCG and unconjugated estriol with controls: no need to adjust as with alpha-fetoprotein. J Soc Gynecol Investig 1996;3(1):20.

43. Spencer K, Cicero S, Atzei A, et al. The influence of maternal insulin-dependent diabetes on fetal nuchal translucency thickness and first-trimester maternal serum biochemical markers of aneuploidy. Prenat Diagn 2005;25:927–9.

44. Spencer K, Cowans NJ, Spencer CE, et al. A re-evaluation of the influence of maternal insulin-dependent diabetes on fetal nuchal translucency thickness and first-trimester maternal serum biochemical markers of aneuploidy. Prenat Diagn 2010;30:937–40.

45. Savvidou MD, Syngelaki A, Muhaisen M, et al. First trimester maternal serum free b-human chorionic gonadotropin and pregnancy-associated plasma protein A in pregnancies complicated by diabetes mellitus. BJOG 2012;119:410–6.

46. Ball S, Wright D, Sodre D. Temporal effect of Afro-Caribbean Race on Serum Pregnancy-Associated Plasma Protein-A at 9–13 Weeks' Gestation in Screening for Aneuploidies. Fetal Diagn Ther 2012;31:162–9.

47. Madsen H, Ekelund C, Torring N, et al. Impact of type 1 diabetes and glycemic control on fetal aneuploidy biochemical markers. Acta Obstet Gynecol Scand 2011. http://dx.doi.org/10.1111/j.1600-0412.2011.01212.x.

48. Gurram P, Benn P, Campbell W, et al. First Trimester Screening Markers In Women with pregestational diabetes mellitus: is a correction factor needed? Society of Maternal Fetal Medicine 33rd annual pregnancy meeting. February 11–16, 2013, San Francisco, CA. Abstract #596.

49. Kuc S, Wortelboer EJ, Koster MP, et al. Prediction of macrosomia at birth in type-1 and 2 diabetic pregnancies with biomarkers of early placentation. BJOG 2011; 118(6):748–54.

50. Ong CY, Liao AW, Spencer K, et al. First trimester maternal serum free b human chorionic gonadotrophin & pregnancy associated plasma protein A as predictors of pregnancy complications. BJOG 2000;107:1265–70.

51. Pedersen JF, Sorensen S, Molsted-Pedersen L. Serum levels of human placental lactogen, pregnancy-associated plasma protein A and endometrial secretory protein PP14 in first trimester of diabetic pregnancy. Acta Obstet Gynecol Scand 1998;77(2):155–8.

52. Pellitero S, Reverter J, Pizarro E. Pregnancy-Associated Plasma Protein-A levels are related to glycemic control but not to lipid profile or hemostatic parameters in Type 2 Diabetes. Diabetes Care 2007;30:3083–5.

53. Palomaki GE, Kloza EM, Lambert-Messerlian GM. DNA sequencing of maternal plasma to detect Down syndrome: an international clinical validation study. Genet Med 2011;13:913–20.

54. Ashoor G, Poon L, Nicolaides K, et al. Fetal fraction in maternal plasma cell-free DNA at 11–13 weeks' gestation: effect of maternal and fetal factors. Fetal Diagn Ther 2012;31(4):237–43.

55. Tarhouny S, Hadhoud K, Ebrahem M, et al. Assessment of cell-free DNA with microvascular complication of type II diabetes mellitus, using PCR and Elisa. Nucleosides Nucleotides Nucleic Acids 2010;29(3):228–36.

Anemia in Pregnancy

Kari M. Horowitz, MD[a],*, Charles J. Ingardia, MD[b],
Adam F. Borgida, MD[b]

KEYWORDS

- Anemia • Pregnancy • Hemoglobin • Iron • Folate

KEY POINTS

- Physiologic anemia occurs in pregnancy because plasma volume increases more quickly than red cell mass.
- Anemia in pregnancy is defined as hemoglobin and hematocrit lower than 11% and 33% in the first trimester, 10.5% and 32% in the second trimester, and 11% and 33% in the third trimester.
- An increase of 60 mg of elemental iron daily is recommended in the second and third trimesters because an average diet cannot meet the increased iron demand in pregnancy.
- Iron deficiency anemia accounts for 75% of all anemia in pregnancy.
- It is recommended to screen for and treat iron deficiency anemia in pregnancy because treatment to maintain maternal iron stores may be beneficial to neonatal iron stores.

INTRODUCTION

Numerous adaptations occur in women to accommodate pregnancy. One of the most profound changes is a complex interaction among the renal, hematologic, and endocrine systems to prepare for the expected blood loss that occurs at the time of delivery. Fluid retention begins early in pregnancy with a lag in the production of red blood cells (RBCs) causing a "physiologic anemia" of pregnancy in most women. With a focus on singleton gestations this article discusses the physiologic changes in the hematologic system. Also discussed are this physiologic anemia and other common causes of anemia in pregnancy.

HEMODYNAMIC PHYSIOLOGY OF PREGNANCY
Plasma Volume Changes

In response to early renal homeostatic changes, maternal blood volume begins to increase by 6 weeks of gestation. As a result of free body water retention, the maternal

[a] Department of Maternal Fetal Medicine, University of Connecticut Health Center, 263 Farmington Avenue, Farmington, CT 06030, USA; [b] Department of Maternal Fetal Medicine, Hartford Hospital, 85 Jefferson Street, Suite 625, Hartford, CT 06102, USA
* Corresponding author.
E-mail address: khorowitz@resident.uchc.edu

Clin Lab Med 33 (2013) 281–291
http://dx.doi.org/10.1016/j.cll.2013.03.016
0272-2712/13/$ – see front matter © 2013 Elsevier Inc. All rights reserved.

volume can rapidly increase likely because of changes in the renin-angiotensin-aldosterone system causing a change in the osmotic set-point.

Plasma volume continues to rise until the third trimester when it plateaus at 32 to 34 weeks. The average pregnancy has nearly a 50% increase in blood volume, which occurs from an expansion of plasma volume and RBC mass.

Red Cell Mass Changes

Whereas free body water can be retained rapidly by the kidneys, the production of red cells cannot occur as quickly. Because of this lag of increased red cell production, there is a disproportionate increase in intravascular volume causing the "physiologic anemia of pregnancy." The red cell mass increases by approximately 25% (300 mL) by the last month of pregnancy.[1]

PHYSIOLOGIC ANEMIA OF PREGNANCY

Maternal hemoglobin levels decline progressively from 6 weeks gestation to approximately 35 weeks gestation, then increase in the month before delivery (**Fig. 1**). In the absence of iron supplementation, the nadir is approximately 10.5 g/dL at 27 to 30 weeks of gestation.

The Centers for Disease Control and Prevention has published levels of hemoglobin and hematocrit to define anemia as less than the fifth percentile of a healthy reference population. These are 11% and 33% in the first trimester, 10.5% and 32% in the second trimester, and 11% and 33% in the third trimester.[1]

Iron Requirements in Pregnancy

Most women of reproductive age have marginal iron stores. This has been shown in iron assessments of bone marrow in healthy young women. Given the demand for increased red cell mass in pregnancy, iron needs are increased. Because an average diet cannot meet the increased iron demand in pregnancy, the Institute of Medicine recommends an increase of 60 mg of elemental iron daily in the second and third trimesters.[2]

Physiologic retention of fluid early in pregnancy may lead to anemia being a very common diagnosis. It is important to recognize laboratory changes that may indicate true iron deficiency. The red cell mass, hemoglobin, and hematocrit are all relatively lower in pregnancy. The mean corpuscular volume (MCV) and mean corpuscular

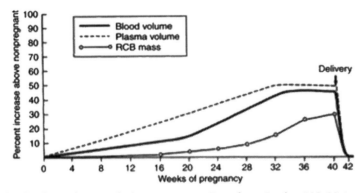

Fig. 1. Blood volume changes during pregnancy. *Data from* Gordon MC. Maternal physiology. In: Gabbe SG, Niebyl JR, Simpson JL, et al, editors. Obstetrics: normal and problem pregnancies. Philadelphia: Churchill Livingstone; 2007.

hemoglobin (MCH) should not change with normal iron. Changes in these indices should heighten the suspicion of the diagnosis of anemia related to iron deficiency.[3]

CLASSIFICATION OF ANEMIAS

There are several methods of classification of anemia: pathogenesis, clinical presentation, and red cell morphology.

Pathogenesis Classification

Pathogenesis classification is divided into two causes relating to bone marrow production: hyporegenerative and regenerative. In hyporegenerative anemia there is failure to increase either erythrocyes or reticulocytes despite increase in erythropoietin. This is caused by alteration of the pluripotent stem cells, which results in a pancytopenia. This alteration displaces normal hematopoesis. This can be the result of myelodysplasia, leukemia, fibrosis, and several infectious or hereditary disorders.

Regenerative anemia occurs in response to loss of erythrocytes (acute or chronic). There is an increased production of erythropoietin that subsequently increases erythrocytes and reticulocytes.

The reticulocyte count is helpful in differentiating causes of anemia with decreased bone marrow response from those where there is an appropriate bone marrow response. This can be particularly helpful when the MCV is normal. Reticulocytes are measured as the absolute number per millimeter or as the proportion of the total number of erythrocytes. Because reticulocytes are released early and have a longer lifespan than mature RBCs, another method to more accurately assess production is the reticulocyte production index (RPI), which corrects for these confounding factors. RPI is calculated by the following formula: reticulocyte count × hemoglobin observed/normal hemoglobin × 0.5. Normal values range from 1% to 2%.

Clinical Presentation Classification

Clinical presentation is classified as acute (eg, acute blood loss, hemolysis) or chronic (eg, infection, chronic disease).

Red Cell Morphology Classification

The World Health Organization classification by red cell morphology (normocytic, microcytic, and macrocytic) is more widely used because of its relationship to more easily understood laboratory analysis of red cell indices. MCV is used to differentiate these anemias. In this classification anemias are divided into microcytic (MCV <82 fL); normocytic (MCV = 82–98 fL); or macrocytic (MCV >98 fL).

MCV is related to MCH, which reports the mean hemoglobin per RBC (normal range, 27–32 pg). Microcytic anemias are also hypochromic, and most macrocytic anemias are hyperchromic.

The mean MCH concentration reports on the average hemoglobin in each RBC as a percentage (normal, 32%–36%), which varies little in most anemias and provides little additional clinical usefulness. Because the MCV represents an average of the total RBC population analyzed, it does not provide information about the homogeneity of the RBC population. Normally RBCs are a standard size (6–8 μg), but in certain disorders the larger portion of cells are not in the normal cell size range. This aspect can be analyzed through the red cell distribution width. As the RBC population exceeds the normal range in RBC size there is an increase of the red cell distribution width (anisocytosis). The normal range for the red cell distribution width is 11% to 15%. Red cell distribution width and MCV together can often be used to differentiate anemias of mixed causes from those with a single cause.

MICROCYTIC ANEMIA

Microcytic anemias arise as a result of hemoglobin synthesis failure or insufficiency. The cause of these anemias falls into three broad categories: (1) heme synthesis deficiency, (2) globin synthesis deficiency, and (3) sideroblastic defects. The anemias associated with these categories include the following:

Heme synthesis deficiency
- Iron deficiency
- Anemia of chronic disease

Globin synthesis deficiency
- α-Thalassemia
- β-Thalassemia
- Sickle cell disease
- Hemoglobin E defect
- Hemoglobin C defect

Sideroblastic defects
- Hereditary sideroblastic anemia
- Acquired sideroblastic anemia

The impact of these disorders in pregnancy is discussed in detail next and elsewhere in this issue.

NORMOCYTIC ANEMIA

Normocytic anemias arise when there is anemia in the setting of normal RBC indices. In normal pregnancy the increase in blood volume may lead to a "dilutional anemia." In the truly anemic patient there is increased blood loss or destruction; failure of bone marrow function (aplastic anemia); nutritional deficiency; renal failure; or hemolysis. Chronic disease may also be associated with a normocytic anemia. Hereditary disorders of RBC membranes (spherocytosis, elliptocytosis) and red cell enzyme deficiencies (glucose-6-phosphate dehydrogenase [G6PD], pyruvate kinase) can also lead to a normocytic anemia.

In regenerative anemia (hemolysis and bleeding) and hyporegenerative anemias (aplasia, chronic disease, nutritional deficiency) the reticulocyte activity, as measured through the corrected RPI, can be diagnostic. In hemolysis other parameters are elevated including lactic dehydrogenase, indirect bilirubin, and haptoglobin levels.

MACROCYTIC ANEMIA

Macrocystic anemias are classified as megaloblastic and nonmegaloblastic. Megaloblastic anemias are related to vitamin B_{12} or folate deficiencies and are characterized by hypersegmented neutrophils. Neutrophils normally develop more segments with aging (usually less than four segments). Hypersegmented neutrophils are those with six or more segments. These anemias also have macro-ovalocytic RBCs. In nonmegablastic anemia these characteristic features are absent.[4,5] The etiologies include the following:

- Megaloblastic
  - Nutritional deficiency
  - Anticonvulsant use

○ Enteral malabsortion
○ Primary bone marrow disorders
○ HIV medications
○ Inherited disorders
• Nonmegaloblastic
○ Medication side effects
○ Hypothyroidism
○ Hepatic disease
○ Splenectomy

SPECIFIC ANEMIAS
Iron Deficiency Anemia

Iron deficiency anemia accounts for 75% of all anemias in pregnancy. Symptoms include easy fatigue, lethargy, and headaches. It is associated with increased risk of low birth weight, preterm delivery, perinatal mortality, lactation failure, and postpartum depression.

Risk factors include diets poor in iron-rich foods (shellfish, beef, turkey, enriched cereals, beans, lentils); diets poor in iron absorption enhancers (orange juice, grapefruit juice, strawberries, broccoli, peppers); diets rich in foods that diminish iron absorption (diary, soy, spinach, coffee, tea); pica; gastrointestinal disease affecting absorption; menorrhagia; and short pregnancy interval. The Centers for Disease Control and Prevention recommends screening for and treating iron deficiency anemia in pregnancy because in addition to maternal benefits, treatment to maintain maternal iron stores may be beneficial to neonatal iron stores.[6]

Laboratory evaluation reveals a microcytic, hypochromic anemia with low plasma iron, high total iron-binding capacity, and low ferritin. The typical diet includes 15 mg elemental iron per day. During pregnancy, the recommended daily iron consumption is 60 mg of elemental iron. The most common treatment is 325-mg tablets iron sulfate taken one to three times a day, which each contain 65 mg elemental iron. Sustained-release and enteric-coated preparations dissolve poorly and are less effective. Reticulocytosis is typically seen in 7 to 10 days. Hemoglobin can rise by as much as 1 g per week in severely anemic women. Absorption can be improved by adding 500 mg of ascorbic acid. Side effects of oral iron include nausea, vomiting, diarrhea, and constipation. These symptoms are related to the dose of iron. Iron therapy should be continued to replete iron stores for 6 months after symptoms resolve.[7,8]

Parenteral iron is available for patients with malaborption syndrome and severely anemic patients who refuse oral iron supplementation. Iron dextran, ferric gluconate, and iron sucrose are the formulations available in the United States. Iron dextran can be given intramuscularly or intravenously. Anaphylactic reactions have been reported in 1% of patients receiving iron dextran. Ferric gluconate and iron sucrose are given intravenously. The pharmacist can calculate the dose of parenteral iron required based on hemoglobin deficit and lean body weight. Intravenous iron therapy has been shown to replete iron stores and raises hemoglobin levels faster than oral iron, but no long-term benefits have been observed.[9,10] Erythropoietin with or without iron supplementation can safely be used to treat severe iron deficiency anemia in pregnancy. When compared with iron supplementation alone, the addition of erythropoietin to iron supplement has been shown to increase reticulocyte count and hematocrit faster, and decrease the time required to reach target hemoglobin levels.[11,12]

Megaloblastic Anemia

Megaloblastic anemia is the second most common nutritional anemia seen in pregnancy. It is most commonly caused by folate deficiency, but it may also be caused by vitamin B_{12} deficiency. These deficiencies are caused by poor nutrition or decreased absorption. Folate and vitamin B_{12} deficiencies are becoming increasingly common in pregnancy because of an increased number of pregnancies after bariatric surgery.

Folate deficiency presents with symptoms of anemia, rough skin, and glossitis. The complete blood count can show macrocytic, normocytic, or normochromic anemia with hypersegmentation of polymorphonuclear leukocytes. The reticulocyte count may be normal or low. White blood cell and platelet counts may also be decreased. Folate levels are low and vitamin B_{12} levels are normal. The recommended treatment is 1 mg oral folate daily. Parenteral folic acid at the same dose may be used in cases of malabsorption. A reticulocyte response is seen in 2 to 3 days.

Vitamin B_{12} deficiency may present with neurologic defects from damage to the posterior columns of spinal cord in addition to symptoms of anemia. The most common causes of vitamin B_{12} deficiency are autoimmune inhibition of intrinsic factor production (pernicious anemia); inadequate production of intrinsic factor after gastrectomy; and malaborption syndrome. Laboratory features are similar to folate deficiency, except folate levels are normal and vitamin B_{12} levels are low. Treatment is 1 mg intramuscular vitamin B_{12} every day for 1 week, followed by once a week for 4 weeks, and then once a month thereafter. Reticulocyte response is seen after 3 to 5 days of therapy.[7]

Sideroblastic Anemia

Sideroblastic anemia is a diverse group of disorders with a common defect in heme biosynthesis and defective iron use. The disorder may be hereditary or acquired. Acquired sideroblastic anemia is associated with malignancies; inflammatory disorders; and drugs and toxins including ethyl alcohol, lead, and isonicotinic acid. It may also be idiopathic with no identifiable cause.

The hallmark of sideroblastic anemia is the ringed sideroblast. Sideroblasts are marrow erythroid precursors. The rings are perinuclear iron representing deposits of iron phosphate that have not been used in heme synthesis. Sideroblastic anemia is diagnosed by ringed sideroblasts found on bone marrow biopsy.

Recommended treatment begins with correcting the underlying disorder or removing the causative agent. Patients are managed with periodic transfusions of washed erythrocytes to maintain hemoglobin in the 9 to 10 range. Treatment includes 100 to 200 mg of vitamin B_6 per day and oral folate supplementation of 1 to 2 mg per day. Sideroblastic anemia is also associated with myelodysplastic syndromes, so patients should be monitored for the development of acute leukemia.[13]

Hereditary Spherocytosis and Elliptocytosis

Hereditary spherocytosis is the most common form of inherited hemolytic anemia. It is still rare with a prevalence of about 1 in 5000. Hereditary spherocytosis is a spectrum of related hematologic disorders characterized by spherocytes, anemia, hemolysis, and jaundice. Molecular defects in the RBC cytoskeleton caused by deficiencies in membrane proteins lead to increased red cell fragility. Inheritance is autosomal-dominant with variable penetrance. Hemolytic crisis can be precipitated by various conditions including infection, trauma, and pregnancy. Diagnosis is suspected based on family history and findings of hyperproliferative anemia and confirmed by osmotic fragility test.

Pregnant women who have not previously had a splenectomy should be monitored for hemolytic crisis and treated with folate supplementation. Hemolytic crisis is treated with transfusion or splenectomy. Splenectomy may be performed during pregnancy to control hemolysis and treat severe anemia. Hereditary spherocytosis does not contribute to perinatal morbidity or mortality in absence of severe anemia. Perinatal outcomes are generally good with no increase in complications as compared with the general population.[7,14]

Hereditary elliptocytosis (autosomal-dominant inheritance) is a milder hemolytic anemia caused by structural defects in the RBC wall. The signs and symptoms are similar but less severe than hereditary spherocytosis. Cases of hereditary elliptocytosis in pregnancy are treated with supportive therapy, including treatment of any underlying condition, folate supplementation, and transfusions if needed.[7]

Autoimmune Hemolytic Anemia

Autoimmune hemolytic anemia is caused by warm-reactive and cold-reactive antibodies. Warm-reactive antibodies are IgG directed against Rh system. They are seen in association with hematologic malignancies; lupus; viral infections; and drug ingestion (penicillin and methyldopa). Cold-reactive antibodies are IgM; are anti-i or anti-Ip; and are seen in association with mycoplasma infections, mononucleosis, and lymphoreticular neoplasms. In many cases, no precipitating event is found. Cases of pregnancy-induced hemolytic anemia with spontaneous remission after pregnancy have been reported. Mild transient hemolysis lasting 1 to 2 months can be seen in infants born to mothers with hemolytic anemia.[15]

Laboratory evaluation shows a hyperproliferative macrocytic anemia. Peripheral blood smear is significant for microcytes, polychromatophilia, poikilocytosis, and normoblasts. Diagnosis is confirmed by positive direct Coombs test.

Treatment is directed toward stopping hemolytic process and correcting the underlying disease. Blood transfusions, corticosteroids, immunosuppression, and splenectomy are the most common treatments. Eighty percent of patients with warm-reactive antibodies respond to corticosteroids. Splenectomy is effective in 60% of patients. Patients who are unresponsive to steroids and splenectomy can undergo a trial immunosuppression. Treatment of cold-reactive antibodies depends on the severity of the disease. Patients with mild anemia may simply need to avoid cold temperatures. Corticosteroids and splenectomy are not effective treatments for cold-reactive antibodies. In severe anemia, a trial of immunosuppression or plasmapheresis may be needed.[7,16]

G6PD Deficiency

G6PD deficiency is the most common hereditary RBC enzyme deficiency. G6PD reduces nicotinamide adenine dinucleotide phosphate while oxidizing glucose-6-phosphate, aiding in the detoxification of free radicals and peroxides. G6PD provides the only means of generating the reduced form of nicotinamide adenine dinucleotide phosphate, and its deficiency makes RBCs vulnerable to oxidative damage. All tissues express the G6PD gene, but the effects of its deficiency are most severe in RBCs.

The G6PD gene is located on the X chromosome. Males carrying the defective gene suffer hemolysis, especially if exposed to drugs that stress the pentose phosphate pathway. Individuals are generally hematologically normal unless they are exposed to precipitating drugs, or have metabolic disturbances to precipitate acute episode of hemolysis. Drugs that can induce hemolysis include the following:

- Acetanilide
- Doxorubicin

- Methylene blue
- Nalidixic acid
- Nitrofurantoin
- Phenazopyridine
- Primaquine
- Sulfamethoxazole

Female heterozygotes are generally unaffected, but may have G6PD activity levels that fall in range of affected males. G6PD deficiency most commonly affects Africans, Mediterranean populations, Sephardic Jews, Asiatic Jews, and some Asian populations. Most African Americans carry a variant that causes mild hemolytic anemia. The Mediterranean variant causes a more severe anemia and may be precipitated by fava beans.[17]

It is unusual for G6PD deficiency to affect pregnancy. Woman should be careful to avoid known precipitants of hemolysis including sulfa drugs and some antimalarials. If a hemolytic episode occurs during pregnancy, the precipitating medication should be discontinued, any infections should be treated, and patients should be supported with transfusion if necessary. Affected male infants of female carriers have increased incidence of hyperbilirubinemia.[18] The incidence of severe jaundice is 11% in newborns with G6PD deficiency, but may be up to 50% if the infant has an affected sibling.[7]

Aplastic Anemia

Aplastic anemia is characterized by pancytopenia in the presence of hypoplastic bone marrow. If untreated, aplastic anemia leads to death by infection or bleeding. There are three possible causes for this disease: (1) there may be insufficient stems cells resulting in an intrinsic defect or a reduction in the number of stems after exposure to a noxious agent, (2) a suppressor substance that inhibits stem cell maturation may be present, and (3) an autoimmune reaction can cause the death of stem cells.

Agents and medications that can lead to marrow aplasia include

- Benzene
- Ionizing radiation
- Nitrogen mustard
- Antimetabolites
- Antimitotic agents
- Toxic chemicals
- Chloramphenicol
- Anticonvulsants (carbamazepine, phenytoin)
- Analgesics
- Gold salts
- Paroxysmal nocturnal hemoglobinuria (discussed later)

Many other agents have also been implicated in cases of aplastic anemia, and in 50% of cases no causative agent can be found.[7,19] There have also been reported cases of pregnancy-associated aplastic anemia. Cases are classified as pregnancy induced if they are identified after the onset of pregnancy, no other cause can be identified, there is a decrease in all blood cell counts, and there is hypoplastic bone marrow.[20,21]

Patients with aplastic anemia present with symptoms related to severe anemia, bleeding, and infection. Laboratory evaluation reveals pancytopenia with hypoproliferative reticulocyte count. Bone marrow biopsy shows hypoplastic bone marrow with normoblastic erythropoiesis. The mortality rate is 50% in cases of severe aplastic anemia. Bone marrow transplant is the treatment of choice with a 50% to 70% long-term survival rate.[7,20]

Supportive therapy (see later) is the recommended treatment of aplastic anemia during pregnancy, because bone marrow transplant in pregnancy is contraindicated. With supportive treatments, maternal mortality rate is less than 15% and more than 90% survive in remission. The maternal risks in pregnancy are caused by infections and hemorrhage. The goal of supportive treatment is to maintain hemoglobin levels through periodic transfusions, prevent and treat infection, and stimulate hematopoiesis. This is done by using intravenous immunoglobulin, colony-stimulating factors, and steroids.[21,22] There are reports of women treated for aplastic anemia with immunosuppression before pregnancy. Half of all pregnancies were uncomplicated; however, 33% become transfusion dependent during pregnancy, 19% experienced a relapse, and deaths occurred because of severe disease and thrombosis.[22] Successful pregnancies have also been reported after bone marrow transplant after high-dose cyclophosphamide and total body irradiation regimens. Total body irradiation is associated with an increased risk of spontaneous abortion. There is also an increased incidence of preterm labor and low-birth-weight infants, but there does not seem to be an increased incidence of congenital anomalies.[23]

PAROXYSMAL NOCTURNAL HEMOGLOBINURIA

Paroxysmal nocturnal hemoglobinuria (PNH) is a rare, nonhereditary hematopoietic disorder characterized by nighttime hemolysis with dark morning urine. PNH is caused by a somatic mutation of the phosphatidylinositol glycan class A gene on the X chromosome. Phosphatidylinoitsol glycan class A encodes for the glycosyltransferase enzyme. This enzyme catalyzes the first step in production of phosphatidylinositol-anchored complement regulatory proteins, which protect against complement activation. Deficiencies of these proteins cause the RBCs to become susceptible to compliment lysis, resulting in intravascular hemolysis.

PNH begins insidiously. There is variability in the severity and presentation of the disease, and there is no familial tendency. The disease usually manifests in adulthood beginning with skin pallor, periodic dark urine, and severe fatigue. Diagnosis is based on flow cytometry confirming the deficiency of glycophophatidylinositol-anchored membrane proteins on erythrocytes, leukocytes, and platelets. Exacerbations of PNH are precipitated by infection, menstruation, transfusion, surgery, and iron ingestion. Complications of PNH include the following:

- Intravascular hemolysis
- Neutropenia
- Thrombocytopenia
- Infections
- Aplastic anemia
- Venous thrombosis
- Embolism

Thrombosis accounts for 50% of deaths outside of pregnancy, often involving intra-abdominal vessels including hepatic and mesenteric veins. If untreated, median survival is 12 years with transformation into acute leukemia; progression to marrow aplasia; or most commonly death from blood loss, infection, or thrombosis.

In pregnancies complicated by PNH, there is up to a 20% maternal mortality rate. Half of all infants are delivered premature because of complications. The most serious complication is thromboembolism, which occurs in 12% of patients. Of patients who developed thromboembolism, 75% developed Budd-Chiari syndrome or hepatic vein thrombosis, which carries a 50% mortality rate. The most common complication of PNH in pregnancy is anemia or hemolysis, occurring in 75% of patients.[24] Thrombocytopenia can also occur, and there is an increased risk of infection caused by leukopenia. Thromboprophylaxis is recommended, although still high risk of a thromboembolic event despite treatment.[25]

The definitive treatment for PNH is bone marrow transplant. Therapies for PNH in pregnancy include iron therapy, transfusions, and corticosteroids. Iron can be given orally to replace lost iron; however, it may lead to erythropoiesis and precipitate complement lysis. If hemolysis occurs after iron supplementation, erythropoiesis should be suppressed by treatment with transfusions or corticosteroids. Use of corticosteroids is also controversial because in some patients steroids can quickly stop hemolysis by inhibiting components of the complement pathway, but steroids may also suppress inflammation, which may stimulate complement. The treatment of acute episodes is aimed at decreasing hemolysis. Women with PNH who become pregnant should be monitored closely with attention to anemia and early detection of infection, and should be treated with thromboprophylaxis.[24] Women with a history of a thrombotic event should be treated with therapeutic anticoagulation.[25] Detailed guidelines for anticoagulant use in pregnancy are discussed elsewhere in this issue.

REFERENCES

1. Pritchard JA. Changes in the blood volume during pregnancy and delivery. Anesthesiology 1965;26:393.
2. Centers for Disease Control (CDC). CDC criteria for anemia in children and childbearing-aged women. MMWR Morb Mortal Wkly Rep 1989;38:400.
3. Institute of Medicine. Iron deficiency anemia: recommended guidelines for the prevention; detection, and management among US children and women of childbearing age. Washington, DC: Institute of Medicine; 1993.
4. Tefferi A. Anemia in adults: a contemporary approach to diagnosis. Mayo Clin Proc 2003;78:1274–80.
5. Tefferi A, Hanson CA, Inwards DJ. How to interpret and pursue an abnormal complete blood count in adults. Mayo Clin Proc 2005;80:923–36.
6. Centers for Disease Control and Prevention. Recommendations to prevent and control iron deficiency in the United States. MMWR Recomm Rep 1998; 47(RR-3):1–29.
7. Creasy RK, Resnik R, Iams JD, et al. Anemia in pregnancy. In: Creasy, Resnik, Iams, editors. Creasy & Resnik's maternal-fetal medicine principles and practice. 6th edition. Philadelphia: Saunders Elsevier; 2009. p. 855–84.
8. American College of Obstetricians and Gynecologists. Anemia in pregnancy. ACOG practice bulletin No. 95. Obstet Gynecol 2008;112:201–7.
9. Bhandal N, Russell R. Intravenous versus oral iron therapy for postpartum anaemia. BJOG 2006;113:1248–52.
10. Freossler B, Cocchiaro C, Saadat-Gilani K, et al. Intravenous iron sucrose versus oral iron ferrous sulfate for antenatal and postpartum iron deficiency anemia: a randomized trial. J Matern Fetal Neonatal Med 2012. [Epub ahead of print].
11. Breymann C, Visca E, Huch R. Efficacy and safety of intravenously administered iron sucrose with and without adjuvant recombinant human erythropoietin for the treatment of iron-deficiency anemia during pregnancy. Am J Obstet Gynecol 2001;184:662–7.

12. Krafft A, Breymann C. Iron sucrose with and without recombinant erythropoietin for the treatment of severe postpartum anemia: a prospective, randomized, open-label study. J Obstet Gynaecol Res 2011;37:119–24.

13. Barton JR, Shaver DC, Sibai BM. Successive pregnancies complicated by idiopathic sideroblastic anemia. Am J Obstet Gynecol 1992;166:576–7.

14. Maberry MC, Mason RA, Cunningham FG, et al. Pregnancy complicated by hereditary spherocytosis. Obstet Gynecol 1992;79:735.

15. Kumar R, Advani AR, Sharah J, et al. Pregnancy induced hemolytic anemia: an unexplained entity. Ann Hematol 2001;80:623–6.

16. Sacks DA, Platt L, Johnson CS. Autoimmune hemolytic anemia during pregnancy. Am J Obstet Gynecol 1981;140:942–6.

17. Beutler E. Glucosse-6-phosphate dehydrogenase deficiency. N Engl J Med 1991;324:169–74.

18. Weng YH, Chou YH, Lien RI. Hyperbilirubinemia in healthy neonates with glucose-6-phosphate dehydrogenase deficiency. Early Hum Dev 2003;71:129–36.

19. Snyder TE, Lee LP, Lynch S. Pregnancy-associated hypoplastic anemia: a review. Obstet Gynecol Surv 1991;46:264.

20. Deka D, Malhotra N, Sinha A, et al. Pregnancy associated aplastic anemia: maternal and fetal outcome. J Obstet Gynaecol Res 2003;29:67–72.

21. Kwon JY, Lee Y, Shin JC, et al. Supportive management of pregnancy-associated aplastic anemia. Int J Gynaecol Obstet 2006;95:115–20.

22. Tichello A, Socie G, Marsh J, et al. Outcome of pregnancy and disease course among women with aplastic anemia treated with immunosuppression. Ann Intern Med 2002;137:164–72.

23. Sanders JE, Hawley J, Levy W, et al. Pregnancies following high-dose cyclophosphamide with or without high-dose busulfan or total-body irradiation and bone marrow transplantation. Blood 1996;87:3045–52.

24. Fieni S, Bonfanti L, Gramellini D, et al. Clinical management of paroxysomal nocturnal hemoglobinuria in pregnancy: a case report and updated review. Obstet Gynecol Surv 2006;61:593–601.

25. Ray JG, Burows RF, Ginsberg JS, et al. Paroxysomal nocturnal hemoglobinuria and the risk of venous thrombosis: review and recommendations for management of the pregnant and nonpregnant patient. Haemostasis 2000;30:103–17.

Current Management of Sickle Cell Disease in Pregnancy

Biree Andemariam, MD[a],*, Sabrina L. Browning, MD[b]

KEYWORDS

- Sickle cell disease • Sickle cell anemia • Hemoglobinopathy • Anemia • Pregnancy
- Management

KEY POINTS

- Women with sickle cell disease (SCD) are living longer and with an improved quality of life. As a result, they are typically reaching the reproductive years and may decide to have children.
- Pregnancy in women with SCD is complicated and there is an increased risk of fetal and maternal complications compared to women without SCD.
- Management of SCD during pregnancy should be provided by a multidisciplinary team of health care personnel with expertise in the unique challenges that arise in patients with SCD during pregnancy. At a minimum, this team should include a hematologist with specific training in managing patients with hemoglobinopathies and a maternal-fetal medicine specialist.
- Opiate analgesics are safe to use in pregnant patients with SCD.
- Patients on prophylactic blood transfusion before pregnancy can continue this regimen. However, initiating prophylactic transfusion just for the pregnancy has not been validated.

INTRODUCTION

Owing to medical advancements and the introduction of innovative therapies, individuals with inherited disorders of the hemoglobin molecule such as sickle cell disease (SCD) are now living longer[1] and with an enhanced quality of life. As a result of this increased life expectancy,[2] it is imperative to increase practitioner knowledge regarding the complicated interplay of pregnancy and hemoglobinopathy in women with SCD, who are now more regularly reaching child-bearing age. Pregnancy in SCD is complex, because individuals with this disease generally experience a higher

The authors have nothing to disclose.
[a] Division of Hematology-Oncology, Lea Center for Hematologic Disorders, Adult Sickle Cell Clinical and Research Center, University of Connecticut Health Center, 263 Farmington Avenue, MC 1628, Farmington, CT 06030, USA; [b] Yale University School of Medicine, 333 Cedar Street, New Haven, CT 06510, USA
* Corresponding author.
E-mail address: andemariam@uchc.edu

rate of both maternal and fetal complications and often a worsening of their sickle cell–related complications as well.[3,4] In an effort to minimize these issues, optimal medical management during this potentially problematic period should involve hematologists and maternal-fetal medicine specialists.[5,6] It is critical that the management of patients with SCD during pregnancy be attentive and thorough, starting from the period of preconception and throughout postpartum care.

SCD: EPIDEMIOLOGY, PATHOPHYSIOLOGY, AND THE CLINICAL PICTURE
What is SCD and Who Does It Affect?

SCD is a term that comprises a group of genetic disorders, inherited in an autosomal recessive manner, that result in the production of the abnormal red blood cell (RBC) hemoglobin molecule referred to as hemoglobin S (hb S). This classification includes homozygous sickle cell anemia, hemoglobin SS (hb SS), the most common and usually most clinically severe of the sickle hemoglobinopathies, and the variant heterozygous disorders such as the pairing of hb S with hemoglobin C or a single allele for β-thalassemia.[7] The combination of sickle cell anemia and α-thalassemia is also incorporated into the SCD grouping. SCD is the most frequently inherited blood disorder, impinging on the lives of millions on a global level, most notably individuals of African, Mediterranean, and Hispanic descent. This alteration in the normal genetic framework likely has its evolutionary origins stemming from the relative resistance to malaria conferred on individuals who are carriers of a single sickle cell gene. Although the prevalence of SCD in the United States is not firmly established, recent estimates indicate there may be up to 100,000 people living in the United States[8,9] with this disease.

Pathophysiology of SCD

SCD is a consequence of a single base pair change in the β-globin gene that alters the protein framework and normal structure of adult RBC hemoglobin. A point mutation replaces the hydrophilic glutamic acid with a hydrophobic valine in the sixth position of the amino acid chain for β-globin. This mutation yields an irregular structure that interacts with other hemoglobin S molecules to form polymers in states of decreased oxygen tension.[10] These stiff, rodlike polymers cause recurrent damage to the RBC membrane and are responsible for the characteristic "sickled" shape of the erythrocytes in this disease. Repeated injury to the RBC is the causative factor in the chronic hemolytic destruction of these blood cells with consequent decrease in the normal RBC life span[11] and resultant severe anemia, both distinctive pathologic features in SCD.[10] The inflexible, irregularly shaped sickled cells lack the capacity shown by normal RBCs to travel smoothly through small blood vessels, resulting in frequent blockage of blood flow and decreased perfusion to vital body tissues distal to the occlusion.[11] Intermittent, unpredictable episodes of severe bodily pain called vasoocclusive crises are the hallmark of the disease. Many sickle-related sequelae occur at least partially as a consequence of obstruction of the microvasculature and the ensuing decreased delivery of oxygen and nutrients. Other more recently elucidated factors contributing to the vasculopathy of SCD[12,13] include the following:

- A proinflammatory environment in patients with SCD with enhancement in number and function of white blood cells and both increased plasma levels and gene expression of proinflammatory mediators such as tumor necrosis factor-α and interleukin-8.[12]
- Increased adhesion of the fragile, sickle-shaped RBCs to endothelial cells, circulating leukocytes, and blood platelets.[13]

Clinical Features and Potential Complications Associated with SCD

The irregular hb S molecule in SCD is responsible for multiorgan disease sequelae that are varied and widespread throughout the body. Patients can have an extensive, chronic, and often debilitating nature of this genetic illness that is challenging for patients and their families. The presence and severity of these complications can differ significantly among patients, even those with the same homozygous hb SS genotype.[14] A twin study[15] of 9 monozygotic pairs (6 homozygous hb SS, 3 hemoglobin SC) found that both the frequency and the severity of complications differed significantly between these patients with SCD despite their equivalent genetic makeup. This genotype-phenotype mismatch is responsible for the mixed and unpredictable clinical picture observed by health professionals caring for patients with SCD.

The potential comorbidities associated with SCD arise from the complicated pathophysiology[7,11] due to:

- A chronic hemolytic anemia secondary to the increased fragility and decreased deformability of RBCs.
- Repeated vasoocclusive crises with tissue hypoxia.
- Chronic end-organ damage.

Therefore, the clinical pathology of SCD can be divided into these 3 main categories. Each leads to significant comorbid sequelae that render SCD a potentially widespread systemic disease (**Box 1**).

SCD AND PREGNANCY
A Historical Perspective

The first report in the literature of pregnancy in women with SCD was published in 1924 by Sydenstricker[17] who briefly described 2 cases of pregnant women with sickle cell anemia. Almost 2 decades after this report, Kobak and colleagues[18] described the negative effects associated with SCD and pregnancy. They identified an increased tendency for pregnancies in patients with SCD to result in spontaneous abortion or stillbirth and a propensity toward pregnancy-related complications such as premature labor. In addition, maternal mortality was increased (33%). Investigators of several case reports and small case series published shortly thereafter confirmed these increased complications in mothers with SCD and their fetuses. However, data remained scarce because of the rarity of pregnancy in patients with SCD. With the report by Turner[19] in 1951, only 24 pregnant women with SCD had been documented in the literature.

Maternal and Fetal Risks in SCD

Despite continued efforts to better comprehend and quantify the risks and complications faced by women with SCD during pregnancy, multiple obstacles remain and likely contribute to the varied published results. However, as the survival of patients with this inherited hemoglobinopathy continues to increase, it is crucial to examine the occurrence of maternal and fetal morbidity and mortality experienced by individuals with SCD during pregnancy. In general, agreement exists that the clinical course of pregnancy in SCD is erratic and is associated with greater risks for fetus and mother compared with pregnant women with normal hemoglobin genotypes.[4] **Table 1** shows findings obtained in key published studies to date on outcomes in SCD during pregnancy.

Although these valuable investigations examined large numbers of pregnant patients with SCD and were conducted across numerous clinical locations, the resulting

---

Box 1
Potential complications associated with SCD

Anemia

- Acute anemia (parvovirus B19 infection, splenic sequestration, hyperhemolysis)
- Chronic intravascular hemolytic anemia with related complications
  - Pulmonary hypertension (from nitric oxide depletion)[16]
  - Gallbladder disease (pigment gallstones)
  - Transfusion-related complications
    - Iron overload (cardiomyopathy, endocrinopathy, hepatopathy)
      - Iron chelation therapy toxicity (ototoxicity, nephrotoxicity)
    - Transfusion-transmitted viral infections (HIV, hepatitis B, hepatitis C)
    - RBC alloimmunization
    - Poor venous access from repeated venipuncture
  - Extramedullary hematopoiesis

Vasoocclusion

- Painful crises
- Stroke
- Sickle cell retinopathy
- Acute chest syndrome
- Avascular necrosis
- Chronic leg ulcerations

Chronic organ damage

- Lung disease (ie, asthma)
- Functional asplenia, with resulting infectious risk caused by encapsulated bacteria
- Renal disease (renal papillary necrosis, glomerular disease)

Abbreviation: HIV, human immunodeficiency virus.

---

data continue to vary significantly. Some of these studies were retrospective and many differed in their definitions for specific obstetric and fetal complications, thus further complicating the interpretation of the data on the risk of SCD in pregnancy. For example, in several small studies performed in the United States there were no documented maternal deaths in the women with SCD.[20,22] However, data collected recently from a large inpatient US database[3] showed more than a 5-fold increase in maternal mortality compared with pregnant women without SCD (see **Table 1**). In addition, a study in Jamaica published in 2011 by Asnani and colleagues[25] revealed that during a 9-year period (1998–2007) mortality in pregnant women with SCD represented 9.3% of the total number of deaths reported to the Jamaican maternal mortality surveillance system (Ministry of Health, Jamaica). The maternal mortality for women with SCD in this study[25] was 718.8 deaths per 100,000 subjects, which yielded an odds ratio of approximately 11 when compared with the deaths that occurred in mothers without SCD. The higher death rates reported in studies of SCD populations in less developed areas of the world may be related to less advanced or accessible obstetric and disease-specific care. Therefore, despite the acknowledged decline in the rate of death during pregnancy for women with SCD in the past 40 years, it is imperative that the hazards of pregnancy on individuals with this inherited hemoglobinopathy continue to be evaluated. The need for comprehensive education and specialized management for pregnant women with SCD is universal and is emphasized by the potentially dangerous effects of pregnancy in patients with SCD.[26]

To fully comprehend the adverse impact of pregnancy on women with SCD, the unique response of these already anemic individuals to the physiologic changes of pregnancy must be kept in mind.[4] Although alterations in normal physiology are advantageous to healthy pregnant women, they can be harmful to mothers with SCD in whom exacerbations of their inherited blood disorder and associated comorbidities often arise during pregnancy. These physiologic variations in several organ systems that develop during pregnancy are likely involved in the complications and additional organ dysfunction associated with pregnancy in SCD, and they are as follows:

- Physiologic anemia. The placenta and developing fetus require an increased amount of oxygen. In response to this increased demand, there is typically an increase in blood volume to enhance oxygen delivery to the fetus. However, in women with SCD, this increased volume of blood plasma occurs in the setting of reduced RBC survival related to their hemolytic anemia. This change can consequently worsen anemia in patients with SCD who may already have significantly decreased hemoglobin levels.[26]
- Increased oxygen consumption. More oxygen is consumed by the placenta and growing fetus, so pregnant women with SCD are more frequently exposed to low oxygen states, which may lead to exacerbation of their SCD.
- Increased glomerular filtration rate.[27] Increased activation of the renin-angiotensin-aldosterone system.
- Increased minute ventilation.[27] Minute ventilation increases from 7.5 L/min to approximately 10.5 L/min.
- Increased heart rate, stroke volume, and cardiac output.[27]

Another important potential maternal complication is the development of venous thromboembolic events during the gravid period. James and colleagues[28] showed that women with SCD are 6.7 times more likely to develop a venous thromboembolism during pregnancy than their healthy matches with normal hemoglobin structure (odds ratio 6.7, 95% confidence interval 4.4–10.1).[28] However, the use of prophylactic anticoagulation has not been rigorously studied in pregnant women with SCD and therefore is not the standard of care.

To date, published evidence has shown a wide range of clinical outcomes for a pregnant mother with SCD and her fetus. The outcomes are variable, ranging from a normal pregnancy to one complicated by many different adverse outcomes.[3,21,22] Improvements in the well-being of the expectant mother with SCD and her baby during pregnancy have been observed and likely are attributed to improved prenatal and intrapartum care. There is significant value to continued investigation into both the pregnancy-related and SCD-related complications experienced by these patients during pregnancy.

MANAGEMENT OF SCD IN PREGNANCY

The need for dedicated and intensive care for these patients during pregnancy is well established.[23] This care should preferably be implemented before conception and should be continued throughout gestation and the postpartum period. Moreover,

Table 1
Maternal and fetal morbidity and mortality in women with SCD during pregnancy

Study Information	Number of SCD Subjects/Deliveries	Maternal Mortality	Fetal Mortality	Significant Complications
Koshy et al,[20] 1988 Prospective RCT Multicenter (United States)	N = 189 (100 hb SS, 66 hb SC, 23 sickle cell β-thalassemia)	0%	Stillbirths, 5.7% in hb SS Neonatal death, 1.9% in hb SS Perinatal death, 7.6% in hb SS	Women had increased rates of infection, preeclampsia, preterm delivery
Cooperative Study of Sickle Cell Disease Smith et al,[21] 1996 Multicenter Prospective Cohort (United States)	N = 445 (320 hb SS, 77 hb SC, 48 sickle cell β-thalassemia)	2 (0.45%) maternal deaths occurred (both with hb SS genotype)	Stillbirths, 0.7% Miscarriages, 6.5% (no increase compared with rates in general African American population) Elective abortions, 28.8%	21% of infants were SGA; no significant increase in obstetric complications
Sun et al,[22] 2001 Retrospective (1980–1999) Single institution (United States)	N = 127 deliveries (69 to hb SS women, 58 to hb SC)	0%	No significant difference in fetal deaths between women with SCD (hb SS or hb SC) and women with normal hemoglobin genotype	Increased risk of IUGR, antepartum hospitalization, postpartum infection, preterm labor, and premature rupture of membranes
Serjeant et al,[23] 2004 Cohort Single institution (Jamaica)	N = 94 pregnancies in 52 subjects with hb SS	2 (2.1%) hb SS maternal deaths reported	Increased rate of spontaneous abortions (36%) compared with normal hemoglobin controls (10%) Stillbirths, 7.1% (did not reach statistical significance)	Significantly lower mean birth weight in subjects with SCD and larger proportion of babies born premature

| Villers et al,[3] 2008 Retrospective database study: Nationwide Inpatient Sample (2000–2003) Multicenter (United States) | N = 17,952 deliveries to women with SCD | 10 (0.05%) maternal deaths reported (6 times greater than the rate for women without SCD) | There was no significant increase in intrauterine fetal death in subjects with SCD compared with controls with normal hemoglobin genotype (odds ratio 1.1, P = .62) | Significantly increased morbidity including pneumonia, cerebral vein thrombosis, DVT, sepsis, postpartum infection, pregnancy-induced hypertension, eclampsia, placental abruption, preterm labor |
| Al Kahtani et al,[24] 2012 Retrospective (2001–2010) Single institution (Saudi Arabia) | N = 392 subjects with hb SS | 2 reported maternal deaths (0.5%), not statistically significant (P = .11) | Increased rates of stillbirths (4.8%), neonatal deaths (2.6%), and higher perinatal death rates (77.7 per 1000 deliveries) in SCD group | Increased frequency of antepartum hospital admissions, preeclampsia, and preterm labor. There were also higher rates of low birth weights and IUGR |

Abbreviations: DVT, deep vein thrombosis; hb SC, hemoglobin SC disease; hb SS, hemoglobin SS sickle cell anemia; IUGR, intrauterine growth restriction; RCT, randomized controlled trial; SGA, small for gestational age.

the model management of SCD in pregnancy ideally is delivered with an interdisciplinary team approach,[29] a team that includes:

1. A hematologist with advanced knowledge in care of patients with SCD
2. A maternal-fetal medicine specialist with expertise in high-risk pregnancy management
3. Additional specialists responsible for the maintenance of associated underlying comorbidities (see **Box 1**)
4. Other providers such as social workers with experience in managing the potential psychosocial obstacles imposed by this chronic condition on the daily lives of patients and their families

Preconception Management

With significant progress in the management of individuals with SCD stemming from the use of novel therapeutic regimens and preventative measures such as penicillin prophylaxis in children, aggressive immunization strategies, and stroke screening,[1,30] girls born with SCD are increasingly likely to reach their reproductive years. With their inherited hemoglobinopathy no longer serving as a decisively prohibiting factor, these young women are therefore faced with decisions regarding starting a family. Discussion and education regarding the numerous concerns surrounding pregnancy in SCD should be initiated early for these young women, their partners, and their family members.

Objectives for patient education include:

- Establishing a shared understanding of the patient's goals and wishes regarding having children[5,29]
- A discussion about the potential complications of pregnancy in SCD
- Ensuring that patients have a clear understanding of these potential challenges
- Ensuring that patients are knowledgeable regarding the need for more vigilant and frequent monitoring during and after pregnancy

Crucial to achieving proper care of patients with SCD is the determination of a definitive genotype and subsequently an accurate diagnosis of a specific sickle cell hemoglobinopathy. Although this may be known in most patients, any confusion should trigger confirmation through a hemoglobin electrophoresis study, because it has been determined that risks for mother and fetus are not equivalent among different genotypes.[4,6] In women with SCD planning to conceive, it is vital that information be provided on partner screening and assessment of the offspring's risk of inheriting SCD based on the determination of the genetic makeup of the partner. Even if the patient's partner does not carry the mutation for the abnormal hb S molecule (ie, does not have sickle cell anemia or sickle cell trait hb AS), various other mutated adult hemoglobin molecules may be carried unknowingly by the father of the baby and, when paired with the genes of the mother with SCD, may result in an affected child with one of the heterozygous sickle cell variants.[26,31] The risk of passing a sickle hemoglobinopathy, inherited in autosomal recessive fashion, along to the child can be summarized as follows:

- hb SS patient + hb SS partner → 100% risk of sickle cell anemia (hb SS) in baby
- hb SS patient + carrier sickle cell trait hb AS partner → 50% risk of sickle cell anemia in baby
- hb SS patient + partner with 1 normal hb A allele and 1 hb C allele → 50% likelihood of baby with hb SC disease

- hb SS patient + partner with β-thalassemia trait → 50% likelihood of baby with hb S–β-thalassemia

When determining the genotype of both the individual with SCD and her partner it is crucial to use accurate diagnostic tests. The proper diagnostic approach involves obtaining:

- A complete blood count (CBC)
- Mean corpuscular volume of RBCs
- A hemoglobin electrophoresis for quantification of hemoglobin subtypes (notably hemoglobin C as well as hemoglobin A2 if there is suspicion for simultaneous inheritance of β-thalassemia or other variants of SCD)

The available sickle cell solubility tests, such as Sickledex, should not be used for screening of partners or for confirming a patient's diagnosis before attempting pregnancy because this test is incapable of identifying any other adult hemoglobins besides the hemoglobin S molecule (such as hemoglobin C or β-thalassemia trait). Therefore the true genetic risk held by the partner can easily be overlooked.[4–6] The aforementioned laboratory evaluations allow a complete investigation into the partner's hemoglobinopathy trait status.

Couples found to be at risk of having an affected child should be offered genetic counseling with information provided regarding their reproductive options including prenatal screening and preimplantation genetic diagnosis.[32] Preimplantation genetic diagnosis refers to the testing of deoxyribonucleic acid (DNA) in embryos created in vitro.[33] Three days after fertilization is complete, a blastomere cell is removed from the embryo and can be analyzed either through a polymerase chain reaction test or by haplotyping the genome. This genetic testing of embryos then allows couples to select the embryos without SCD to be implanted into the mother. This technique may be preferred by couples who are unwilling to terminate a pregnancy of a fetus with SCD identified prenatally because of moral or religious beliefs.[34,35] Oyewo and colleagues[36] examined the results of 16 preimplantation genetic diagnosis cycles performed at a tertiary care center in London between 2002 and 2007. Of the embryos that were transferred during these procedures, approximately 18% resulted in live births. In addition, there were several barriers to the more widespread use of preimplantation genetic diagnosis :

- Cost
- Ethical dilemmas
- Lack of patient awareness of this option
- A poor understanding of the severity of SCD because of its clinical variability

The availability of a preimplantation genetic diagnosis for SCD reproductive planning has also given parents the option to conceive a subsequent child who is human leukocyte antigen (HLA)–matched and can serve as an appropriate bone marrow donor for the older sibling.[34,35] In 2008, the European Society for Human Reproduction and Embryology reported on the idea of using preimplantation genetic diagnosis to select embryos free of SCD that are also HLA-matched to a couple's living child affected with SCD. A successfully implanted embryo with such features has the capability to serve as a stem cell donor for an affected sibling. In the largest study of preimplantation genetic diagnosis for disorders of the hemoglobin molecule, conducted by Kuliev and colleagues,[35] 395 cycles of preimplantation diagnosis yielded a total of nearly 100 deliveries of healthy babies with normal hemoglobin genotype. Of the 33% of these in whom typing for HLA yielded perfect matches to siblings who were suffering with an inherited hemoglobinopathy, 12 individuals at the time of publication had already successfully donated or were involved in plans to donate their stem cells (retrieved from an umbilical cord blood sample) to their affected sister or brother.

Another major goal of the management of women with SCD before conception is to achieve maximization of their sickle cell care before pregnancy in an effort to minimize the medical, sickle-related, and pregnancy-related complications that may arise during pregnancy. This optimization of management, including proper coverage by specialists, is key to effective preconception care and should be performed in any woman with SCD who plans to conceive.[37] It is constructive for this task to include an evaluation of the end-organ complications and dysfunction that can occur. A systematic review of their current medication regimen, with directed patient education concerning the potential teratogenic effects and harms associated with commonly used medications (**Box 2**), should be part of the initial patient encounter.

Hydroxyurea, the first and only disease-modifying therapy approved by the US Food and Drug Administration for SCD, has proved to be a central component to the treatment of adults with SCD.[39] The beneficial effects observed in patients with SCD taking this medication have been linked to its ability to increase the level of fetal hemoglobin through poorly understood mechanisms. In the Multicenter Study of Hydroxyurea for Sickle Cell Anemia (MSH),[40] a key multicenter randomized controlled trial (RCT), hydroxyurea yielded a statistically significant decrease in the number of painful crises. In addition, the researchers reported a decrease in the frequency of acute chest syndrome and number of transfusions. A 7-year follow-up study[41] also showed a significant mortality benefit during active treatment with hydroxyurea. With resultant greater use of hydroxyurea in clinical practice, it is increasingly pertinent to explore the harms of exposing a fetus to this medication in utero.

Hydroxyurea is a known teratogen. The National Toxicology Program has acknowledged evidence on the developmental impairment observed in the fetuses of mice and rats with maternal use of hydroxyurea during the gestational period.[41] A case series involving 31 individuals receiving hydroxyurea for several different illnesses[42] showed (1) growth abnormalities in 2 of the fetuses, and (2) an increased number of pregnancies that delivered before reaching full term. Hydroxyurea can also negatively influence spermatogenesis in men, as suggested by decreased numbers of sperm produced and disrupted sperm motility in male mice exposed to this medication.[43] Although hydroxyurea has been found to help decrease the number of pain crises experienced by individuals with SCD, many patients still require opioid analgesic

---

Box 2
Medications with potential teratogenicity commonly used in SCD

Hydroxyurea (Hydrea)
- Cessation at least 6 months before conception or instantly on pregnancy confirmation[38]

Angiotensin-converting enzyme inhibitors/angiotensin receptor blockers
- Cessation before conception

Injectable iron chelation therapy, deferoxamine
- Avoid during pregnancy (there may be some potential for safe use during second and third trimester[26])

Oral iron chelators
- Avoid during pregnancy

medications for their often debilitating chronic pain and for the intermitted pain crises that can still ensue. Although the potential for a baby born to a mother on this analgesic regimen to exhibit opioid withdrawal should be considered, there have not been any identified links to birth defects or long-term clinical sequelae. Therefore, these medications are generally continued during pregnancy in women with SCD.[26,44]

Along with the elimination of potentially teratogenic medications from the therapeutic regimen of women with SCD before conception, attention should be paid to health maintenance or preventative measures that may enhance the health status of these patients before pregnancy. All patients with SCD should have:

- Administration of the influenza vaccine yearly
- Vaccination against *Streptococcus pneumoniae* once with a booster at 5 years
- Annual echocardiographic screening to assess for pulmonary hypertension (referral to a pulmonologist for further evaluation is appropriate if the tricuspid regurgitant jet velocity is greater than 2.5 m/sec)
- Comorbid asthma identified and optimized
- Screening blood work for liver and kidney function, iron overload status, and RBC alloantibodies conducted before conception

Prenatal Care

Once conception has occurred, focus must shift to the close monitoring of mother and fetus to identify and manage any acute SCD-related or obstetric complications that develop. Rahimy and colleagues[45] discovered that implementation of an active prenatal care program in The Republic of Benin, West Africa, for women with SCD, proved to be beneficial with an improvement in the well-being of these women during pregnancy and more positive results with regard to their fetal outcomes and delivery. They reported on 111 pregnancies from 108 pregnant women with SCD and provided them with education and the necessary tools in the prevention of malaria and early recognition of infectious complications before week 28 of their pregnancies.[45] Using this strategy, the women with SCD had a mortality comparable with women without SCD (maternal mortality of 1.8% in SCD group vs overall maternal mortality of 1.2% for the maternity unit in the study hospital). This study shows that concerted antenatal management can have a positive impact on pregnancy outcomes.

A pregnant woman with SCD seeking prenatal diagnosis of her fetus for SCD can be offered several options. The American College of Obstetricians and Gynecologists (ACOG)[6] in their 2007 Practice Bulletin offers several means for genetic diagnosis:

- Chorionic villus sampling at 10 to 12 weeks' gestation with evaluation of chorionic villi DNA
- Amniocentesis after 15 weeks' gestation with evaluation of DNA in amniotic fluid cells

In addition, a new and unique noninvasive method for prenatal diagnosis involves the use of digital polymerase chain reaction on cell-free DNA obtained from maternal plasma.[46] In a study of this noninvasive prenatal diagnostic test, an accurate sickle cell genotype was identified in 75% and 82% of female and male fetuses, respectively. The ACOG guidelines[6] identify the 2 invasive options but emphasize that the full use of these techniques has been limited by patient apprehension, typically ethical or cultural in nature. They also recognize the increased likelihood of patients to put aside these concerns if they already have a child with SCD, because they have a greater interest in learning the hemoglobin genotype of the unborn child. Even when prenatal diagnosis is performed in this group, it seems that the decision making often ceases once disease status is recognized in the fetus without frequent movement toward elective termination of the pregnancy. For example, almost 75% of families with a known hb SS fetus diagnosed prenatally chose to carry the baby to term.[47] Despite these data, the presentation of genetic counseling and associated education and testing to women with SCD are critical components to comprehensive care.

Prenatal care: maternal management

The collaborative management central to effective care of pregnant women with SCD is designed to minimize both pregnancy-related complications and morbidity secondary to acute sickle cell–related problems with an end goal to optimize the safety and well-being of the unborn fetus. According to Hassel,[5] pregnant women with SCD should visit their obstetrician every other week in the first 2 trimesters to monitor for various obstetric complications with the objective of identifying them in their early stages and treating them successfully. Prenatal management must also include frequent monitoring for the development of symptomatic anemia as well as factors that can serve as triggers for the major manifestation of SCD, the painful vasoocclusive crisis. Therefore:

- These patients should be cognizant of the importance of avoiding dehydration, rigorous physical activity, stress, and cold temperatures
- Pregnancy-related nausea should also be controlled, thereby reducing the likelihood of developing dehydration, which could trigger a vasoocclusive episode[48]
- Blood pressure monitoring: an increase in blood pressure should prompt attentive observation, because these women are capable of developing pregnancy-induced hypertension (preeclampsia)
- Laboratory evaluation: a CBC and measurement of reticulocyte count can help assess hemolytic activity and worsening of anemia during pregnancy
- Pregnant women with SCD should continue to take prenatal vitamins and additional folic acid supplementation (ACOG Clinical Management Guidelines[6]) throughout the pregnancy
- Consideration should be given to the use of vitamins void of iron in patients with SCD who have a diagnosis of iron overload[49]

There are features of prenatal care in patients with SCD that are controversial and there are mixed findings across various studies of their benefit. One of these issues is the use of prophylactic RBC transfusion therapy, which was shown in an RCT to have no benefit in terms of reduction in pregnancy-related complications or fetal growth impairment. Koshy and colleagues[20] randomized pregnant women with SCD to a group receiving an aggressive program of routine RBC transfusion or a group receiving transfusions for acute exacerbations or complications related to their SCD. No difference was found between the groups in the frequency of obstetric and pregnancy-related problems. However, there was a significant decrease in the number of painful vasoocclusive crises ($P<.05$) experienced by the women who received the transfusions prophylactically. These data were supported by findings of 2 other studies. A retrospective study of the usefulness of prophylactic transfusion[50] found a decrease in the percentage of pregnancies with pain crises by approximately 33%. A small retrospective cohort study conducted in Brazil[51] found that prophylactic erythrocytapheresis administered to pregnant women with SCD during their third trimester reduced the risk of intrauterine growth restriction and oligohydramnios. Although other studies have reported advantageous fetal outcomes with prophylactic maternal transfusion, including a reduction in perinatal mortality and fetal growth abnormalities, a Cochrane Review from 1996[52] declared insufficient evidence to state for or against routine transfusions during pregnancy for women with SCD. In general practice, routine prophylactic transfusion in pregnant women who were not already on a transfusion program before conception is not the standard of care.

The approach and treatment of potential acute complications of SCD during pregnancy are as follows:

- Acute painful vasoocclusive crisis
  - Patients should be evaluated quickly by a multidisciplinary team and treated with pain medication regimen, fluids, and supplemental oxygen as appropriate and parallel to the treatment of painful sickle cell crisis in nonpregnant sickle cell individuals.
  - Early identification of infections is required, with appropriate treatment targeted at suspected causal organisms.
  - Opiates for pain relief may be used as in patients with SCD who are not pregnant, because no known relationship to congenital deformations or toxicity during pregnancy has been identified. Use of opiates chronically to treat pain in SCD can lead to neonatal abstinence syndrome after delivery but the severity of this syndrome has been found to be discordant with dosages in pregnant women with SCD on methadone for chronic pain treatment.
  - Meperidine hydrochloride is generally avoided in patients with SCD with a history of seizures or reduced renal function secondary to the seizure risk (wide-ranging risk reported from 1%–12%)[53] associated with normeperidine (a metabolite of the medication).[29,32,53]
  - Pregnant patients with SCD must be monitored for sequelae of vasoocclusion including splenic sequestration and acute chest syndrome. Although there is no absolute contraindication to exchange transfusion therapy in pregnancy, consultation by hematology is encouraged and careful attention to volume status during the procedure should be used.
- Acute anemia
  - Obtain reticulocyte count and monitor for reticulocytopenia; consider need for transfusion of RBCs.
- Urinary tract infections
  - Higher risk of urinary infections:
    - Lower urinary tract (up to 40% of pregnancies)
    - Upper urinary tract (approximately 8% of pregnancies complicated by pyelonephritis)

Several additional sickle-related complications, such as acute chest syndrome, acute stroke, and parvovirus B19 infection, can occur in the pregnant patient with SCD and the approach to managing these conditions is identical to that used in nonpregnant patients with SCD with these same complications.

Most women with SCD have been transfused at some point in their lives. As a result, many of these patients develop RBC alloantibodies and this may be further compounded by the independent risk of alloimmunization in pregnancy.[54] A report of 30 women with SCD during pregnancy, all of whom had received transfusions before or during the pregnancy, found that approximately 20% of these women produced alloantibodies while pregnant. The significance of this is in the danger to the fetus of a mother with alloantibodies, if these antibodies are of the type that can cause hemolytic disease of the newborn. The methods to minimize this risk include pretransfusion matching of antigens between donor and recipient RBCs.[55] A comprehensive transfusion history with known alloantibodies should be obtained from women with SCD, ideally even before conception. The routine initial prenatal blood type and antibody screen also identifies at-risk pregnancies for alloimmunization. In addition, for those patients undergoing prophylactic or indicated transfusions, the type and cross-match procedure should identify potential problems with alloimmunization.

Fetal surveillance

With evidence in the literature recognizing the risk of fetal growth impairment complicating pregnancies in women with SCD, close fetal growth monitoring is a part of the comprehensive prenatal care. This growth surveillance initiates fetal growth ultrasounds beginning at 18 weeks, with serial follow-up scans on a monthly basis. Starting at 32 to 34 weeks, the twice-weekly nonstress tests/biophysical profiles are used to assess placental function with regard to adequate oxygenation of the fetus. Interpretation of these placental function tests should be cautious if the patient is actively participating in a therapeutic regimen that includes narcotic pain medications, which can suppress fetal activity and yield results that seem abnormal even though the fetus is well oxygenated.[5] Others have recommended the use of umbilical artery Doppler at approximately 28 to 30 weeks[56] for quantification of flow state in this artery to assess uteroplacental oxygen and nutrient delivery. Although evidence for the benefits of antenatal surveillance is limited, the ACOG Practice Bulletin guidelines[6] (2007) state that these examinations are sensible owing to the understood risk for preterm labor, stillbirth, and growth impairment in pregnancy complicated by SCD.

Intrapartum Care

Since SCD is considered a high-risk condition in pregnancy, delivery between 38 and 40 weeks' gestation is key and can help avoid potential consequences of late pregnancy and minimize harm to the infant. Delivery should occur vaginally unless obstetric issues prevent this from occurring, because SCD does not serve as a contraindication for vaginal delivery. During labor, women with SCD should be given fluids intravenously to prevent the development of dehydration.[57] The anesthesiologist should be advised that the pain medication doses required by pregnant women with SCD during labor may be in excess of those typically required in healthy obstetric patients, given the development of higher tolerance to opioids used chronically to treat their sickle cell pain.

The logistics of delivery in patients with SCD with hip replacements as a result of avascular necrosis must be considered, because adjustments to the typical positions assumed by the woman during delivery may be necessary. In addition, harvesting of hematopoietic stem cells from the umbilical cord blood of the newborn baby should be considered because these cells could potentially be used as a curative allogeneic stem cell transplantation donor source for an older or subsequent sibling with SCD. This option should preferably be discussed before labor and delivery so that arrangements for stem cell harvesting at the time of delivery can be arranged.

Postpartum Care

SCD-related complications in pregnant women do not end with delivery of the baby. Unique challenges can arise in the postpartum period. First, despite concerns about risks of dehydration exacerbating SCD crisis, women with SCD should be encouraged to breast-feed because there are no data to support that breast-feeding is associated with an increase in crisis frequency. Instead, the decision to breast-feed should be determined by evaluating risks of delaying the reintroduction of any SCD-specific medications typically known to cross into breast milk. It is known that hydroxyurea is transferred into breast milk,[4,58] and therefore it is recommended that this drug be withheld while a mother is breast-feeding. If the mother has a history of frequent vasoocclusive crisis episodes and would benefit from hydroxyurea therapy, then cessation of breast-feeding may be discussed with the mother. Studies of iron chelation therapies have found that these medications likely are excreted in the breast milk as well and should be avoided in lactating mothers. Although opioids can be detected in breast milk, there seems to be no danger to the baby associated with this exposure.[59] Nevertheless, the child's pediatrician should be alerted of this exposure so that close monitoring for side effects can be initiated. In conclusion, women with SCD should be educated on the numerous advantages of breast-feeding and these advantages should be weighed against any risks associated with the delay of introduction of SCD-related therapies.

A common clinical question during postpartum care for women with SCD is what contraceptive methods are safe. According to the Green-top guidelines from the United Kingdom published in 2011,[60] contraceptive methods using progesterone, including the progesterone-only birth control pill, injectable contraceptives, and intrauterine devices containing levonorgestrel, should be used in women with SCD in the postnatal period. These guidelines state that estrogen-containing contraceptive methods should instead be used as second-line options for birth control. A systematic review on contraceptive use in women with SCD found that progestin-only and combined oral birth control pills did not increase the likelihood of vasoocclusion.[61] However, this review failed to include thromboembolic disease as an outcome of contraceptive use and scarcity of data resulted in no comments regarding the danger associated with intrauterine devices. Further study regarding the risk of hormonal contraception on thrombosis in SCD is needed.[62]

SUMMARY

The management of pregnancy in women with SCD involves enhanced understanding of the interaction between the pathophysiology of SCD and the normal physiologic changes of pregnancy. Specialized clinical comanagement between hematologists and obstetricians is therefore paramount. A team-based approach with observant monitoring for the various complications that can arise allows early and practical treatment of these potential problems and can lead to better outcomes during these high-risk pregnancies. Since the number of individuals with SCD reaching adulthood will continue to increase, continued investigation should be conducted to increase knowledge of the complications and effective interventions for management of SCD in pregnancy.

REFERENCES

1. Prabhakar H, Haywood C Jr, Molokie R. Sickle cell disease in the United States: looking back and forward at 100 years of progress in management and survival. Am J Hematol 2010;85:346–53.
2. Platt OS, Brambilla DJ, Rosse WF, et al. Mortality in sickle cell disease: life expectancy and risk factors for early death. N Engl J Med 1994;330(23): 1639–44.
3. Villers MS, Jamison MG, De Castro LM, et al. Morbidity associated with sickle cell disease in pregnancy. Am J Obstet Gynecol 2008;199:125.e1–5.
4. Rogers DT, Molokie R. Sickle cell disease in pregnancy. Obstet Gynecol Clin North Am 2010;37:223–37.
5. Hassel K. Pregnancy and sickle cell disease. Hematol Oncol Clin North Am 2005;1:803–16.

6. American College of Obstetricians and Gynecologists. ACOG Practice Bulletin No. 78: hemoglobinopathies in pregnancy. Obstet Gynecol 2007;109:229–37.

7. Rees DC, Williams TN, Gladwin MT. Sickle-cell disease. Lancet 2010;376: 2018–31.

8. Brousseau DC, Panepinto JA, Nimmer M, et al. The number of people with sickle-cell disease in the United States: national and state estimates. Am J Hematol 2010;85:77–8.

9. Hassel KL. Population estimates of sickle cell disease in the U.S. Am J Prev Med 2010;38:S512–21.

10. Bunn FH. Pathogenesis and treatment of sickle cell disease. N Engl J Med 1997; 337(11):762–9.

11. Serjeant GR. Sickle-cell disease. Lancet 1997;350:725–30.

12. Lanaro C, Franco-Penteado CF, Albuqueque DM, et al. Altered levels of cytokines and inflammatory mediators in plasma and leukocytes of sickle cell anemia patients and effects of hydroxyurea therapy. J Leukoc Biol 2009;85(2): 235–42.

13. Adam SS, Hoppe C. Potential role for statins in sickle cell disease. Pediatr Blood Cancer 2013;60(4):550–7.

14. Fertrin KY, Costa FF. Genomic polymorphisms in sickle cell disease: implications for clinical diversity and treatment. Expert Rev Hematol 2010;3(4): 443–58.

15. Weatherall MW, Higgs DR, Weiss H, et al. Phenotype/genotype relationships in sickle cell disease: a pilot twin study. Clin Lab Haematol 2005;27(6): 384–90.

16. Gladwin MT, Vichinsky E. Pulmonary complications of sickle cell disease. N Engl J Med 2008;359(21):2254–65.

17. Sydenstricker VP. Further observations on sickle cell anemia. J Am Med Assn 1924;83:12–7.

18. Kobak AJ, Stein PJ, Daro AF. Sickle-cell anemia in pregnancy. A review of the literature and report of six cases. Am J Obstet Gynecol 1941;41(5):811–23.

19. Turner CM. Sickle cell anemia in pregnancy. Resumé of literature, with a case report. J Natl Med Assoc 1951;43(3):165–8.

20. Koshy M, Burd L, Wallace D, et al. Prophylactic red-cell transfusions in pregnant patients with sickle cell disease. A randomized cooperative study. N Engl J Med 1988;319(22):1447–52.

21. Smith JA, Espeland M, Bellevue R, et al. Pregnancy in sickle cell disease: experience of the cooperative study of sickle cell disease. Obstet Gynecol 1996; 87(2):199–204.

22. Sun PM, Wilburn W, Raynor BD, et al. Sickle cell disease in pregnancy: twenty years of experience at Grady Memorial Hospital, Atlanta, Georgia. Am J Obstet Gynecol 2001;184(6):1127–30.

23. Serjeant GR, Loy LL, Crowther M, et al. Outcome of pregnancy in homozygous sickle cell disease. Obstet Gynecol 2004;103(6):127–85.

24. Al Kahtani MA, AlQahtani M, Alshebaily MM, et al. Morbidity and pregnancy outcomes associated with sickle cell anemia among Saudi women. Int J Gynaecol Obstet 2012;119(3):224–6.

25. Asnani MR, McCaw-Binns AM, Reid ME. Excess risk of maternal death from sickle cell disease in Jamaica: 1998-2007. PLoS One 2011;6(10):1–9.

26. Naik RP, Lanzkron S. Baby on board: what you need to know about pregnancy in the hemoglobinopathies. Hematology Am Soc Hematol Educ Program 2012;(2012):208–14.

27. Chang J, Streitman D. Physiologic adaptations to pregnancy. Neurol Clin 2012; 30(3):781–9.
28. James AH, Jamison MG, Brancazio LR, et al. Venous thromboembolism during pregnancy and the postpartum period: incidence, risk factors, and mortality. Am J Obstet Gynecol 2006;194(5):1311–5.
29. Howard J, Oteng-Ntim E. The obstetric management of sickle cell disease. Best Pract Res Clin Obstet Gynaecol 2012;26(1):25–36.
30. Rappaport VJ, Velazquez M, Williams K. Hemoglobinopathies in pregnancy. Obstet Gynecol Clin North Am 2004;31:287–317.
31. Koshy M. Sickle cell disease and pregnancy. Blood Rev 1995;9:157–64.
32. Oteng-Ntim E, Nazir S, Singhal T, et al. Sickle cell disease in pregnancy. Obstet Gynaecol Reprod Med 2012;22(9):254–63.
33. Cooper AR, Jungheim ES. Preimplantation genetic diagnosis: indications and controversies. Clin Lab Med 2010;30:519–31.
34. Bodurtha J, Strauss JF. Genomics and perinatal care. N Engl J Med 2012;366: 64–73.
35. Kuliev A, Pakhalchuk T, Verlinksky O. Preimplantation genetic diagnosis for hemoglobinopathies. Hemoglobin 2011;35:547–55.
36. Oyewo A, Salubi-Udu J, Khalaf Y, et al. Preimplantation genetic diagnosis for the prevention of sickle cell disease: current trends and barriers to uptake in a London teaching hospital. Hum Fertil 2009;12(3):153–9.
37. Rizack T, Rosene-Montella K. Special hematologic issues in the pregnant patient. Hematol Oncol Clin North Am 2012;26:409–32.
38. Brawley OW, Cornelius LJ, Edwards LR, et al. National Institutes of Health Consensus Development Conference statement: hydroxyurea treatment for sickle cell disease. Ann Intern Med 2008;148(12):932–8.
39. Lanzkron S, Strouse JJ, Wilson R. Systematic review: hydroxyurea for the treatment of adults with sickle cell disease. Ann Intern Med 2008;148(12):939–55.
40. Charache S, Terrin ML, Moore RD, et al. Effects of hydroxyurea on the frequency of painful crises in sickle cell anemia: Investigators of the Multicenter Study of Hydroxyurea in Sickle Cell Anemia. N Engl J Med 1995;332(20):1317–22.
41. Steinberg MH, Barton F, Castro O, et al. Effect of hydroxyurea on mortality and morbidity in adult sickle cell anemia: risks and benefits up to 9 years of treatment. JAMA 2003;289(13):1645–51.
42. Thauvin-Robinet C, Maingueneau C, Robert E, et al. Exposure to hydroxyurea during pregnancy: a case series. Leukemia 2001;15(8):1309–11.
43. Berthaut I, Guignedoux G, Kirsch-Noir F, et al. Influence of sickle cell disease and treatment with hydroxyurea on sperm parameters and fertility of human males. Haematologica 2008;93(7):988–93.
44. Kellogg A, Rose CH, Harms RH, et al. Current trends in narcotic use in pregnancy and neonatal outcomes. Am J Obstet Gynecol 2011;204(3):259.e1–4.
45. Rahimy MC, Gangbo A, Adjou R, et al. Effect of active prenatal management on pregnancy outcomes in sickle cell disease in an African setting. Blood 2000; 95(5):1685–9.
46. Barrett AN, McDonnell TC, Chan KC, et al. Digital PCR analysis of maternal plasma for noninvasive detection of sickle cell anemia. Clin Chem 2012;58(6): 1026–32.
47. Alter BP. Prenatal diagnosis of hematologic diseases, 1986 update. Acta Haematol 1987;78:137–41.
48. Barfield WD, Barradas DT, Manning SE. Sickle cell disease and pregnancy outcomes: women of African descent. Am J Prev Med 2010;38:S542–9.

49. Adegoke AA, Kongnyuy EJ. Iron supplementation for sickle cell disease during pregnancy (Protocol). Cochrane Database of Systematic Reviews 2011;12: 1–11.

50. Ngo C, Kayem G, Habibi A. Pregnancy in sickle cell disease: maternal and fetal outcomes in a population receiving prophylactic partial exchange transfusions. Eur J Obstet Gynecol Reprod Biol 2010;152:128–42.

51. Gilli SC, De Paula SC, Biscaro FP. Third-trimester erythrocytapheresis in pregnant patients with sickle cell disease. Int J Gynaecol Obstet 2007;96(1):8–11.

52. Okusanya BO, Oladapo OT. Prophylactic versus selective blood transfusion for sickle cell disease in pregnancy (Protocol). Cochrane Database of Systematic Reviews 2013;2:1–8.

53. Ballas SK, Bauserman RL, McCarthy WF, et al. Hydroxyurea and acute painful crises in sickle cell anemia: effects on hospital length of stay and opioid utilization during hospitalization, outpatient acute care contacts, and at home. J Pain Symptom Manage 2010;40(6):870–82.

54. Moise KJ Jr, Argoti PS. Management and prevention of red cell alloimmunization in pregnancy: a systematic review. Obstet Gynecol 2012;120(5):1132–9.

55. Vichinsky EP, Luban NL, Wright E, et al. Prospective RBC phenotype matching in a stroke-prevention trial in sickle cell anemia: a multicenter transfusional trial. Transfusion 2001;41:1086–92.

56. Maulik D, Mundy D, Heitmann E, et al. Evidence-based approach to umbilical artery Doppler fetal surveillance in high-risk pregnancies: an update. Clin Obstet Gynecol 2010;53(4):869–78.

57. Simms-Stewart D, Thame M, Hemans-Keen A. Retained placenta in homozygous sickle cell disease. Obstet Gynecol 2009;114(4):825–8.

58. Sylvester RK, Lobell M, Teresi ME, et al. Excretion of hydroxyurea into milk. Cancer 1987;60(9):2177–8.

59. Keegan J, Parva M, Finnegan M, et al. Addiction in pregnancy. J Addict Dis 2010;29(2):175–91.

60. Royal College of Obstetricians and Gynaecologists (RCOG). Management of sickle cell disease in pregnancy. Green-top guideline, no.61. Agency for Healthcare Research and Quality 2011.

61. Haddad LB, Curtis KM, Legardy-Williams JK, et al. Contraception for individuals with sickle cell disease: a systematic review of the literature. Contraception 2012;85:527–37.

62. Gomez A, Grimes DA, Lopez LM, et al. Steroid hormones for contraception in women with sickle cell disease. Cochrane Database of Systematic Reviews 2007;2:1–11.

Diagnosis and Management of Neonatal Alloimmune Thrombocytopenia in Pregnancy

Noel K. Strong, MD*, Keith A. Eddleman, MD

KEYWORDS

- NAIT • Maternal • Fetal • Neonatal • Alloimmune • Alloimmunization
- Thrombocytopenia • HPA

KEY POINTS

- Neonatal alloimmune thrombocytopenia (NAIT) is the most common cause of severe thrombocytopenia and intracranial hemorrhage in the term newborn.
- The most common human platelet alloantigens (HPAs) implicated in NAIT are HPA-1a in the white population and HPA-4a in Asian populations.
- A diagnosis of NAIT should be considered for any neonate with unexplained thrombocytopenia.
- Head ultrasound or magnetic resonance imaging should be performed promptly on all neonates with suspected NAIT to exclude intracranial hemorrhage.
- Neonatal therapy should be initiated before laboratory confirmation in cases of suspected NAIT.
- Prenatal management of a woman with a prior delivery of an infant with NAIT uses a combination of IVIG or prednisone depending on a severity scale of the index NAIT case.

INTRODUCTION

Fetal or neonatal alloimmune thrombocytopenia (NAIT) is the most common cause of severe thrombocytopenia in an otherwise healthy newborn. It occurs in approximately 1 in 1000 live births. NAIT is analogous to Rhesus (Rh) alloimmunization in pathophysiology. It is caused by the placental transfer of maternal alloantibodies against fetal platelet antigens inherited from the father. The transplacental transfer of maternal alloantibodies against fetal platelet antigens leads to the destruction of fetal antigen-positive platelets. Presentation of NAIT varies from an incidentally detected mild thrombocytopenia in a well newborn to life-threatening in utero or postnatal intracranial hemorrhage (ICH). Unlike Rh alloimmunization, it may present unexpectedly in a first pregnancy in 40% to 60% of cases.[1] It has often been observed to be more severe

Icahn School of Medicine at Mount Sinai, Department of Obstetrics, Gynecology and Reproductive Science, 5 East 98th Street, 2nd Floor, New York, NY 10029, USA
* Corresponding author.
E-mail address: noel.strong@mssm.edu

Clin Lab Med 33 (2013) 311–325
http://dx.doi.org/10.1016/j.cll.2013.03.024
0272-2712/13/$ – see front matter © 2013 Elsevier Inc. All rights reserved.

labmed.theclinics.com

in subsequent pregnancies. As such it is important that the diagnosis of NAIT be considered in the work-up of all cases of neonatal thrombocytopenia to determine the risk to future pregnancies and corresponding management plans. This article discusses the pathogenesis and incidence of NAIT, and the antenatal and postnatal management of this condition.

DEFINITION OF NEONATAL THROMBOCYTOPENIA

Historically, neonatal thrombocytopenia has been defined as a platelet count of less than 150×10^9/L and occurs in approximately 0.5% to 0.9% of newborns.[2] This value is based on the definition used in adults to represent the lower fifth percentile. More recent studies have demonstrated that in neonates the fifth percentile is lower than the standard adult value of 150,000/μL.[3] In 2009, the Intermountain Healthcare group reviewed the platelet counts of 34,146 neonates gestational ages 22 to 42 weeks on the first 3 days of life. The study found that in preterm infants less than or equal to 32 weeks gestational age the fifth percentile was 104×10^9/L and in late preterm and term infants the fifth percentile was 123×10^9/L. Regardless of which definition is used to define thrombocytopenia, it seems widely agreed that severe neonatal thrombocytopenia is defined as a platelet count of less than 50×10^9/L. Severe neonatal thrombocytopenia occurs in 0.12% to 0.24% of newborns (**Table 1**).

Table 1 Neonatal thrombocytopenia		
Thrombocytopenia	Platelet Count	% of Newborns
Mild	100–150 $\times$ 10^9/L	0.8
Moderate	50–100 $\times$ 10^9/L	0.5
Severe	<50 $\times$ 10^9/L	0.2

Standard ranges used to define mild, moderate, and severe thrombocytopenia are defined in the article.

DIFFERENTIAL DIAGNOSIS OF NEONATAL THROMBOCYTOPENIA

Causes of thrombocytopenia can be classified into disorders of increased destruction, including consumption, or decreased production as shown in **Boxes 1–3**.

PATHOGENESIS

Pregnancies in which there is an incompatibility between the platelet antigen of the mother and her fetus are "at risk" for NAIT. In such pregnancies, passage of the antigen-positive fetal platelets into the circulation of the antigen-negative mother may result in the maternal immunization. Subsequently, maternal antiplatelet IgG alloantibodies are produced and directed against the "foreign" or fetal platelet antigen. These maternal IgG platelet alloantibodies pass transplacentally into the fetal circulation and bind the fetal platelets. The antibody-coated platelets pass through the reticuloendothelial system and are rapidly removed from the circulation by phagocytes (**Fig. 1**). The severity of the resulting fetal-neonatal thrombocytopenia is determined by several variables including

- Concentration of maternal IgG alloantibodies
- Subclass of maternal IgG alloantibodies

Box 1
Increased consumption

Immune mediated

    Autoimmune

    Alloimmune

    Drug induced

Peripheral consumption

    Hypersplenism

    Kasabach-Merritt syndrome (giant hemangioma)

    Disseminated intravascular coagulation

    Necrotizing entercolitis

Miscellaneous

    Neonatal cord injury

    Von Willebrand disease

Box 2
Decreased production

Infiltrative disorders

TAR syndrome

Wiskott-Aldrich syndrome

Congenital leukemia

Osteopetrosis

Box 3
Mixed causes

Infection

Congenital (TORCH)

Acquired (bacterial sepsis)

Extracorporeal membrane oxygenation

Exchange transfusions

Aneuploidy (T21 and T18)

Drug toxicity

- Concentration of antigen on the fetal-neonatal platelets
- Activity of the phagocytes in the reticuloendothelial system
- Ability of fetal-neonatal bone marrow to compensate for the rapid destruction of fetal platelets

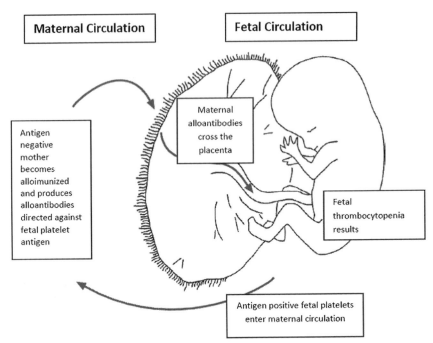

Fig. 1. Pathophysiology of NAIT. After exposure of antigen-positive fetal platelets to antigen-negative maternal circulation, IgG alloantibodies reactive against the fetal platelet antigen form. These alloantibodies cross the placenta and attach to antigen-positive fetal platelets, causing accelerated destruction of these platelets by phagocytes as they pass through the fetal reticuloendothelial system resulting in thrombocytopenia. (*Data from* Blanchette VS, Johnson J, Rand M. The management of alloimmune neonatal thrombocytopenia. Baillieres Best Pract Res Clin Haematol 2000;13(3):365–90.)

HUMAN PLATELET ALLOANTIGENS AND NAIT

Human platelet alloantigens (HPAs) are glycoproteins (GP) found on the surface of platelets. An alloantigen is an antigen that is present in a portion of the population and absent in the rest of that population. There are 24 platelet-specific alloantigens that have been identified. They are named using the HPA system by number in the order in which they were first described. Of the platelet-specific alloantigens, six are grouped into biallelic systems (HPA-1, -2, -3, -4, -5, and -15). Within this nomenclature the platelet alloantigens are further defined according to the frequency in which they appear within the population, with "a" designating the high-frequency alloantigen and "b" designating the low-frequency alloantigen (**Table 2**).[2]

Of the HPAs described, only a small number are responsible for most clinically significant NAIT. Antibodies to platelet antigen HPA-1a are the most commonly implicated antibodies in the white population and are responsible for approximately 80% of the cases of NAIT in this population. Antibodies directed against HPA-5b, HPA-1b, HPA-3a, and HPA-9b (9%, 4%, 2%, and 2% of cases, respectively) are implicated in the remainder of cases within this population.[2,4] Within the Asian population, antibodies directed against

HPA-4a (80% of cases) and HPA-3a (15% of cases) account for most cases. NAIT tends to be clinically more severe in cases with alloantibodies against HPA-1a.[5] HPA-1 antigens are expressed on platelet GPIIIa. Anti–HPA-1a antibodies have been implicated in impaired platelet aggregation, which may explain the severity of bleeding symptoms.[6]

Table 2
Human platelet alloantigens

Antigen	Other Names	Glycoprotein Location	Amino Acid Change	Phenotype Frequency
HPA-1a (P1A1) HPA-1b (P1A2)	P1A, Zw	GPIIIa	Leu <-> Pro33	72% a/a 26% a/b 2% b/b
HPA-2a (Kob) HPA-2b (Koa)	Ko, Sib	GPIb	Thr <-> Met145	85% a/a 14% a/b 1% b/b
HPA-3a (P1A1) HPA-3b (P1A1)	Bak, Lek	GPIIb	Ile:Ser843	37% a/a 48% a/b 15% b/b
HPA-4a (P1A1) HPA-4b (P1A1)	Pen, Yuk	GPIIIa	Arg:Gln143	>99.9% a/a <0.1% a/b <0.1% b/b
HPA-5a (P1A1) HPA-5b (P1A1)	Br, Hc, Zav	GPIa	Glu:Lys505	80% a/a 19% a/b 1% b/b
HPA-6bw		GPIIIa	Arg:Gln489	<1% b/b
HPA-7bw		GPIIIa	Pro <-> Ala407	<1% b/b
HPA-8bw		GPIIIa	Arg:Cys636	<0.1% b/b
HPA-9bw		GPIIb	Val:Met837	<1% b/b
HPA-10bw		GPIIIa	Arg:Gln62	1% b/b
HPA-11bw		GPIIIa	Arg:His633	<0.5% b/b
HPA-12bw		GPIb	Gly:Glu15	1% b/b
HPA-13bw		GPIa	Met:Thr799	<1% b/b
HPA-14bw	Oea	GPIIIa	Del:Lys611	1% b/b
HPA-15a (P1A1) HPA-15b (P1A1)	Gov	CD109	Tyr:Ser703	35% a/a 42% a/b 23% b/b
HPA-16bw	Duva	GPIIIa	Thr:Ile140	<1%
NA	NAKa	CD36 (GPIV)		99.8

Phenotypic frequencies for antigens shown are for white populations only.

Data from McQuilten ZK, Wood EM, Savoia H, et al. A review of pathophysiology and current treatment for neonatal alloimmune thrombocytopenia (NAIT) and introducing the Australian NAIT registry. Aust N Z J Obstet Gynaecol 2011;51:191–8.

INCIDENCE

NAIT is a relatively rare disorder. The reported incidence in prospective studies varies from 1 in 500 to 1 in 5000 livebirths.[1,5,7] The frequency of NAIT in whites is lower than would be expected given that the incidence of HPA-1a negativity in mothers is approximately 2%. Seventy-five percent of white males are homozygous (HPA-1a/1a) and 25% are heterozygous. Given these percentages after the index pregnancy, 85% of couples would be at risk for NAIT. However, only 10% of HPA-1a–negative mothers exposed to HPA-1a–positive platelets during pregnancy become immunized. This may be related to the presence or absence of specific anti–HLA-2 antigens. Studies have demonstrated that other factors, such as HLA type, can modulate severity of disease in offspring.[8–10] Increased risk in HPA-1a–negative mothers expressing HLA-B8, HLA-DR3, and HLA-DR52a antigens has been observed. The presence of HLA-DRB3*0101 allele in HPA-1a–negative women increases the NAIT risk as much as 140-fold.[10]

CLINICAL AND LABORATORY DIAGNOSIS

The diagnosis of NAIT is based on clinical and laboratory features. Diagnostic criteria include thrombocytopenia; fetomaternal incompatibility for a platelet antigen; maternal alloantibodies reactive against fetal (or paternal) platelet antigen; and a clinical response to antigen-negative (compatible) but not antigen-positive (incompatible) platelets.

The history of a previously affected infant or fetus provides strong supportive evidence for the diagnosis of NAIT. In neonates, platelet counts less than 100×10^9/L should be considered abnormally low and should prompt work-up for an underlying cause.

CLINICAL PRESENTATION

The typical infant with NAIT is full-term with normal birth weight. Affected infants are firstborns 40% to 60% of the time. Thrombocytopenia is generally unexpected and often severe. One series reports a median platelet count of 19×10^9/L on Day 1 of life. Consistent with the frequent finding of severe thrombocytopenia, hemorrhagic symptoms are often observed. NAIT should be suspected in a thrombocytopenic neonate with extensive purpura or visceral hemorrhage but no evidence of sepsis, skeletal anomalies, or other systemic diseases that may cause thrombocytopenia, including maternal idiopathic thrombocytopenic purpura. Although affected infants may have no symptoms, many exhibit bleeding symptoms including evidence of ICH.[11] In a case series of 88 infants with NAIT resulting from anti–HPA-1a antibodies, 90% had purpura, 66% had hematomas, 30% had gastrointestinal bleeding, and 14% had ICH (**Table 3**).[12] Looking across several studies, central nervous system hemorrhage has been reported to occur in 8% to 22% of cases (**Table 4**).[13] The greatest risk for ICH exists when the platelet count is less than 20×10^9/L (**Fig. 2**). Fetuses or neonates with siblings that had ICH are at highest risk for ICH. In these cases ICH tends to occur earlier than in the sibling. An intraparenchymal bleed can occur as early as 16 weeks gestational age because IgG alloantibodies can cross the placenta as early as Week 14 of pregnancy, and fetal GPs are expressed on platelets starting at 16 weeks gestational age.[7] For all hemorrhagic complications, including ICH, bleeding and symptoms may be delayed, because the platelet count usually falls further during the first several days of life. Death or neurologic impairment occurs in up to 25% of infants. Platelet counts recover to normal in 1 to 2 weeks.[12]

Table 3
Incidence of hemorrhagic symptoms in infants with NAIT

Hemorrhagic Symptoms	N	%
Petechiae/purpura	79	90
Hematoma	58	66
Gastrointestinal	26	30
Melena	24	27
Hematemesis	2	2
Hemoptysis	7	8
Hematuria	3	3
Retinal hemorrhage	6	7
Central nervous system hemorrhage	12	14
No symptoms	9	10

Data from Kaplan C, Murphy MF, Kroll H, et al. Feto-maternal alloimmune thrombocytopenia: antenatal therapy with IVIgG and steroids—More questions than answers. European Working Group on FMAIT. Br J Haematol 1998;100:62.

Table 4
Frequency of ICH in infants with NAIT

Investigator	Study Period	Number of NAIT Cases	Number of Cases with ICH (%)
Pearson et al	1945–1963	55	12 (22)
Blanchette	1977–1985	15	3 (20)
Mueller-Eckhardt et al	1977–1988	88	12 (14)
Uhrynowska et al	1981, not reported	46	5 (11)
Muller et al	1985	84	7 (8)
Total		288	39 (14)

Data from Blanchette VS, Johnson J, Rand M. The management of alloimmune neonatal thrombo-cytopenia. Baillieres Best Pract Res Clin Haematol 2000;13(3):365–90.

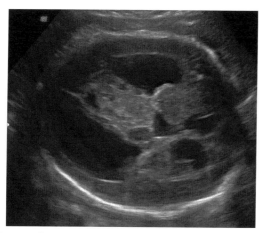

Fig. 2. Ultrasound image of intracranial hemorrhage. The figure demonstrates an organized clot that appears echogenic on ultrasound, and bilateral intraventricular enlargement to point to hemorrhage would be useful to the reader.

LABORATORY DIAGNOSIS

The laboratory diagnosis of NAIT requires demonstration of fetomaternal platelet surface antigen incompatibility and the presence of maternal alloantibodies reactive against fetal-paternal platelet antigen. Among the most frequently used techniques to confirm these findings are the platelet suspension immunofluorescence test, shown in **Fig. 3**, and the monoclonal antibody-specific immobilization of platelet antigens assay.[14] Platelet typing of the parents and neonate can also be determined by either genotyping or enzyme-linked immunoabsorbent assay. In some cases these tests may fail to yield the diagnosis because private or undescribed HPA antigens may be responsible for NAIT.[13,14]

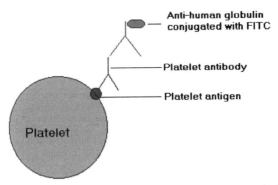

Fig. 3. Platelet suspension immunofluorescence test (PSIFT). Maternal platelets are incubated with control anti–HPA-1a serum allowing antigen-antibody complex formation. The antigen-antibody complexes are then labeled with antihuman globulin labeled with a flurochrome (fluorescin isothiocynate [FITC]), which can be detected by flow cytometry. (*Data from* Risson D, Davies M, Williams B. Review of neonatal alloimmune thrombocytopenia. J Paediatr Child Health 2012;48:816–22.)

MANAGEMENT

The mother of a fetus with NAIT is unaffected and asymptomatic. In contrast to Rh alloimmunization, NAIT develops 40% to 60% of the time in the first pregnancy of an at-risk couple. Alternatively, NAIT should be suspected in the fetus of a couple with previously affected offspring. Unexplained fetal deaths in the maternal history or fetal hydrocephalus or bleeding in previous pregnancies may alert the physician to the possibility of NAIT. Evidence of a bleed or hydrocephalus on a routine screening pregnancy ultrasound may also prompt work-up for NAIT. Thrombocytopenia may worsen as the gestation progresses. Platelet counts can fall by more than 10 × 1000/mL^3 per week. With each subsequent affected pregnancy, thrombocytopenia tends to occur earlier in gestation and tends to be more severe. A history of antenatal ICH in a sibling is predictive of early onset, more severe disease in the subsequent child.[13]

POSTNATAL MANAGEMENT

In many cases of NAIT there is no history of a previously affected sibling and thrombocytopenia is unexpected. Firstborns make up 40% to 60% of NAIT cases. In these cases, other known causes of thrombocytopenia must be quickly excluded and appropriate therapy initiated promptly, because the risk of postnatal ICH is significant if left untreated. Treatment should be initiated based on clinical diagnosis before immunologic confirmation for best outcomes.

When clinically significant thrombocytopenia is identified in a neonate without an apparent cause, the first step of the work-up is to confirm the presence of thrombocytopenia by examination of the peripheral smear and repeat venous blood sample. In neonates with confirmed thrombocytopenia a careful maternal history should be obtained and a thorough neonatal examination should be performed. Examination and history should focus on narrowing the differential diagnosis as described in **Boxes 1–3**. The maternal history should include inquiry into medications taken in pregnancy; hypertensive disorders of pregnancy; history of idiopathic thrombocytopenic purpura; or collagen-vascular disorders (ie, systemic lupus erythematous). Neonatal examination should carefully focus on such things as limb abnormalities, cutaneous hemangiomas, hepatosplenomegaly, and other findings that might indicate another cause for thrombocytopenia besides NAIT. A maternal platelet count and fetal coagulation profile and TORCH work-up should also be obtained; in the absence of findings that indicate a different cause, NAIT should be considered the likely diagnosis until proved otherwise. At this point, a neonatal head ultrasound should be performed. Blood from both parents should be collected for antigen typing and maternal serum should be tested for the presence of platelet-specific and HLA alloantibodies. **Fig. 4** illustrates the algorithm described for diagnosis.

Appropriate therapy for infants with suspected NAIT and severe thrombocytopenia or hemorrhagic manifestations should be commenced as soon as possible and not delayed until after confirmatory tests are complete. The most effective treatment for such infants is the transfusion of antigen-negative compatible platelets. The most reliable source for compatible platelets is the mother. This is because the putative platelet antigen is lacking on her platelets. However, if maternal platelets are used, they must be plasma depleted by centrifugation or washing to remove maternal alloantibodies. If maternal platelets are unavailable or deemed inappropriate, antigen-negative platelets may be obtained from another family member or unrelated blood donor.[15] Management while awaiting compatible antigen-negative platelet includes a high-dose corticosteroid course, exchange transfusion, IVIG infusion, or a trial of random donor platelets. IVIG or glucocorticoid therapy may increase platelet counts rapidly, although a substantial increase of platelet counts usually does not occur until after 24 to 72 hours.[7] In cases with severe bleeding, platelets should be transfused. Repeated platelet transfusions may be required. Platelet counts usually increase rapidly after transfusion.

PRENATAL MANAGEMENT

In cases where the possibility of NAIT is suspected before delivery because of a history of previously affected sibling, the finding of hydrocephalous or intracranial bleed on ultrasound in the current pregnancy or the finding of maternal platelet alloantibodies on serum testing warrants prenatal testing. The existence of fetomaternal platelet antigen incompatibility can be confirmed by first genotyping for paternal platelet antigens. In cases that remain at risk, fetal platelet genotyping can be obtained by chorionic villus sampling or amniocentesis. Studies looking at fetal platelet genotyping by cell-free fetal DNA in maternal plasma are ongoing but may provide a noninvasive route for diagnosis in the near future.[16] Reference laboratories for platelet genotyping in the United States include Blood Center of Wisconsin and Puget Sound Blood Center.

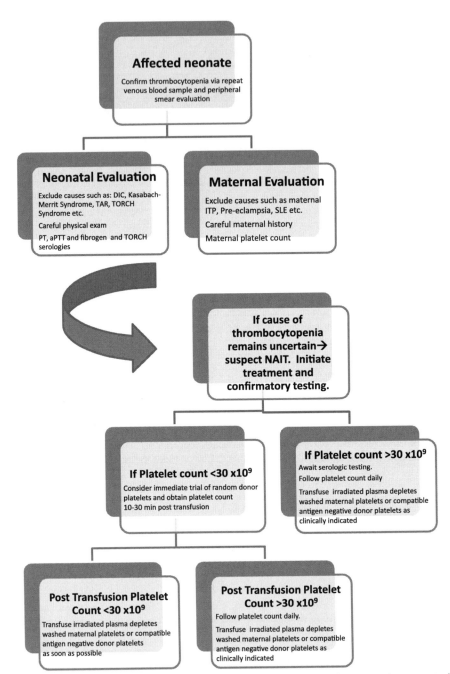

Fig. 4. Algorithm for management of unexpected neonatal thrombocytopenia, suspected NAIT. (*Data from* Blanchette VS, Johnson J, Rand M. The management of alloimmune neonatal thrombocytopenia. Baillieres Best Pract Res Clin Haematol 2000;13(3):365–90.)

The treatment options for suspected NAIT include maternal IVIG administration; glucocorticoids; serial in utero platelet transfusions; in utero IVIG administration; and early delivery (after 32 weeks of gestation). Choice of treatment regimen is usually directed by perceived risk of NAIT. The risk for NAIT has been stratified into standard risk, high risk, and highest or very high risk based on prior clinical history as shown in **Table 5**.[17–20] For cases at standard risk treatment should consist of either maternal IVIG administration at a dosage of 1 g/kg/wk starting at 20 weeks gestational age or prednisone at a dose of 0.5 mg/kg daily starting at 20 weeks gestational age. For cases at high risk, therapy with IVIG and high-dose corticosteroids should be instituted. A regimen of maternal IVIG administration at a dosage of 1 g/kg/wk and prednisone at a dose of 1 mg/kg daily should be instituted at 20 weeks gestational age. In cases that are at very high risk maternal IVIG administration at a dosage of 2 g/kg/wk should be started at 12 weeks gestational age. Fetal blood sampling (FBS) should then be performed at 20 weeks gestational age and if the fetus is found to be thrombocytopenic prednisone at a dose of 1 mg/kg daily should be added (**Fig. 5**).[17–22] In patients who do not respond to IVIG and glucocorticoid administration, serial matched platelet transfusions may be used. Matched platelet transfusions only transiently increase the fetal platelet count because the transfused platelets also are targeted.[1] Treatment regimens should be continued until delivery. In severely thrombocytopenic fetuses, early delivery with cesarean section may help reduce the risk of ICH.[6]

Table 5	
Approach to risk assessment for women with history of NAIT in prior pregnancy	
Clinical Features of Prior Pregnancy	**Risk of Baby with Severe NAIT**
Previous sibling with antenatal ICH	Highest or very high risk
Previous sibling with in utero fetal death	Highest or very high risk
Previous sibling with peripartum ICH	High risk
Previous sibling with isolated thrombocytopenia, no ICH	Standard risk

Data from McQuilten ZK, Wood EM, Savoia H, et al. A review of pathophysiology and current treatment for neonatal alloimmune thrombocytopenia (NAIT) and introducing the Australian NAIT registry. Aust N Z J Obstet Gynaecol 2011;51:191–8.

FBS AND IN UTERO PLATELET TRANSFUSION

FBS can be used to diagnose and determine the severity of thrombocytopenia, allow in utero transfusion, and measure response to and direct therapy.[21]

Most centers prefer to undertake these procedures in an operating room setting on the labor and delivery unit or in an ultrasound unit in close proximity to an operating room because serious complications (eg, prolonged bradycardia) may necessitate an emergent cesarean delivery if the fetus is considered viable, greater than 24 weeks gestational age. Some providers may consider an antenatal steroid course before the procedure to promote fetal lung maturity in the case that an emergent delivery becomes necessary. Patients are usually instructed to avoid oral intake for 6 to 8 hours before the procedure and intravenous access is secured before the procedure.

Before the procedure the abdomen is prepared and draped, after which the cord insertion site at the placenta is identified using ultrasound guidance. A 22-gauge amniocentesis needle is then introduced into the umbilical vein at the cord insertion site under continuous real-time ultrasound visualization. In contrast to intrauterine transfusion of red blood cells, a smaller caliber needle is used to minimize the risk of bleeding from the puncture site because the risk for fetal exsanguination is increased twofold over cordocentesis in other conditions.[18,23]

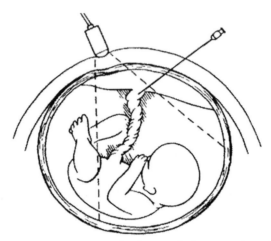

Fig. 5. Fetal blood sampling or in utero platelet transfusion procedure. After cleansing the mother's abdomen with antiseptic, a long, thin needle is inserted into the mother's uterus guided by ultrasound into blood vessels of the umbilical cord. Fetal blood is sampled for fetal platelet count. Using the same technique fetal platelet transfusion can be accomplished.

An initial sample of blood is withdrawn for hematologic evaluation. In addition to determining the platelet count, mean corpuscular red cell volume can be assessed as a method of affirming that fetal, as opposed to maternal, blood has been obtained (mean corpuscular volume >100 μL suggests fetal red blood cells). After withdrawing a blood sample, a short-acting paralytic agent is used to minimize fetal movement and prevent tearing of the umbilical vein. The decision to transfuse platelets should not be undertaken on an empiric basis because the infusion of platelets when the fetal platelet count is normal can result in thrombocytosis, hypercoagulability, and fetal death.

Antigen-negative platelets (from a blood group O donor) should be processed and available at the bedside to treat significant thrombocytopenia and reduce the risk of puncture site bleeding. Alternatively, maternal platelets can be obtained by apheresis 48 hours before the procedure and washed to remove the offending antibody.

If platelet transfusion is decided on, the primary operator should visualize the transfused platelets streaming away from the needle as they mix with fetal blood in the umbilical vein throughout the transfusion. The fetal heart rate should be monitored periodically to check for bradycardia. At the end of the platelet infusion, a second blood sample should be obtained to determine the final platelet count and the needle is removed. In cases where transfusion is decided against, some providers infuse a small aliquot (3–5 mL) of platelets to serve as a plug at the site of puncture to reduce postprocedural blood loss. At the completion of all procedures the site of puncture should be visualized to determine if there is excessive bleeding or streaming.

The volume of platelet transfusion is determined using the following equation:

Volume transfused (mL)

$$= \frac{\text{Fetoplacental Volume (mL)} \times (\text{target final} - \text{initial platelet count}) \times 2}{\text{Platelet count of transfused concentrate}}$$

The fetoplacental volume is calculated by multiplying the ultrasound estimate of fetal weight in grams by 0.14. The factor of 2 is used in the numerator of the equation to allow for possible platelet sequestration in the fetal spleen or liver. Because the half-life of platelets is only about 3 days, the target final fetal platelet count is 300,000 to 500,000/μL to achieve a nadir platelet count of 30,000 to 50,000/μL at the time of the next transfusion.[24] Transfusions are generally repeated weekly because of the limited half-life of transfused platelets. Although no clear gestational age threshold for delivery can be garnered from the literature, delivery after 32 weeks of gestation seems prudent if serial transfusions are being performed.

FBS and in utero platelet transfusion carries with it significant procedure-associated risks including bleeding, premature delivery, and death. It has been estimated that FBS and in utero platelet transfusion has a fetal loss rate of 1.3% per procedure and 5% to 8% per affected pregnancy. Serial in utero platelet transfusion was investigated by Overton and colleagues[25] in 2002. This study included 12 pregnancies that underwent a total of 84 transfusions. In this cohort two intrauterine fetal deaths were observed resulting in a fetal loss rate of 1.2% per procedure and 8.3% per pregnancy. However, no ICH was observed in survivors. Given these reported rates of fetal loss, the role of FBS and in utero platelet transfusion in the management of NAIT has diminished and is generally limited to use in highest risk and refractory cases.

MODE OF DELIVERY

There is no consensus on the most appropriate mode of delivery. A prospective study of 200 cases of NAIT identified 17 cases of postnatal ICH, all of which occurred within 24 hours of delivery, suggesting perhaps the trauma of delivery as a triggering factor. In support of this theory a large screening study out of Norway found a lower rate of NAIT-related adverse events with the use of early cesarean delivery when compared with historical controls. Van den Akker and colleagues[26] reported on 32 pregnancies affected by NAIT managed with IVIG who underwent cesarean delivery only for obstetric indications. In contrast to the previously mentioned studies this group found no difference in outcomes of ICH or death between those delivered vaginally and those delivered by cesarean section, even in the setting of severe thrombocytopenia.[27]

In the absence of clear evidence for a preferential mode of delivery some suggest using a delivery algorithm based perceived risk as outlined in **Table 5**. In this scheme those at high and highest risk should be considered candidates for cesarean delivery. It seems most generally accepted, however, that vaginal delivery only be allowed for those patients whose fetuses have a platelet count greater than 50×10^9/L at the time of delivery (or >100×10^9/L at 32 weeks gestational age) as assessed by FBS. As previously described, FBS carries significant risks for bleeding, premature or emergent delivery, and fetal loss, so many may opt to forgo FBS and true fetal platelet count remains unknown. For cases where fetal platelet count is unknown, cesarean section before term is commonly recommended, although evidence supporting this practice is lacking. In all cases, delivery should occur in a tertiary care center secondary to the risk for ICH and need for platelet transfusion.

REFERENCES

1. Letsky EA, Greaves M. Guidelines on the investigation and management of thrombocytopenia in pregnancy and neonatal alloimmune thrombocytopenia. Maternal and Neonatal Haemostasis Working Party of the Haemostasis and Thrombosis Task Force of the British Society for Haematology. Br J Haematol 1996;95:21.
2. McQuilten ZK, Wood EM, Savoia H, et al. A review of pathophysiology and current treatment for neonatal alloimmune thrombocytopenia (NAIT) and introducing the Australian NAIT registry. Aust N Z J Obstet Gynaecol 2011;51:191–8.
3. Wiedmeier SE, Henry E, Sola-Visner MC, et al. Platelet reference ranges for neonates, defined using data from over 47,000 patients in a multihospital healthcare system. J Perinatol 2009;29:130.
4. Mueller-Eckhardt C, Kiefel V, Grubert A, et al. 348 cases of suspected neonatal alloimmune thrombocytopenia. Lancet 1989;1:363.
5. Bishop JF, Matthews JP, Yuen K, et al. The definition of refractoriness to platelet transfusions. Transfus Med 1992;2:35.
6. Jolly MC, Letsky EA, Fisk NM. The management of fetal alloimmune thrombocytopenia. Prenat Diagn 2002;22:96.
7. Kaplan C. Alloimmune thrombocytopenia of the fetus and the newborn. Blood Rev 2002;16:69.
8. Grainger JD, Morrell G, Yates J, et al. Neonatal alloimmune thrombocytopenia with significant HLA antibodies. Arch Dis Child Fetal Neonatal Ed 2002;86:F200.
9. Davoren A, McParland P, Crowley J, et al. Antenatal screening for human platelet antigen-1a: results of a prospective study at a large maternity hospital in Ireland. BJOG 2003;110:492.
10. Williamson LM, Hackett G, Rennie J, et al. The natural history of fetomaternal alloimmunization to the platelet-specific antigen HPA-1a (PIA1, Zwa) as determined by antenatal screening. Blood 1998;92:2280.
11. Murphy MF, Hambley H, Nicolaides K, et al. Severe fetomaternal alloimmune thrombocytopenia presenting with fetal hydrocephalus. Prenat Diagn 1996;16: 1152.
12. Kaplan C, Murphy MF, Kroll H, et al. Feto-maternal alloimmune thrombocytopenia: antenatal therapy with IVIgG and steroids. More questions than answers. European Working Group on FMAIT. Br J Haematol 1998;100:62.
13. Blanchette VS, Johnson J, Rand M. The management of alloimmune neonatal thrombocytopenia. Baillieres Best Pract Res Clin Haematol 2000;13(3):365–90.
14. Risson D, Davies M, Williams B. Review of neonatal alloimmune thrombocytopenia. J Paediatr Child Health 2012;48:816–22.
15. Ouwehand WH, Smith G, Ranasinghe E. Management of severe alloimmune thrombocytopenia in the newborn. Arch Dis Child Fetal Neonatal Ed 2000;82: F173.
16. Scheffer P, Ait Soussan A, Verhagen O, et al. Noninvasive fetal genotyping of human platelet antigen-1a. BJOG 2011;118:1392–5.
17. Symington A, Paes B. Fetal and neonatal alloimmune thrombocytopenia: harvesting the evidence to develop a clinical approach to management. Am J Perinatol 2011;28:137–44.
18. Silver RM, Porter TF, Branch DW, et al. Neonatal alloimmune thrombocytopenia: antenatal management. Am J Obstet Gynecol 2000;182(5):1233–8.
19. Porcelijn L, Kanhai HH. Fetal thrombocytopenia. Curr Opin Obstet Gynecol 1998; 10:117.

20. Birchall JE, Murphy MF, Kaplan C, et al. European collaborative study of the antenatal management of fetomaternal alloimmune thrombocytopenia. Br J Haematol 2003;122(2):275–88.
21. Berkowitz RL, Bussel JB, McFarland JG. Alloimmune thrombocytopenia: state of the art 2006. Am J Obstet Gynecol 2006;195(4):907–13.
22. Weiner E, Zosmer N, Bajoria R, et al. Direct fetal administration of immunoglobulins: another disappointing therapy in alloimmune thrombocytopenia. Fetal Diagn Ther 1994;9:159.
23. Radder CM, Brand A, Kanhai HH. Will it ever be possible to balance the risk of intracranial haemorrhage in fetal or neonatal alloimmune thrombocytopenia against the risk of treatment strategies to prevent it? Vox Sang 2003;84:318–25.
24. Murphy MF, Waters AH, Doughty HA, et al. Antenatal management of fetomaternal alloimmune thrombocytopenia: report of 15 affected pregnancies. Transfus Med 1994;4:281–92.
25. Overton T, Duncan K, Jolly M, et al. Serial aggressive platelet transfusion for fetal alloimmune thrombocytopenia: platelet dynamics and perinatal outcome. Am J Obstet Gynecol 2002;186(4):826–31.
26. Van Den Akker E, Oepkes D, Brand A, et al. Vaginal delivery for fetuses at risk of alloimmune thrombocytopenia? BJOG 2006;113:781–3.
27. Ghevaert C, Campbell K, Walton J, et al. Management and outcome of 200 cases of fetomaternal alloimmune thrombocytopenia. Transfusion 2007;47:901–10.

Maternal Thrombocytopenia in Pregnancy: Diagnosis and Management

Tracy M. Adams, DO[a,b,*], M. Baraa Allaf, MD[a,b],
Anthony M. Vintzileos, MD[a,b]

KEYWORDS

- Thrombocytopenia • Pregnancy • Immune thrombocytopenia
- Thrombotic thrombocytopenic purpura • HELLP syndrome

KEY POINTS

- Thrombocytopenia affects 7% to 10% of pregnancies.
- Around 70% of thrombocytopenia in pregnancy is caused by gestational thrombocytopenia, which is a benign phenomenon.
- ITP is the most common cause of thrombocytopenia at less than 20 weeks gestation and the focus of treatment is to increase platelet counts to prevent spontaneous bleeding and to ensure a safe delivery.
- TTP is a rare but life-threatening disease that should be suspected with thrombocytopenia and MAHA, and treatment with IVIG should begin immediately to prevent death.
- Preeclampsia, HELLP syndrome, and AFLP are obstetric causes of thrombocytopenia in pregnancy. Delivery is the treatment of choice for these disorders; however, it does not guarantee a cure, and postpartum supportive care is often warranted.

INTRODUCTION

Thrombocytopenia in pregnancy is defined as a platelet count of less than 150×10^9/L and can be caused by either diminished production or increased destruction of platelets. Thrombocytopenia is a common finding in pregnancy and affects approximately 7% to 10% of pregnancies.[1] Some studies suggest that the platelet count in normal pregnancy is lower than that in the nonpregnant state; however, most women still maintain platelet levels in the normal range.[2,3] Thrombocytopenia is classified as mild when platelet counts are between 100 and 150×10^9/L, moderate when platelets are between 50 and 100×10^9/L, and severe if platelet counts fall lower than 50×10^9/L.

Although most cases of thrombocytopenia in pregnancy do not result in adverse outcomes, the underlying pathology can sometimes be life threatening; therefore,

[a] Stony Brook University Hospital, 101 Nicolls Road, Stony Brook, NY 11794, USA; [b] Department of Obstetrics and Gynecology, Winthrop University Hospital, 259 First Street, Mineola, NY 11501, USA
* Corresponding author.
E-mail address: Tadams@winthrop.org

Clin Lab Med 33 (2013) 327–341
http://dx.doi.org/10.1016/j.cll.2013.01.002
0272-2712/13/$ – see front matter © 2013 Elsevier Inc. All rights reserved.

when thrombocytopenia is diagnosed in pregnancy the woman should undergo further clinical and laboratory assessment to determine the cause. Thrombocytopenia can have medical and obstetric causes. The causes of thrombocytopenia in pregnancy are summarized in **Tables 1** and **2** according to frequency, severity, and timing of presentation (<20 vs >20 weeks gestation).

DIFFERENTIAL DIAGNOSIS

The differential diagnosis for thrombocytopenia is extensive; however, a thorough history and physical examination can help significantly to narrow the diagnosis. If the low platelet count was seen on automated complete blood count a manual count should first be ordered to rule out pseudothrombocytopenia. This phenomenon occurs because of platelet clumping caused by the addition of anticoagulant ethylenediaminetetraacetic acid to the sample. If clumps are seen on manual count, a repeat complete blood count using citrate as an anticoagulant instead may improve the sample.

A detailed history inquiring about medications, alcohol and drug use, and eating habits could quickly narrow the differential. The history should also include a risk assessment for HIV and hepatitis. Key questions regarding the symptoms of systemic lupus erythematosus (SLE) or antiphospholipid antibody syndrome can also help to determine if these entities are responsible for the thrombocytopenia.

A thorough review of the complete blood count with differential and a comprehensive metabolic panel can help to determine if a primary marrow disorder or liver disease is the cause. **Table 3** identifies distinguishing factors between thrombotic thrombocytopenia purpura (TTP); hemolytic uremic syndrome (HUS); hemolysis elevated liver enzymes, low platelet (HELLP) syndrome; preeclampsia and eclampsia; immune thrombocytopenia (ITP); and gestational thrombocytopenia (GT).

Table 1
Causes of thrombocytopenia in pregnancy at less than 20 weeks gestation

Causes According to Decreasing Frequency	Causes According to Decreasing Severity
Autoimmune thrombocytopenia	Thrombotic thrombocytopenia Purpura/hemolytic uremic syndrome
Gestational thrombocytopenia	Heparin-induced thrombocytopenia
Pseudothrombocytopenia (artifactual or dilutional)	Infection (HIV, viral disease, bacterial disease with sepsis)
Drug-induced refer to **Box 2**	Primary marrow disorder
Connective tissue disorder (systemic lupus erythematosus and antiphospholipid antibody syndrome)	Connective tissue disorders
Primary bone marrow disorder (acute leukemia, aplastic anemia, myelodysplasia)	Other drug-induced refer to **Box 2**
Infection (HIV, viral disease, bacterial disease with sepsis)	Hypersplenism
Hypersplenism (liver disease, Epstein-Barr virus, lymphoproliferative disorder)	Alcoholism, malnutrition, folate or B_{12} deficiency
Alcoholism, malnutrition, folate or B_{12} deficiency	Autoimmune thrombocytopenia
Thrombotic thrombocytopenia Purpura/hemolytic uremic syndrome	Gestational thrombocytopenia
	Pseudothrombocytopenia

Table 2
Causes of thrombocytopenia in pregnancy at greater than 20 weeks gestation

According to Decreasing Frequency	According to Decreasing Severity
Gestational thrombocytopenia	Acute fatty liver/TTP/HUS
Autoimmune thrombocytopenia	Heparin-induced thrombocytopenia
Pseudothrombocytopenia	Preeclampsia or HELLP syndrome
Preeclampsia or HELLP syndrome	Infection (HIV, viral disease, bacterial disease with sepsis)
Drug-induced refer to **Box 2**	Primary bone marrow disorder (acute leukemia, aplastic anemia, myelodysplasia)
Connective tissue disorder (SLE and antiphospholipid antibody syndrome)	Connective tissue disorder (SLE, and antiphospholipid antibody syndrome)
TTP/HUS	Drug-induced refer to **Box 2**
Acute fatty liver	Hypersplenism (liver disease, EBV, lymphoproliferative disorder)
Primary bone marrow disorder (acute leukemia, aplastic anemia, myelodysplasia)	Alcoholism, malnutrition, folate or B_{12} deficiency
Infection (HIV, viral disease, bacterial disease with sepsis)	Autoimmune thrombocytopenia
Hypersplenism (liver disease, EBV, lymphoproliferative disorder)	Gestational thrombocytopenia
Alcoholism, malnutrition, folate, or B_{12} deficiency	Pseudothrombocytopenia

Abbreviations: EBV, Epstein-Barr virus; HELLP, hemolysis elevated liver enzymes, low platelets syndrome; HUS, hemolytic uremic syndrome; SLE, systemic lupus erythematosus; TTP, thrombotic thrombocytopenic purpura.

GESTATIONAL THROMBOCYTOPENIA

GT is the leading cause of thrombocytopenia during pregnancy. It occurs in up to 5% to 8% of pregnant women and accounts for more than 70% of maternal thrombocytopenia.[4,5] Unlike ITP, the degree of thrombocytopenia in GT is usually mild to moderate, typically remaining greater than $70 \times 10^9/L$, and about two-thirds being 130 to $150 \times 10^9/L$.[5] Patients are asymptomatic with no evidence of bleeding and

Table 3
Distinguishing factors of causes of thrombocytopenia in pregnancy

Characteristic	Preeclampsia	HELLP	HUS	TTP	ITP	GT
Onset	>20 wk	>20 wk	Postpartum	Throughout	Throughout	>20 wk
MAHA	±	+	+	+	−	−
Coagulopathy	±	+	−	−	−	−
Hypertension	+	+	+	−	−	−
Renal dysfunction	+	+	+	±	−	−
Hepatic dysfunction	±	+	±	±	−	−
Neurologic involvement	±	±	±	+	−	−
Abdominal symptoms	±	+	±	±	−	−

Abbreviations: GT, gestational thrombocytopenia; HELLP, hemolysis elevated liver enzymes, low platelets syndrome; HUS, hemolytic uremic syndrome; ITP, idiopathic thrombocytopenic purpura; MAHA, microangiopathic hemolytic anemia; TTP, thrombotic thrombocytopenic purpura.

report no history of thrombocytopenia outside pregnancy. It has extremely low risk of fetal thrombocytopenia.[6] The platelet count usually returns to normal within 2 to 12 weeks postpartum. **Box 1** summarizes the characteristics of GT.

There are significant differences between GT and ITP in the onset time of thrombocytopenia, the lowest platelets level, and the postpartum recovery.[7] If the platelet count is less than 70×10^9/L, the most likely diagnosis is ITP. However, it is not possible to distinguish between the more severe form of GT and ITP until the postpartum period, because both are diagnoses of exclusion.[1] In general, the detection of thrombocytopenia before 28 weeks' gestation and a platelet count less than 50×10^9/L highly suggests a diagnosis of ITP.[8]

The pathogenesis of GT is not understood. It may occur as a result of an acceleration of increased platelet destruction that occurs during pregnancy or because of the reduced lifespan of platelets during pregnancy.[9,10]

GT does not seem to have negative implications for either mother or fetus. No risk for fetal hemorrhage or bleeding complications is observed.[11] Therefore, the only special care required for these women is assessment of platelet counts close to term, and follow-up platelet counts postpartum.

Management

GT requires no treatment and routine prenatal care is appropriate.[12] Platelet count should be monitored every 4 weeks; more frequent monitoring as pregnancy advances depends on the rate of decline. Weekly platelet counts starting at 36 weeks are reasonable if the platelet counts fall lower than 70×10^9/L.

The mode of delivery is determined by obstetric and maternal indications. Epidural anesthesia is considered to be safe in women with GT who have platelet counts higher than 50 to 80×10^9/L.[13]

In the postpartum period a normal neonatal platelet count and a restoration of normal maternal platelet values after delivery confirms the diagnosis of GT. Should thrombocytopenia persist the patient should be evaluated by a hematologist. Recurrence of GT in subsequent pregnancies is common, and the patient should be informed of this after her initial diagnosis is made.

IMMUNE THROMBOCYTOPENIC PURPURA

ITP occurs in 1 in 1000 to 1 in 10,000 pregnancies, and is responsible for 3% of all thrombocytopenia at delivery.[14,15] Although an uncommon entity in pregnancy, ITP is the most common cause of platelet dysfunction before 20 weeks gestation.[16] The

---

Box 1
Characteristics of GT

1. Mild to moderate thrombocytopenia ($>70 \times 10^9$/L)

2. Asymptomatic with no history of abnormal bleeding

3. No history of thrombocytopenia outside pregnancies

4. Occurs in mid-second or third trimester

5. No fetal or neonatal thrombocytopenia

6. Complete postpartum resolution

7. Recur in subsequent pregnancies

8. Detected on routine prenatal screening with no specific diagnostic tests

recent international consensus group defines ITP as a platelet count of less than 100×10^9/L in the absence of any other causes for the thrombocytopenia.[17] ITP is an autoimmune process in which there is impaired platelet production and increased platelet destruction. The main site of platelet destruction is the spleen. Around two-thirds of patients with ITP in pregnancy have pre-existing disease, whereas only one-third are diagnosed in pregnancy.[18]

Maternal Presentation

In adults the onset of ITP is usually insidious with no identifiable precipitating factors. Many people are asymptomatic and only diagnosed incidentally by routine laboratory assessment, such as done in pregnancy. If symptoms are present they can range from minimal bruising to serious bleeding from multiple sites including the mucosa, gastrointestinal tract, and intracranial hemorrhage. Spontaneous bleeding is usually not a concern unless the platelet count falls lower than 20×10^9/L. It is believed that ITP is not affected by pregnancy; however, pregnancy, particularly delivery and the postpartum period, can be affected by thrombocytopenia, the major concern being uncontrolled hemorrhage.

Neonatal Presentation

Maternal IgG antiplatelet antibodies can cross the placenta, and studies indicate that 12% to 15% of infants born to these mothers develop severe thrombocytopenia.[12,19] Severe neonatal thrombocytopenia can manifest as petechiae, ecchymoses, melena, and on rare occasions intracranial hemorrhage. Severe hemorrhage caused by neonatal thrombocytopenia is a rare event, and has not been associated with mode of delivery; therefore, cesarean delivery in women with ITP should be reserved for obstetric indications.[19,20] Invasive fetal procedures that can cause bleeding, such as placement of a scalp electrode, forceps, or vacuum delivery, should be avoided because of these concerns. Maternal characteristics including platelet count, presence of antiplatelet antibody, antecedent history of autoimmune thrombocytopenia, and corticosteroid therapy have not proved to be predictive of severe neonatal thrombocytopenia.[19]

Diagnosis

ITP first presenting in pregnancy can represent a diagnostic challenge. It is a diagnosis of exclusion, and specific diagnostic tests are used to rule out other causes of thrombocytopenia. The physician should:

- Perform a thorough history and physical examination
- Patients should have a complete blood count with reticulocyte count, peripheral blood film
- Patients should be screened for HIV, hepatitis C virus (HCV), and *Helicobacter pylori*

Special differential diagnostic considerations in the pregnant woman are for HELLP syndrome, preeclampsia, acute fatty liver of pregnancy (AFLP), obstetric hemorrhage, antiphospholipid antibody syndrome, folate deficiency, and GT. Bone marrow examination is not required in pregnancy, and antiplatelet immunoglobulin measurement has no value in the diagnosis of ITP in pregnancy, because some crossover can be seen with GT.[16] It may be impossible to distinguish GT from ITP during pregnancy, because resolution postpartum may be the only distinguishing factor between the two entities.

Management

Management of ITP in pregnancy should take a multidisciplinary approach and include an obstetrician, maternal fetal medicine specialist, hematologist, obstetric anesthesiologist, and neonatologist. Treatment should be started in a woman in the first and second trimesters if she is symptomatic or if the platelet counts fall lower than 20×10^9/L, because of the risk of spontaneous bleeding. In the third trimester consideration must be given to the bleeding risk at delivery and the possibility of receiving regional anesthesia. Platelet counts may fall in the third trimester; frequent monitoring in the third trimester is warranted so that preparations can be made for delivery.[21] A platelet count of greater than 50×10^9/L is generally accepted as safe for invasive procedures and delivery.[22]

The minimum platelet count to allow administration of regional anesthesia is controversial, however, because of the theoretical risk of epidural hematoma formation and subsequent neurologic injury.[23] The American National Red Cross, the French Society of Anesthesia, and the British Committee for Standards in Haematology in guidelines for the management of ITP suggest a minimum platelet count of 80×10^9/L to administer epidural anesthesia.[24–26] However, many obstetric anesthesiologists administer regional anesthesia at lower levels based on individual risks and benefits. Therefore, patients with ITP should have consultation with an obstetric anesthesiologist proximal to the time of delivery to review all anesthetic options.

First-line Therapy

Corticosteroids

The two main primary treatment options for ITP in pregnancy are corticosteroids and intravenous immune globulin (IVIG). The first-line therapy is low-dose prednisone (10–20 mg/day),[17] which could be increased to 1 to 1.5 mg/kg/d if needed. A response usually occurs within 3 to 7 days, and platelet counts reach their maximum in 2 to 3 weeks.[22] The dose is then adjusted to maintain a platelet count at which the patient has no symptoms, or higher than 50×10^9/L. Low-dose prednisone is generally accepted as safe treatment in pregnancy; however, it may exacerbate hypertension, hyperglycemia, and osteoporosis, and may cause excessive weight gain and psychosis. Discontinuation should be done with a taper to avoid precipitation of an adrenal crisis.

Intravenous immune globulin

If corticosteroids are ineffective, or if a faster rise in platelet count is required, IVIG should be used. Response to IVIG therapy is expected to occur within 6 to 72 hours. IVIG is a temporary treatment and 70% of patients have pretreatment platelet counts within 30 days; repeat infusions may be repeated as needed to maintain an adequate platelet count for delivery.[17,27,28] The regimen of IVIG treatment that has been shown to have greatest increase in platelets is 1 g/kg given as one or two infusions over 2 days.[17] Headache is a common side effect of this treatment. Rarely, renal failure and thrombosis result from IVIG treatment.

Additional Therapies

Intravenous anti-D treatment has been found safe and effective in the second and third trimesters for Rh (D)-positive pregnant women who have never had a splenectomy.[29,30] The dose is 50 to 75 μg/kg. Response is usually seen in 4 to 5 days. Common side effects are hemolytic anemia, fever, and chills. Rare side effects include intravascular hemolysis, disseminated intravascular coagulation (DIC), renal failure, and death. The neonates of treated women should be observed for neonatal jaundice, anemia, and direct antiglobulin test positivity.[17]

In refractory cases of ITP, combination of IVIG with high-dose methylprednisone (1000 mg) has been suggested.[21] Platelet transfusion in combination with IVIG therapy has been associated with decreased bleeding and a rapid increase in platelet counts in some patients.[31,32]

Other medical treatments for ITP that are safe in pregnancy include azathioprine, cyclosporin A, and rituximab. Azathioprine has been found useful in patients with a splenectomy at a dose of 150 mg/day.[33] Cyclosporin A has been successful in patients who fail first-line therapy. In one study, 80% of patients who failed therapy with steroids and IVIG responded to treatment with cyclosporin A.[34]

Surgical management of ITP is a splenectomy. Eighty percent of patients respond to splenectomy and 66% of patients who respond require no additional therapy for at least 5 years.[35–37] Splenectomy can be performed safely in pregnancy and often a laparoscopic approach is used. After splenectomy pregnant women require vaccination against infections with *Streptoccus pneumoniae*, *Haemophilus influenza, and Neisseria meningitides.*

Treatment of a patient with ITP should be a collaboration between the obstetrician, hematologist, and obstetric anesthesiologist. Therapy should be based on the patient's symptoms and platelet count if they are close to term, and the decision between oral prednisone and IVIG therapy should be based on the severity of the symptoms and how rapidly the increase in platelet count is required. There are therapies available for refractory ITP, which should be tailored to meet the individual's needs.

THROMBOTIC THROMBOCYTOPENIC PURPURA

TTP is a rare disorder occurring in 1 in 25,000 pregnancies.[1] It is a severe disease caused by a deficiency of von Willebrand cleaving protein ADAMTS13. When von Willebrand factor molecules are not cleaved platelet aggregation occurs, which causes thrombi in the microcirculation. TTP can be congenital or acquired immune. In congenital TTP there is a genetic cause for ADAMTS13 deficiency, but in acquired immune TTP there are antibodies directed against ADAMTS13, which causes its deficiency.[38,39]

TTP is seen more commonly in females than in males with a 3:1 ratio.[1] Diagnosis is first made in pregnancy in 5% to 25% of TTP cases because pregnancy can be a precipitating factor.[40] TTP can be difficult to diagnose when presenting for the first time in pregnancy because it shares many characteristics with pregnancy-related disorders. **Table 3** highlights many distinguishing factors between ITP and these disorders.

Clinical Presentation

TTP has classically been associated with the pentad of (1) thrombocytopenia, (2) microangiopathic hemolytic anemia (MAHA), (3) renal dysfunction, (4) neurologic disorders, and (5) fever. It has been noted, however, that renal dysfunction and fever are frequently absent, and neurologic disorders are not seen in up to 35% of patients. Therefore, revised diagnostic criteria state the presence of thrombocytopenia, and microangiopathic anemia alone should raise suspicion for TTP.[41] Clinical symptoms of TTP are variable because they are representative of multiorgan thromboses. Thrombocytopenia can present asymptomatic. Neurologic symptoms are variable and range from headache to coma and are often transient. Renal dysfunction can manifest as proteinuria or microhematuria. Patients can present with chest pain or severe abdominal pain suggesting cardiac and gastrointestinal involvement. In addition, many patients have nonspecific symptoms, such as arthralgia and myalgia fatigue and jaundice.

Diagnosis

The diagnosis is based on presenting history of symptoms, physical examination, and complete blood count with a peripheral smear.[40] ADAMTS13 assays are used for diagnosis confirmation and to monitor for possible relapse every 3 to 4 months (discussed later).

Laboratory Assessment

On complete blood cell count thrombocytopenia and anemia are present. The median platelet count at presentation is 10 to 30 $\times$ 10^9/L, and median hemoglobin levels are 8 to 10 g/dL.[40] On the peripheral smear schistocytes are seen and represent red blood cell destruction. Haptoglobin should be low, and reticulocyte count and lactate dehydrogenase should be high. The coagulation profile (prothrombin time, partial thromboplastin time, and fibrinogen) is usually normal, which can be helpful in distinguishing from other microangipathies. Elevated troponin T has been seen in 50% of cases of acute idiopathic TTP, which is alarming because coronary artery occlusion can lead to sudden death.[42]

ADAMTS13 Assay

Treatment should be started as soon as a patient presents with MAHA and thrombocytopenia (preferably within 4–8 hours).[40] Treatment should not be delayed until the results of the ADAMTS13 assay are available. Before starting treatment of suspected TTP, however, blood should be drawn to measure ADAMTS13 activity; if it is less than 5% the diagnosis of TTP is established.[43] ADAMTS13 activity has been reported as decreased in normal pregnancy, but not to less than 5%.[44]

Management

The treatment of choice for suspected or confirmed acute TTP is daily plasma exchange therapy. This therapy has been shown to reduce mortality rates from 90% down to 10% to 20%,[40] and this is why prompt initiation of treatment is so important. In addition to removing autoantibodies, plasma exchange increases ADAMTS13 levels. Because TTP can be difficult to distinguish from the pregnancy-related microangiopathies, if diagnosis is made in the third trimester delivery is often beneficial because it is the definitive treatment of pregnancy-related disease. If, however, TTP is diagnosed early in pregnancy regular plasma exchange therapy has led to progression of pregnancies with delivery of live infants.[40,45]

Plasma exchange is the treatment of choice for pregnant and nonpregnant patients. Although no optimal regimen has been identified the most recent guidelines recommend starting daily exchange with 1.5 $\times$ plasma volume exchange with solvent- or detergent-treated fresh frozen plasma (FFP), decreasing to a 1 $\times$ plasma volume exchange when the laboratory values stabilize, and continuing treatment for at least 2 days after the platelet count rises higher than 150 $\times$ 10^9/L. For refractory disease corticosteroids or rituximab may be added to plasma exchange to improve outcomes. Red blood cell transfusion and folate supplementation should be given as needed. When platelets are higher than 50 $\times$ 10^9/L begin thromboprophylaxis. After treatment patients should be started on corticosteroids for maintenance.[40]

Pregnant patients with TTP should be followed by a maternal fetal medicine specialist, and serial fetal monitoring for growth and antenatal surveillance with maternal and fetal Doppler studies should be performed. The patient should also be followed closely for the development of preeclampsia because she is at an increased risk of ischemic placental disease.

Future Pregnancies

Recurrence of TTP in subsequent pregnancies has been reported as high as 50%.[46] Baseline ADAMTS13 levels may be helpful in predicting which women will relapse, and if the activity is reduced to less than 10%, initiation of elective therapy may reduce microvascular thrombosis and improve pregnancy outcome.[40]

HEMOLYTIC UREMIC SYNDROME

HUS is a MAHA that can be difficult to distinguish from TTP. The incidence is not separated from that of TTP and is reported at 1 in 25,000 pregnancies. HUS is characterized by primary renal involvement. Usually HUS is precipitated by infection; however, there is an atypical form associated with pregnancy. The onset of pregnancy associated HUS is typically postpartum, which can be helpful in differentiating this from TTP. Patients present with acute renal failure, varying degrees of thrombocytopenia, and MAHA. In addition to the timing ADAMTS13 deficiency of less than 5% can help distinguish the two because the activity is not severely reduced in HUS.

MANAGEMENT

Treatment should be initiated with plasma exchange before the results of the ADAMTS13 assay for suspected TTP. Pregnancy-related HUS does not generally respond well to plasma exchange therapy, and 76% of patients with this disease develop end-stage renal disease.[47] Eculizumab has been used for treatment of pregnancy-related HUS and seems to be safe and effective at restoring kidney function.[48,49] It is currently approved for this use in the United States.

THROMBOCYTOPENIA RELATED TO OBSTETRIC DISORDERS

These disorders include preeclampsia and eclampsia, HELLP syndrome, and AFLP. There is overlap between these obstetric disorders with the common feature of thrombocytopenia.

Preeclampsia and HELLP

Preeclampsia is a hypertensive disorder of pregnancy. The minimum diagnostic clinical findings are persistent hypertension (systolic blood pressure of $\leq$140 or diastolic blood pressure $\leq$90) and proteinuria ($\leq$1+ or 300 mg/d). In severe preeclampsia there are abnormal hepatic, renal, and hematologic laboratory findings, of which thrombocytopenia is a finding. Preeclampsia is a common cause of thrombocytopenia during the third trimester of pregnancy and is reported to cause as much as 21% of maternal thrombocytopenia.[1]

Moderate thrombocytopenia may be one of the earliest manifestations of preeclampsia, often preceding other laboratory findings of this disorder. Unlike preeclampsia, thrombocytopenia is a prominent manifestation of HELLP syndrome, and may be severe, with platelet counts less than 50×10^9 and the patient may develop DIC.

The pathophysiology of thrombocytopenia in these disorders might be related to endothelial damage and release of tissue factor and coagulation activation, which lead to accelerated platelet destruction, platelet activation, and enhanced platelet clearance.[50]

The primary treatment of thrombocytopenia in these conditions is achieved by delivery of the fetus. In cases of severe thrombocytopenia, patients should be stabilized first before delivery, often with blood products, such as FFP and cryoprecipitate. In general, platelet transfusions are less effective because of the ongoing process of platelet destruction.[22] Therefore, platelet transfusions are reserved for severe thrombocytopenia with active bleeding or to increase the platelet count in preparation for an operative delivery.[22]

In general thrombocytopenia recovery begins promptly after delivery and most patients resolve by 3 days postpartum.[51] Progression of thrombocytopenia and hemolysis beyond 3 days postpartum may require treatment with plasma exchange for the presumed diagnosis of TTP,[52] especially in the presence of neurologic symptoms or acute renal failure.

Acute Fatty Liver of Pregnancy

AFLP is a rare and serious disorder with an approximate incidence of 1:7000 to 1:20,000 deliveries.[53] Typically presentation is in the third trimester of pregnancy with nausea, vomiting, right upper quadrant pain, polyuria, polydipsia, and jaundice.

Laboratory findings include low platelet count; a recent study showed 47% of patients with AFLP had platelet count less than 100×10^9/L.[54] Other laboratory findings in AFLP are prolongation of prothrombin time, low fibrinogen, low antithrombin levels, elevated bilirubin levels, elevated white blood cell count, and hypoglycemia. Severe cases often present with jaundice or in acute renal failure with hyperuricemia.

The clinical picture is similar to DIC; however, in AFLP, the laboratory findings are not caused by consumption of the clotting factors but rather by decreased production by the impaired liver. There is a clinical overlap between AFLP and HELLP syndrome and it may be difficult to differentiate them. However, evidence of hepatic insufficiency, such as hypoglycemia, jaundice, or encephalopathy, is suggestive of AFLP.

Management

The medical treatment of AFLP is mainly supportive. The primary treatment is emergent delivery. This should occur after maternal stabilization, which requires glucose infusion and reversal of coagulopathy by administration of blood products, such as FFP, cryoprecipitate, packed red blood cells, and platelets as needed.

THROMBOCYTOPENIA RELATED TO MEDICAL DISORDERS

The medical disorders that cause thrombocytopenia are outlined **Tables 1** and **2.**

Antiphospholipid Syndrome

ITP is a clinical finding associated with antiphospholipid syndrome (APS). The clinical features, diagnosis, and management of APS are discussed elsewhere in this issue. Although not part of the criteria for diagnosis, thrombocytopenia occurs in approximately one-third of patients with APS. The thrombocytopenia is usually mild to moderate and rarely severe enough to cause bleeding.

Management options during pregnancy are similar to those for primary ITP. However, if the patient meets criteria for a diagnosis of primary APS, a combination of low-dose aspirin and prophylactic heparin is helpful in preventing adverse pregnancy outcomes. Moderate thrombocytopenia should not alter decisions about antithrombotic therapy in APS.[55] In patients who have more marked thrombocytopenia, decisions should be individualized. Steroids may be required to boost the platelet count because the mechanism of the thrombocytopenia in APS is the same as in ITP.[1]

Systemic Lupus Erythematosus

Thrombocytopenia less than 100×10^9/L is one of the diagnostic criteria of SLE. The thrombocytopenia of SLE rarely becomes severe. If treatment is required in severe thrombocytopenia, patients may respond to hydroxychloroquine, glucocorticoids, or other immunosuppressive medications used for other manifestations of SLE.

DRUG-INDUCED THROMBOCYTOPENIA

Medication should always be excluded as a possible cause of thrombocytopenia, which occurs through immune destruction or through suppression of platelet production in the bone marrow. Obtain a complete history of drug use, including nonprescription drugs and herbal remedies. Thrombocytopenia typically resolves in 5 to 7 days after stopping the drug. The common medications used in pregnancy that may cause thrombocytopenia are given in **Box 2**.

Heparin-induced thrombocytopenia (HIT) occurs in 1% to 5% of patients receiving unfractionated heparin within the previous 5 to 10 days. HIT is an extremely thrombotic process, despite the low platelet count. Alternative anticoagulation, such as danaparoid, should be started after stopping heparin. Regular monitoring of the platelet count is required in pregnant women receiving unfractionated heparin, to monitor for HIT.[56] It is recommended to obtain a baseline platelet count before starting therapy, then repeat platelet counts on Days 7 and 14 of therapy. HIT should be suspected if the platelet count falls by approximately 50% or more. If the repeat platelet counts are normal, no further testing is necessary. Enzyme-linked immunosorbent assay for heparin-dependent antibodies is sensitive for the diagnosis.

Box 2
Common medications used in pregnancy may cause thrombocytopenia

Analgesics
  Aspirin
  Acetaminophen
  Indocin
Antibiotics
  Ampicillin
  Penicillin
  Bactrim
Others
  Heparin
  Methyldopa
  Digitalis
  Cyclosporin

Thrombocytopenia Associated with Viral Infections

Chronic infection with HIV and HCV are frequent causes of chronic thrombocytopenia. About 10% to 30% of patients infected with HIV or HCV may develop thrombocytopenia and it is more prevalent in patients with advanced disease.[57,58] It is for this reason that patients with thrombocytopenia should be screened for these viruses especially if risk factors are present.

Treatment of HIV- and HCV-related thrombocytopenia should be directed toward antiviral therapy with highly active antiretroviral therapy regimens; for women infected with HCV, suppression of HCV virus should be performed before conception. Otherwise, IVIG may be used during pregnancy to increase the platelet count before delivery. Treatment with corticosteroids should be avoided as long as possible, because it can increase the viral load and cause further immunosuppression and infection.

Disseminated Intravascular Coagulation

DIC is one of the most serious complications that can occur in pregnancy. It is a disease process that occurs secondary to obstetric events, such as placental abruption, fetomaternal hemorrhage, amniotic fluid embolism, uterine rupture, chorioamnionitis, sepsis, and retained fetal products. The clinical manifestations can vary from mild disorders with only laboratory findings to massive hemorrhage with very low fibrinogen and platelet levels. Treatment should be directed toward the underline cause and to stabilization of the patient with blood product replacement.

REFERENCES

1. Myers B. Diagnosis and management of maternal thrombocytopenia in pregnancy. Br J Haematol 2012;158(1):3–15.
2. Boehlen FH. Platelet count at term pregnancy: a reappraisal of the threshold. Obstet Gynecol 2000;95:30.
3. Abbassi-Ghanavati MG. Pregnancy and laboratory administrative data: a reference table for physicians. Obstet Gynecol 2006;114:1326–31.
4. Burrows RF, Kelton JG. Thrombocytopenia at delivery: a prospective survey of 6715 deliveries. Am J Obstet Gynecol 1990;162(3):731–4.
5. Burrows RF, Kelton JG. Fetal thrombocytopenia and its relation to maternal thrombocytopenia. N Engl J Med 1993;329(20):1463–6.
6. Samuels P, Bussel JB, Braitman LE, et al. Estimation of the risk of thrombocytopenia in the offspring of pregnant women with presumed immune thrombocytopenic purpura. N Engl J Med 1990;323(4):229–35.
7. Chen Z, Liang MY, Wang JL. [Etiology and clinical characteristics of pregnancy-emerged thrombocytopenia]. Zhonghua Fu Chan Ke Za Zhi 2011;46(11):834–9 [in Chinese].
8. McCrae KR. Thrombocytopenia in pregnancy: differential diagnosis, pathogenesis, and management. Blood Rev 2003;17(1):7–14.
9. Rákóczi I, Tallián F, Bagdány S, et al. Platelet life-span in normal pregnancy and pre-eclampsia as determined by a non-radioisotope technique. Thromb Res 1979;15(3–4):553–6.
10. Fay RA, Hughes AO, Farron NT. Platelets in pregnancy: hyperdestruction in pregnancy. Obstet Gynecol 1983;61(2):238–40.
11. Kamphuis MM, Oepkes D. Fetal and neonatal alloimmune thrombocytopenia: prenatal interventions. Prenat Diagn 2011;31(7):712–9.

12. Silver RM, Branch DW, Scott JR. Maternal thrombocytopenia in pregnancy: time for a reassessment. Am J Obstet Gynecol 1995;173(2):479–82.
13. Neunert C, Lim W, Crowther M, et al. The American Society of Hematology 2011 evidence-based practice guideline for immune thrombocytopenia. Blood 2011; 117(16):4190–207.
14. Gill KK, Kelton JG. Management of idiopathic thrombocytopenia purpura in pregnancy. Semin Hematol 2000;37:275–89.
15. Segal JP, Powe NR. Prevalence of immune thrombocytopenia: analysis of administrative data. J Thromb Haemost 2006;4(11):237–83.
16. Keeling D, Tait C, Makris M. Guideline on the selection and use of therapeutic products to treat haemophilia and other hereditary bleeding disorders. Haemophilia 2008;14(4):671–84.
17. Provan D, Stasi R, Newland AC, et al. International consensus report on the investigation and management of primary immune thrombocytopenia. Blood 2010; 115(2):168–86.
18. Webert KE, Mittal R, Sigouin C, et al. A retrospective 11 year analysis of obstetric patients with idiopathic thrombocytopenia purpura. Blood 2003;102:4306–11.
19. Payne SR, Resnik R, Moore TR, et al. Maternal characteristics and risk of severe neonatal thrombocytopenia and intracranial hemorrhage in pregnancies complicated by autoimmune thrombocytopenia. Am J Obstet Gynecol 1997;177(1): 149–55.
20. Cook RL, Miller RC, Katz VL. Immune thrombocytopenia in pregnancy: a reappraisal of management. Obstet Gynecol 1998;78(4):578–83.
21. Letsky EA, Greaves M. Guidelines on the investigation and management of thrombocytopenia in pregnancy, and neonatal alloimmune thrombocytopenia. Maternal and Neonatal Haemostasis Working Party of the Haemostasis and Thrombosis Task Force of the British Society for Haemotology. Br J Haematol 1996;95(1):21–6.
22. Silver R, Berkowitz R, Bussel J. Thrombocytopenia in pregnancy practice bulletin, no 6. Chicago: American College of Obestetrics and Gynecology; 1999.
23. van Veen JJ, Nokes TJ, Makris M. The risk of spinal haematoma following neuraxial anesthesia or lumbar puncture in thrombocytopenic individuals. Br J Haematol 2010;148(1):15–25.
24. Miller Y, Bachowski G, Benjamin R, et al. Practice guidelines for blood transfusion: a compilation from recent peer reviewed literature. American National Red Cross 2007. Available at: http://www.redcross.org/services/biomed/profess/pgbtscreen. pdf.
25. Samama CM, Bastien O, Forestier F, et al. Antiplatelet agents in the perioperative period: expert recommendations of the French Society of Anesthesiology and Intensive Care. Can J Anaesth 2002;49(6):s26–35.
26. British committee for Standards in Haematology. Guidelines for the investigation and management of idiopathic thrombocytopenic purpura in adults, children and pregnancy. Br J Haematol 2003;120:574–96.
27. George JN, Woolf SH, Raskob GE, et al. Idiopathic thrombocytopenia purpura: a practice guideline developed by explicit methods for the American Society of Hematology. Blood 1996;88(1):3–40.
28. Bussel JB, Pham LC. Intravenous treatment with gamma globulin in adults with immune thrombocytopenia purpura: a review of the literature. Vox Sang 1987; 52(3):206–11.
29. Michel M, Novoa MV, Bussel JB. Intravenous anti-D as a treatment for immune thrombocytopenia purpura during pregnancy. Br J Haematol 2003;123(1):142–6.

30. Sieunarine K, Shapiro S, Al Obaidi M, et al. Intravenous anti-D immunoglobulin in the treatment of resistant immune thrombocytopenic purpura during pregnancy. BJOG 2007;114(4):505–7.
31. Spahr JE, Rodgers GM. Treatment of immune-mediated thrombocytopenia with concurrent intravenous immunoglobulin and platelet transfusion: a retrospective review of 40 patients. Am J Hematol 2008;83(2):122–5.
32. Carr JM, Kruskall MS, Kaye JA, et al. Efficacy of platelet transfusions in immune thrombocytopenia. Am J Med 1986;80(6):1051–4.
33. Quiquandon I, Fenaux P, Caulier MT, et al. Reevaluation of the role of azathioprine in the treatment of adult idiopathic thrombocytopenic purpura: a report on 53 cases. Br J Haematol 1990;74(2):223–8.
34. Emilia G, Morselli M, Luppi M, et al. Long term salvage therapy with cyclosporin A in refractory idiopathic thrombocytopenic purpura. Blood 2002;99(4): 1482–5.
35. Schwartz J, Leber MD, Gillis S, et al. Long term follow up after splenectomy performed for immune thrombocytopenia purpura. Am J Hematol 2003;72(2): 94–8.
36. Vianelli N, Galli M, de Vivo A, et al. Efficacy and safety of splenectomy in immune thrombocytopenic purpura: long term results of 402 cases. Haematologica 2005; 90(1):72–7.
37. Kojouri K, Vesely SK, Terrell DR, et al. Splenectomy for adult patients with idiopathic thrombocytopenia purpura: a systematic review to assess long term platelet count responses, prediction of response, and surgical complications. Blood 2004;104(9):2623–34.
38. Furlan M, Robles R, Solenthaler M, et al. Acquired deficiency of von Willebrand factor-cleaving protease in a patient with thrombotic thrombocytopenic purpura. Blood 1998;91(8):2839–46.
39. Tsai HM, Lian EC. Antibodies to von Willebrand factor-cleaving protease in acute thrombotic thrombocytopenic purpura. N Engl J Med 1998;339(22):1585–94.
40. Scully M, Hunt BJ, Benjamin S, et al. Guidelines on the diagnosis and management of thrombotic thrombocytopenic purpura and other thrombotic microangiopathies. Br J Haematol 2012;158(3):323–35.
41. Galbusera M, Noris M, Remuzzi G. Thrombotic thrombocytopenic purpura then and now. Semin Thromb Hemost 2006;32(2):81–9.
42. Hughes C, McEwan JR, Longair I, et al. Cardiac involvement in acute thrombotic thrombocytopenic purpura: association with troponin T and IgG antibodies to ADAMTS13. J Thromb Haemost 2009;7(4):529–36.
43. Peyvandi F, Ferrari S, Lavoretano S, et al. von Willebrand cleaving protease (ADAMTS13) and ADAMTS13 neutralizing autoantibodies in 100 patients with thrombotic thrombocytopenic purpura. Br J Haematol 2004;127(4):433–9.
44. Sánchez-Luceros A, Farías CE, Amaral MM, et al. von Willebrand factor-cleaving protease (ADAMTS13) activity in normal non-pregnant women, pregnant and post-delivery women. Thromb Haemost 2004;92(6):1320–6.
45. Ambrose A, Welham RT, Cefalo RC. Thrombotic thrombocytopenic purpura in early pregnancy. Obstet Gynecol 1985;66(2):267–72.
46. Vesely SK, Li X, McMinn JR, et al. Pregnancy outcomes after recovery from thrombotic thrombocytopenic purpura–hemolytic uremic syndrome. Transfusion 2004;44(8):1149–58.
47. Fakhouri F, Roumenina L, Provot F, et al. Pregnancy associated hemolytic uremic syndrome revisited in the era of complement gene mutations. J Am Soc Nephrol 2010;21(5):859–67.

48. Greenbaum L, Babu S, Furman RR, et al. Eculizumab is an effective long- term treatment in patients with atypical hemolytic uremic syndrome resistant to plasma exchange infusion: an extension study. Blood 2005;106:193.
49. Kelly R, Arnold L, Richards S, et al. The management of pregnancy in paroxysmal nocturnal haemoglobinuria on long term eculizumab. Br J Haematol 2010;149(3): 446–50.
50. McCrae KR, Samuels P, Schreiber AD. Pregnancy-associated thrombocytopenia: pathogenesis and management. Blood 1992;80(11):2697–714.
51. Katz VL, Thorp JM Jr, Rozas L, et al. The natural history of thrombocytopenia associated with preeclampsia. Am J Obstet Gynecol 1990;163(4 Pt 1):1142–3.
52. McMinn JR, George JN. Evaluation of women with clinically suspected thrombotic thrombocytopenic purpura-hemolytic uremic syndrome during pregnancy. J Clin Apher 2001;16(4):202–9.
53. Knight M, Nelson-Piercy C, Kurinczuk JJ, et al. A prospective national study of acute fatty liver of pregnancy in the UK. Gut 2008;57(7):951–6.
54. Mellouli MM, Amara FB, Maghrebi H, et al. Acute fatty liver of pregnancy over a 10-year period at a Tunisian tertiary care center. Int J Gynaecol Obstet 2012; 117(1):88–9.
55. Martin JN Jr, Morrison JC, Files JC. Autoimmune thrombocytopenic purpura: current concepts and recommended practices. Am J Obstet Gynecol 1984; 150(1):86–96.
56. Aster RH. Heparin-induced thrombocytopenia and thrombosis. N Engl J Med 1995;332(20):1374–6.
57. Kaslow RA, Phair JP, Friedman HB, et al. Infection with the human immunodeficiency virus: clinical manifestations and their relationship to immune deficiency. A report from the Multicenter AIDS Cohort Study. Ann Intern Med 1987;107(4): 474–80.
58. Godeau B, Chevret S, Varet B, et al. Intravenous immunoglobulin or high-dose methylprednisolone, with or without oral prednisone, for adults with untreated severe autoimmune thrombocytopenic purpura: a randomised, multicentre trial. Lancet 2002;359(9300):23–9.

Guidelines for Use of Anticoagulation in Pregnancy

Kisti P. Fuller, MD*, Garry Turner, MD, Satya Polavarapu, MD, Anne-Marie Prabulos, MD

KEYWORDS

- Pregnancy • Anticoagulation • Acute thrombosis • Breastfeeding
- Heparin-induced thrombocytopenia

KEY POINTS

- For acute thrombosis or thrombosis prophylaxis in pregnancy, use low-molecular-weight heparin (LMWH) as first-line therapy unless contraindicated.
- Follow pregnant patients on therapeutic LMWH with anti–factor Xa levels (target level of 0.6–1 unit/mL 4 hours after dose) every 1 to 3 months. Patients on prophylactic LMWH do not require monitoring unless they have a body mass index greater than 40 or have renal disease.
- Patients with lupus anticoagulant on unfractionated heparin (UFH), or any patient with altered baseline activated partial thromboplastin time levels, should be monitored with anti–factor Xa activity (target 0.3–0.7 units/mL) or protamine titration (target 0.2–0.4 units/mL).
- Hold therapeutic doses of LMWH or UFH for 24 hours before delivery to allow for regional anesthesia and avoid bleeding complications. Restart anticoagulants 4 to 6 hours after vaginal delivery and 6 to 12 hours after cesarean delivery.
- Consider bridging to oral anticoagulants postpartum for patients who require prolonged anticoagulation.
- UFH, LMWH, and warfarin may be used in breastfeeding women.

INTRODUCTION

Venous thromboembolism (VTE) is uncommon during pregnancy, with a prevalence of 0.06%. Although uncommon, VTE is one of the leading causes of maternal mortality and the risk of VTE is increased sixfold in pregnancy.[1] Most patients have no prior history of VTE. During pregnancy, deep venous thrombosis (DVT) most commonly occurs in the lower extremities with the left leg being affected in >80% of cases.[2] Lower

None of the authors have any relationship to disclose.

Department of Maternal-Fetal Medicine, University of Connecticut John Dempsey Hospital, 263 Farmington Avenue, Farmington, CT 06030, USA

* Corresponding author.

E-mail address: kfuller@uchc.edu

Clin Lab Med 33 (2013) 343–356

http://dx.doi.org/10.1016/j.cll.2013.03.018

labmed.theclinics.com

extremity DVT is more common in the antepartum period (75%) versus postpartum; in contrast, pulmonary embolism (PE) is more commonly diagnosed postpartum (61%) and has a significant association with cesarean delivery, age >35, and obesity.[2,3]

Women with a new VTE diagnosed during pregnancy should receive therapeutic anticoagulation for a minimum of 3 months. Following therapy, prophylactic anticoagulation should be used for the remainder of the pregnancy and for 6 weeks postpartum.[1]

Women with a history of a VTE should be screened for thrombophilia and antiphospholipid antibodies even if a transient risk factor was present at the time of the event.[4] The rate of recurrence without antepartum prophylaxis varies from 2.4–6.2% and is dependent on multiple variables.[5,6]

Women with a thrombophilia or VTE associated with hormonal exposure (estrogen containing contraceptives or pregnancy) are at higher risk for recurrence than women with VTE associated with a non-hormonal transient risk factor or women without a thrombophilia.[4–6]

Due to variability in data it is difficult to make absolute recommendations for treatment. ACOG[4] recommends that women without a thrombophilia with prior VTE associated with a non-hormonal transient risk factor be managed with surveillance antepartum and prophylaxis postpartum (another option is to continue surveillance postpartum for low-risk patients). For women with a prior VTE associated with pregnancy or estrogen, ACOG[4] recommends prophylactic LMWH or UFH both antepartum and postpartum. Prophylactic LMWH or UFH is also recommended for women with prior VTE and no associated risk factor. The risks and benefits must be discussed with each individual patient before deciding on a management plan.

- Anticoagulant medications
  - Oral
    - Vitamin K antagonists
      - High-risk patients (such as women with mechanical valves) have an increased risk of thrombosis when on UFH or LMWH versus warfarin.[7] The data regarding this finding are often debated because not all patients in the studies were followed to maintain therapeutic dosing.
      - These medications cross the placenta. Continuation of warfarin throughout pregnancy is associated with adverse outcomes such as increased maternal and fetal bleeding, miscarriage, and fetal malformation.
        - Fetal malformations associated with warfarin are midfacial hypoplasia, stippled epiphyses, limb hypoplasia, and central nervous system anomalies.
        - Discontinuing warfarin before 6 to 8 weeks' gestational age minimizes the risk of embryopathy.[7,8]
      - Warfarin may cause fetal hemorrhagic complications because of the immature fetal liver and low fetal levels of vitamin K–dependent clotting factors. Women taking warfarin should be transitioned to UFH or LMWH 3 weeks before planned delivery to avoid delivery trauma leading to fetal hemorrhage.[9]
      - High-risk women attempting pregnancy have two options. They may continue on warfarin, be advised to keep close records of their menstrual cycle, and take frequent pregnancy tests to facilitate discontinuation of warfarin before 6 to 8 weeks gestational age. The second option is transitioning to LMWH before conception. This option decreases the risk of

early miscarriage but is associated with increased cost, as well as inconvenience and the pain of injections.[10]

- ○ Most patients who are on warfarin before pregnancy are transitioned to therapeutic doses of LMWH.
- ○ An alternative is to give an intermediate dose of LMWH, which is 75% of the normal therapeutic dose.[9] Intermediate dosing has been shown to be effective for DVT prophylaxis in high-risk patients with cancer.[11]

- ■ Thrombin inhibitors
  - • Dabigatran
    - ○ Use in pregnancy is not recommended.[9]
- ■ Factor Xa inhibitors
  - • Rivaroxaban (Xarelto)
  - • Apixaban
    - ○ Use of either in pregnancy is not recommended.[9]
- ○ Parenteral
  - ■ Heparin
    - • Form a complex with antithrombin. This complex rapidly inactivates clotting factors such as thrombin and factor Xa, leading to inhibition of fibrin formation and platelet aggregation.[12,13]
    - • Not absorbed orally, so must be given intravenously or subcutaneous. Subcutaneous administration requires a higher dosage than intravenous administration because of decreased bioavailability.[12]
    - • Heparin does not cross the placenta. It is not associated with increased risk of teratogenicity or fetal bleeding.[9]
    - • Initial treatment of VTE may be intravenous or subcutaneous. Patients who receive intravenous therapy with weight-adjusted dosing have lower rates of recurrent VTE.[12]
      - ○ Intravenous heparin for pregnant patients with acute VTE is initially dosed based on the patient's weight (bolus of 80 units/kg, followed by 18 units/kg/h).[1,12] Dosing is adjusted based on activated partial thromboplastin time (aPTT) drawn every 4 to 6 hours with a goal to maintain aPTT at 1.5 to 2.5 times control.[1]
      - ○ Therapeutic subcutaneous heparin is less commonly used. The initial dose is 333 units/kg followed by 250 units/kg every 12 hours. As with intravenous heparin, adjust dose by checking aPTT 4 to 6 hours after the last dose, with the goal of aPTT 1.5 to 2.5 times control.[4,9]
      - ○ Patients with lupus anticoagulant (LAC), or any patient with altered baseline aPTT levels, on UFH should be monitored with protamine titration (target 0.2–0.4 units/mL) or anti–factor Xa activity (target 0.3–0.7 units/mL) 4 to 6 hours after the dose.[12,14]
      - ○ Some clinicians advocate monitoring all patients on heparin with anti–factor Xa levels. There is significant variation in aPTT results between laboratories. Also, aPTT levels can be affected by conditions such as liver disease, consumptive coagulopathy, and other biological factors. The exception is patients with hyperbilirubinemia and hypertriglyceridemia; anti–factor Xa levels can be inaccurate in these patients and aPTT should be used.[14]
    - • Prophylactic dose
      - ○ First trimester: 5000 to 7500 units every 12 hours
      - ○ Second trimester: 7500 to 10,000 units every 12 hours

- o Third trimester: 10,000 units every 12 hours[4]
- o When clinically indicated, the dose may be adjusted to an anti–factor Xa level (target 0.1–0.3 units/mL)[15]
- Complications associated with heparin
  - o Osteoporosis
    - Heparin binds to osteoblasts, activation factors that increase osteoblast activity are then released.[12]
    - A reduction in bone density has been seen in up to 30% of patients on heparin for longer than 1 month.[15] Heparin-associated bone loss is often reversible and does not require treatment. The dose or length of heparin therapy is not related to the amount of bone loss.[16,17]
  - o Transient increase in transaminases (with the exception of bilirubin)[12]
  - o Skin reactions
    - Bruising, allergic reaction at injection site, skin necrosis[9,12,18]
  - o Heparin-induced thrombocytopenia (HIT)
    - Thrombocytopenia occurs in 5% of pregnancies. For patients taking heparin products, the differential diagnosis should include HIT.
    - HIT type I: occurs within first 2 days after initial heparin. Platelets decrease slightly. Nonimmune mechanism; may be the result of the effect of heparin on platelet activation. Resolves without therapy. Minimal risk of serious bleeding complications. Heparin may be continued.[19]
    - HIT type II: occurs 5 to 10 days after initial heparin; rare after 14 days. Secondary to immunoglobulins against heparin-platelet factor 4 complex. Venous and arterial thrombosis may occur, as well as necrotic skin lesions at injection sites. Heparin should be discontinued immediately.[1,19]
    - When initiating heparin therapy, Linkins and colleagues[19] recommend checking a platelet count every 2 to 3 days from day 4 to 14. If platelet level drops by 50% or greater, heparin should be discontinued. The preferred diagnostic method to confirm a HIT type II reaction is a serotonin release assay or heparin-induced platelet activation.[19,20] Laboratory tests for HIT are not available at all facilities and can be complex. If HIT is suspected, consultation with a hematologist is recommended.
      - For patients with a low risk (<1%) of HIT, platelet counts do not need to be routinely monitored.[19]
      - Pregnant women are at low risk of developing HIT and do not need routine platelet monitoring.[19,21]
    - Patients with a history of a HIT type II reaction may not receive any form of heparin (even the small amounts used for catheter flushes may cause a reaction).[22]
    - Risk of HIT varies among different populations. The rate is higher in patients receiving UFH versus LMWH or other anticoagulants. HIT occurs in 2.7% to 5% of nonpregnant patients taking UFH but is rare in pregnant women.[19,21,23,24] The overall incidence of HIT with LMWH varies from 0.2% to 0.8%.[23,25,26] HIT is rare in patients less than 40 years old and postpartum women. Early onset HIT may be seen in patients who received heparin within the last 100 days.[24,27]

- Avoid HIT by using LMWH when available and, when possible, limit heparin therapy to less than 5 days.[26]
- For pregnant women who develop HIT, danaparoid (factor Xa inhibitor; discussed later) is recommended. Danaparoid does not cross the placenta and rarely causes HIT. Danaparoid is not available in the United States. Fondaparinux has also been used, but danaparoid is preferable if it is available.
  ○ Persistent anticoagulant effect
  - There have been reports of prolonged aPTT persisting in patients for as long as 28 hours after the last dose of therapeutic subcutaneous heparin. This persistent anticoagulant effect is not seen with intravenous heparin.[10]
- LMWH
  - Derived from UFH. Works similarly to heparin by binding antithrombin and inactivating factor Xa. Unlike UFH, most LMWH is not large enough (mean molecular weight of 4000–5000 compared with 15,000 for UFH) to inhibit thrombin. Because of the decreased effect on thrombin, LMWH does not prolong the aPTT.[12,28]
  - LMWH does not cross the placenta. It is not associated with an increased risk of teratogenicity or fetal bleeding.[29,30]
  - In general, LMWH is recommended rather than UFH because of increased bioavailability, long half-life, and decreased incidence of side effects such as thrombocytopenia and osteoporosis.[28]
    ○ UFH may be preferred in some instances. For patients who are hemodynamically unstable and at increased risk for significant bleeding, UFH may be preferred because of its shorter half-life and reversibility.[13]
  - LMWH is excreted by the kidneys and may accumulate in women with reduced creatinine clearance. Women with renal disease (creatinine clearance <30 mL/min) require careful monitoring with anti–factor Xa levels to avoid supertherapeutic levels. UFH depends less on renal excretion and may be considered first-line therapy for these individuals.[9,31,32]
    ○ For enoxaparin, a reduced prophylactic dose of 30 mg once daily should be used for patients with renal disease. Dosing adjustments are not needed for dalteparin or tinzaparin when used for prophylaxis.[31]
    ○ For patients with renal disease on therapeutic LMWH therapy, titrate the dose according to anti–factor Xa levels (discussed later) or consider using heparin. Trough anti–factor Xa levels may also be used to evaluate accumulation of LMWH.[31]
  - Enoxaparin (Lovenox)
    ○ Therapeutic: 1 mg/kg every 12 hours[4,9]
    ○ Prophylaxis: 40 mg once daily[4,9]
  - Dalteparin (Fragmin)
    ○ Therapeutic: 200 units/kg once daily (or 100 units/kg every 12 hours)[4,9]
    ○ Prophylaxis: 5000 units once daily[4,9]
  - Tinzaparin (Innohep)
    ○ Therapeutic: 175 units/kg once daily[4,9]
    ○ Prophylaxis: 4500 units once daily[4,9]
  - Alternative dosing
    ○ For patients with body mass index greater than 40, consider increasing the prophylactic dose by 30% and/or checking an anti–factor Xa level.[31]

- Once-daily dosing has been used to increase compliance. The data available have not shown an increased risk of recurrent VTE, major bleeding, or mortality with once-daily dosing.[9,18,33]
- The dose for once-daily therapy should be the same total daily dose as the twice-daily regimen. (The exception is enoxaparin, which is dosed at 1.5 mg/kg daily vs 1.0 mg/kg twice daily. The once-daily dosing regimen of enoxaparin is not recommended in pregnancy.)

- Monitoring
  - Check anti–factor Xa levels 4 hours after dose. Target anti–factor Xa level for twice-daily dosing is 0.6 to 1 units/mL. Target for prophylaxis is 0.2 to 0.6 units/mL. Target for once-daily dosing is 1.0 to 2.0 units/mL.[12,31]
  - Routine monitoring is recommended every 1 to 3 months for pregnant women on therapeutic anticoagulation, as well as obese women and women with renal disease on therapeutic or prophylactic dosing. Most women do not require adjustment and data have not consistently shown an improvement in safety or efficacy of therapy with routine monitoring.[9] This information has caused some providers to question the need for routine monitoring, which is costly and may be difficult for patients, without any proven improvement in outcome.
- Adverse reactions
  - Similar to heparin but the frequency of HIT, skin reactions, and osteoporosis are lower.[9]
- Reversal
  - LMWH is partially reversed with protamine sulfate, although the clinical significance of the level of neutralization has not been clearly established.[12]

- Factor Xa inhibitors
  - Danaparoid
    - Half-life 25 hours
    - Dose[19]:
      - Initial bolus
        - Less than 60 kg: 1500 units
        - From 60 to 75 kg: 2250 units
        - From 75 to 90 kg: 3000 units
        - Greater than 90 kg: 3750 units
      - Maintenance
        - 400 units/h for 4 hours
        - Then 300 units/h for 4 hours
        - Then 200 units per hour
        - Adjust maintenance dose to anti-Xa level of 0.5 to 0.8 units/mL
    - Effective for prevention of venous thromboembolism but currently is only indicated for use in patients with HIT.[12]
    - Not able to be reversed.
    - Not available in the United States.[12]
  - Fondaparinux (Arixtra)
    - Half-life is 17 to 21 hours. Mostly renal excreted. For patients with renal disease, the dose should be decreased by 50%.[12]
    - Side effects include fever, nausea, anemia, rash, and edema.
    - Dose:
      - Prophylactic: 2.5 mg subcutaneously once daily

- Prophylaxis contraindicated in patients weighing less than 50 kg[12]
  - ○ Therapeutic:
    - Less than 50 kg: 5 mg subcutaneously once daily
    - From 50 to 100 kg: 7.5 mg subcutaneously once daily
    - Greater than 100 kg: 10 mg subcutaneously daily[12]
  - ○ PT and aPTT are not accurate, but anti–factor Xa can be used to measure the activity of fondaparinux. Routine monitoring is not recommended.[12]
  - ○ For patients with renal disease, the dose should be decreased by 50%.[12]
- Pregnant women receiving fondaparinux have been shown to have increased anti–factor Xa levels in the umbilical cord, but it is unknown whether this has an effect on the fetus.[34] Although the US Food and Drug Administration (FDA) has given it a pregnancy risk factor B classification, it should only be used in women with severe allergic reaction to heparin and when danaparoid is unavailable.[24,35] It is often used in women with HIT because fondaparinux does not react with HIT antibodies.[36]
- The effects of fondaparinux are not reversible with protamine sulfate. Recombinant factor VIIa may be helpful for patients on fondaparinux with bleeding complications.[37,38]
- Direct thrombin inhibitors
  - Bivalirudin
    - ○ No published report of its use in pregnancy[9]
  - Lepirudin (recombinant hirudin)
    - ○ Recommended for patients with HIT[19]
    - ○ Intravenous administration only
    - ○ The product was discontinued by the US manufacturer in 2012
  - Argatroban
    - ○ Recommended for patients with HIT and renal disease.[19]
    - ○ Use during pregnancy has been only case reports, all of which were patients initially treated with UFH or LMWH who developed HIT and required continued anticoagulation.[24,39,40]
- ○ Thrombolysis
  - Thrombolytic agents, such as streptokinase, urokinase, and tissue plasminogen activator, have been used in pregnancy with variable success. There seems to be minimal placental crossing of the medications, but other complications, most importantly bleeding, can cause issues for both mother and fetus.[41] Maternal hemorrhage was seen in 8.1% of women who received thrombolytic treatment. There were no cases of fetal hemorrhage. No randomized control studies have been done, so the success rates, morbidity, and overall safety are difficult to determine. The mortality rates seem to be similar to nonpregnant rates for similar situations, suggesting that pregnancy may not have a significant impact on the results of therapy.[42] Thrombotic therapy should only be used for life-threatening thromboembolism.[9]
- Complications and side effects of anticoagulant medications
  - General complications of anticoagulation are bleeding, HIT, osteoporosis, bruising, allergic reaction, and pain.[9]
- Reversal
  - If delivery occurs more than 4 hours after prophylactic or intravenous heparin dose, there is minimal risk for hemorrhagic complications.[43] The anticoagulant effect of high-dose subcutaneous UFH may take up to 24 hours to resolve. In patients who experience bleeding that is thought to be related to anticoagulants or when delivery cannot be

delayed, heparin effects should be reversed (for LMWH, the effect is only partial) with protamine sulfate.

- Protamine sulfate
  - Protamine is administered intravenously. The half-life of protamine is 7 minutes. The amount of protamine needed is based on calculation of the residual heparin level.
  - Intravenous heparin has a half-life of 60 minutes. The protamine dose should be based on the amount of heparin given in the last 2 to 3 hours[43] One milligram of protamine sulfate is required to neutralize 100 units of heparin.[12] The dose of protamine should be adjusted based on the amount of time since discontinuation of intravenous heparin. For patients in whom heparin was stopped immediately, the dose of protamine is 1 mg per 100 units of heparin. One or 2 hours after heparin has been discontinued, the protamine dose should be 0.5 mg or 0.25 mg per 100 units of heparin, respectively.[44] The maximum dose is 50 mg in 10 minutes.
  - Subcutaneous heparin peaks 2 to 4 hours after the dose and has a half-life of 1 to 2 hours; but the duration of action is less clear and may last up to 24 hours. Initial protamine dose should be calculated based on an approximation of remaining UFH in circulation based on the half-life and dose of UFH given. Patients who received heparin subcutaneously may require a prolonged infusion of protamine. The decision for additional doses may be determined by following aPTT levels every 3 hours to determine resolution of anticoagulant effect. If the aPTT remains increased and bleeding continues, an additional dose of protamine 0.5 mg per 100 units of heparin should be given.
  - Neutralization of anticoagulants can be measured with normalization of aPTT.[12] For patients with LAC, measurement of aPTT may be inaccurate. Because an anti-Xa level is not a useful marker to assess bleeding risk, we recommend using clinical assessment of continued bleeding to guide further dosing of protamine in patients with LAC.
  - Protamine reverses some of the effects of LMWH and heparinoids but does not reverse the effects of other nonheparin anticoagulants. Protamine should be given if LMWH was administered within 8 hours. The dose is 1 mg protamine per 1 mg (100 anti-Xa units) of LMWH, with a maximum dose of 50 mg in 10 minutes. If longer than 8 hours has passed since administration of LWMH, a lower dose of protamine can be given (consider 0.5 mg per 100 anti-Xa units). A second dose of protamine, 0.5 mg per 100 anti-Xa units, can be given if bleeding does not resolve.[12,43,44]
  - Side effects of protamine include hypotension, bradycardia, nausea, vomiting, and bronchoconstriction. These risks can be reduced by giving the protamine slowly.[9,12] Hypersensitivity reactions have also been reported. Protamine in excessive doses (6 mg/kg) can lead to an anticoagulant effect caused by platelet aggregation and consumption.[43]
  - Recombinant factor VIIa (rFVIIa)
    - May be useful in reversing the effects of UFH, LMWH, fondaparinux, argatroban, bivalirudin, and warfarin.[37,38,43–45]
    - The dose has not been clearly established. Vavra and colleagues[38] recommend 20 to 120 μg/kg for LMWH, 90 μg/kg for fondaparinux, and 30 to 90 μg/kg for direct thrombin inhibitors.

- o The use of rFVIIa for reversal of anticoagulants is not approved by the FDA.
- o Thrombosis has been associated with the use of rFVIIa.[38] The risk of thrombosis is variable and may be dose related.[45]
- Vitamin K antagonists
  - o Vitamin K may be used either intravenously or orally to reverse the anticoagulant effects of warfarin. Use of oral supplementation is preferred because there is a risk of anaphylaxis with the intravenous form. Subcutaneous vitamin K is not effective for reversal of anticoagulation.[46–48]
  - o The effective oral dose is 1 to 2.5 mg. Higher doses of vitamin K may lead to resistance when restarting warfarin.[46,47,49]
- The duration of therapeutic anticoagulation needed after acute VTE in pregnancy is unclear. For nonpregnant patients, a minimum of 3 months of therapeutic anticoagulation is recommended.[18] Bates and colleagues[9] recommend continuation of therapeutic anticoagulation for the remainder of the pregnancy and postpartum period. Therapy may be stopped at 6 weeks postpartum as long as the minimum of 3 months of therapy has been achieved by that time.
- Timing for delivery
  - Planned delivery at 39 weeks (unless otherwise indicated), in order to time discontinuation of anticoagulants, may be considered.
    - o Therapeutic dosing with twice-daily UFH or LMWH should be stopped 24 hours before induction or cesarean.[4,9,50]
    - o Prophylactic doses should be stopped 12 hours before delivery.[4,51]
    - o Clearance of heparin can be confirmed with normalization of aPTT (see the earlier discussion of neutralization of anticoagulants), with the exception of patients with LAC. For patients on LMWH, an anti-Xa level does not indicate risk of bleeding.[50]
    - o Consult with anesthesia to determine site-specific preferences for placement of regional anesthesia in patients on anticoagulants.
    - o Pneumatic compression devices are recommended for women who have stopped anticoagulant therapy for delivery.
  - Women at high risk of thrombosis recurrence can be switched to therapeutic intravenous UFH. The IV UFH is held 4 to 6 hours before insertion of regional anesthesia and delivery. Women with a proximal DVT or PE within 2 weeks before delivery are considered high risk for recurrence.[9]
  - Elective cesarean delivery is not recommended for women who require anticoagulation. Cesarean delivery should be performed for obstetric indications only.
- Postpartum anticoagulation management
  - Restart UFH or LMWH 4 to 6 hours after vaginal delivery and 6 to 12 hours after cesarean delivery.[4]
  - Bridge with vitamin K antagonists.
    - o Women who only require anticoagulation for 6 weeks postpartum may prefer to continue on LMWH. Transitioning to warfarin requires frequent testing and often requires 1 to 2 weeks before a therapeutic dose is stabilized. Patients requiring longer than 6 weeks of therapy should be transitioned to oral medications.[4,9]
    - o Initial dose of warfarin may be given the night of delivery in stable patients. The initial dose for the first 2 days should be 5 to 10 mg.

The dose should then be adjusted based on the International Normalization Ratio (INR) results. Patients started on the 10-mg dose become therapeutic faster, but this dose is also associated with more of an initial hypercoagulable effect because of a precipitous decline in protein C concentrations. Risk of bleeding, recurrence, and survival are similar for both the 5-mg and 10-mg dose.[52–54]

- o Target for warfarin therapy is an INR 2.0 to 3.0. Continue UFH or LMWH and warfarin until INR is therapeutic (>2.0) for 2 days.[4]

- Breastfeeding
  - Medications must be passed into the breast milk and be absorbed from the infant's gastrointestinal tract to be a potential problem for the baby. Medications that are more likely to pass into breast milk are nonionized, not protein bound, of low molecular weight, and highly lipid soluble.[9]
  - Vitamin K antagonists
    - o Warfarin does not pass into breast milk and may be initiated or continued while breastfeeding.[55]
  - UFH
    - o UFH does not pass into breast milk and may be initiated or continued while breastfeeding.[15,35,56] The preservative-free formulation is recommended for women who are breastfeeding.
  - LMWH
    - o Small amounts of these medications have been detected in breast milk. Because of their low oral bioavailability, they are not likely to have an effect on a nursing infant.[35]
  - Fondaparinux is passed into the breast milk of lactating rats. Because of its composition, it is doubtful that significant amounts would be enterically absorbed by an infant.[57] Because of limited data, caution is recommended for women who are breastfeeding.[9]
  - Thrombin inhibitors
    - o There is little information about these medications and breast feeding. A case report of a woman taking therapeutic lepirudin reported undetectable levels of the medication in her breast milk.[58]
  - Danaparoid is passed into breast milk in low levels but has poor oral bioavailability. Although the manufacturer recommends avoiding breastfeeding, it is unlikely to cause an infant effect and may be continued.
  - Oral thrombin inhibitors and factor Xa inhibitors
    - o Minimal information is known about these medications in lactating women. At the present time, it is not recommended to use these medications while breastfeeding.[9]

CONCLUSION

The recommendations above are based on the current guidelines for anticoagulation in pregnancy for patients with an acute thromboembolism or thromboembolism prevention. These recommendations may also be applicable for patients that require anticoagulant therapy in pregnancy for other reasons, see articles by Lockshin, Odibo and Stout, and Paidas and Hossain elsewhere in this issue.

REFERENCES

1. Creasy RK, Resnik R, Iams JD, et al. Maternal-fetal medicine principles and practice. 6th edition. Philadelphia: Saunders Elsevier; 2009. p. 862–5.

2. Gherman RB, Goodwin TM, Leung B, et al. Incidence, clinical characteristics, and timing of objectively diagnosed venous thromboembolism during pregnancy. Obstet Gynecol 1999;94:730–4.

3. Chisaka H, Utsunomiya H, Okamura K, et al. Pulmonary thromboembolism following gynecologic surgery and cesarean section. Int J Gynaecol Obstet 2004;84:47–53.

4. Thromboembolism in pregnancy. Practice Bulletin No. 123. American College of Obstetrics and Gynecologist. Obstet Gynecol 2011;188:718–29.

5. Brill-Edwards P, Ginsberg JS, Gent M, et al. Safety of withholding heparin in pregnant women with a history of venous thromboembolism. N Engl J Med 2000;343:1439–44.

6. Pabinger I, Grafenhofer H, Kaider A, et al. Risk of pregnancy associated recurrent venous thromboembolism in women with a history of venous thrombosis. J Thromb Haemost 2005;3(5):949–54.

7. Chan WS, Anand S, Ginsberg JS. Anticoagulation of pregnant women with mechanical heart valves: a systematic review of the literature. J Coagul Disord 2010;2:81–8.

8. Schaefer C, Hannemann D, Meister R, et al. Vitamin K antagonists and pregnancy outcome. A multi-center prospective study. Thromb Haemost 1996;95:949–57.

9. Bates SM, Greer IA, Middeldorp S, et al. VET, thrombophilia, antithrombic therapy, and pregnancy. Antithrombotic therapy and prevention of thrombosis, 9th edition: American College of Chest Physicians evidence-based clinical practice guidelines. Chest 2012;141:e691–736.

10. Anderson DR, Ginsberg JS, Burrows R, et al. Subcutaneous heparin therapy during pregnancy: a need for concern at the time of delivery. Thromb Haemost 1991;65(3):248–50.

11. Lee A, Levine M, Baker R, et al. Low-molecular-weight heparin versus a coumarin for the prevention of recurrent venous thromboembolism in patients with cancer. N Engl J Med 2003;349:146–53.

12. Garcia DA, Baglin TP, Weitz JI, et al. Parenteral anticoagulants: antithrombotic therapy and prevention of thrombosis, 9th edition: American College of Chest Physicians evidence-based clinical practice guidelines. Chest 2012;141(Suppl 2):24–43.

13. Rosenberg V, Lockwood C. Thromboembolism in pregnancy. Obstet Gynecol Clin North Am 2007;34:481–500.

14. Vandiver JW, Vondracek TG. Antifactor Xa levels versus activated partial thromboplastin time for monitoring unfractionated heparin. Pharmacotherapy 2012;32(6):546–58.

15. Clark NF, Delate T, Witt DM, et al. A descriptive evaluation of unfractionated heparin use during pregnancy. J Thromb Thrombolysis 2009;27(3):267–73.

16. Dahlman TC. Osteoporotic fractures and the recurrence of thromboembolism during pregnancy and the puerperium in 184 women undergoing thromboprophylaxis with heparin. Am J Obstet Gynecol 1990;97(3):221–8.

17. Douketis JD, Ginsberg JS, Burrows RF, et al. The effects of long-term heparin therapy during pregnancy on bone density. A prospective matched cohort study. Thromb Haemost 1996;75(2):254–7.

18. Kearon C, Akl E, Comerota A, et al. Antithrombotic therapy and prevention of thrombosis, 9th edition: American College of Chest Physicians evidence-based clinical practice guidelines. Chest 2012;141:e419s–94s.

19. Linkins LA, Dans AL, Moores LK, et al. Treatment and prevention of heparin-induced thrombocytopenia: antithrombotic therapy and prevention of thrombosis, 9th edition: American College of Chest Physicians evidence-based clinical practice guidelines. Chest 2012;141:e495S.

20. Sheridan D, Carter C, Kelton JG. A diagnostic test for heparin-induced thrombocytopenia. Blood 1986;67:27.

21. Fausett M, Vogtlander M, Lee R, et al. Heparin-induced thrombocytopenia is rare in pregnancy. Am J Obstet Gynecol 2000;185(1):148–52.

22. Warkentin TE, Sheppard JA, Sigouin CS, et al. Gender imbalance and risk factor interactions in heparin induced thrombocytopenia. Blood 2006;108:2937.

23. Warkentin TE, Levine MN, Hirsh J, et al. Heparin-induced thrombocytopenia in patients treated with low-molecular-weight heparin or unfractionated heparin. N Engl J Med 1995;332:1330–5.

24. Young SK, Al-Mondhiry HA, Vaida SJ, et al. Successful use of argatroban during the third trimester of pregnancy: case report and review of the literature. Pharmacotherapy 2008;28(12):1531–6.

25. Heeger PS, Backstrom JT. Heparin flushes and thrombocytopenia. Ann Intern Med 1986;105:143.

26. Stein PD, Hull RD, Matta F, et al. Heparin-induced thrombocytopenia in hospitalized patients with venous thromboembolism. Am J Med 2009;122:919.

27. Lubenow N, Kempf R, Eichner A, et al. Heparin-induced thrombocytopenia: temporal pattern of thrombocytopenia in relation to initial use or re-exposure to heparin. Chest 2002;122:37.

28. Weitz J. Low-molecular-weight heparins. N Engl J Med 1997;337(10):688–98.

29. Forestier F, Daffos F, Capella-Pavlovsky M. Low molecular weight heparin does not cross the placenta during the second trimester of pregnancy study by direct fetal blood sampling under ultrasound. Thromb Res 1984;34(6):557–60.

30. Forestier F, Daffos F, Rainaut M, et al. Low molecular weight heparin does not cross the placenta during the third trimester of pregnancy. Thromb Haemost 1987;57(2):234.

31. Nutescu EA, Spinler SA, Wittkowsky A, et al. Low-molecular-weight heparins in renal impairment and obesity: available evidence and clinical practice recommendations across medical and surgical settings. Ann Pharmacother 2009;43(6):1064–83.

32. Boneu B, Caranobe C, Sie P. Pharmacokinetics of heparin and low molecular weight heparin. Baillieres Clin Haematol 1990;3(3):531–44.

33. Voke J, Keidan J, Pavord S, et al, British Society of Haematology Obstetric Haematology Group. The management of antenatal venous thromboembolism in the UK and Ireland: a prospective multicenter observational study. Br J Haematol 2007;139:545–58.

34. Dempfle CE. Minor transplacental passage of fondaparinux in vivo. N Engl J Med 2004;350(18):1914–5.

35. Guyatt GH, Akl EA, Crowther M, et al. Executive summary: antithrombotic therapy and prevention of thrombosis, 9th edition: American College of Chest Physicians evidence-based clinical practice guidelines. Chest 2012;141(Suppl 2):7–47.

36. Savi P, Chong BH, Greinacher A, et al. Effect of fondaparinux on platelet activation in the presence of heparin-dependent antibodies: a blinded comparative multicenter study with unfractionated heparin. Blood 2005;105:139–44.

37. Bijsterveld N, Moons A, Boekholdt S, et al. Ability of recombinant factor VIIa to reverse the anticoagulant effect of the pentasaccharide fondaparinux in healthy volunteers. Circulation 2002;106(2):139–44.
38. Vavra K, Lutz M, Smythe M. Recombinant factor VIIa to manage major bleeding from newer parenteral anticoagulants. Ann Pharmacother 2010; 44(4):718–26.
39. Ekbatani A, Asaro LR, Malinow AM. Anticoagulation with argatroban in a parturient with heparin-induced thrombocytopenia. Int J Obstet Anesth 2010;19(1): 82–7.
40. Taniguchi S, Fukuda I, Minakawa M, et al. Emergency pulmonary embolectomy during the second trimester of pregnancy: report of a case. Surg Today 2008;38: 59–61.
41. Pfeifer GW. Distribution and placental transfer of 131-I streptokinase. Australas Ann Med 1970;19:17–8.
42. Turrentine MA, Braems G, Ramirez MM. Use of thrombolytics for the treatment of thromboembolic disease during pregnancy. Obstet Gynecol Surv 1995;50(7): 534–41.
43. Levi M, Eerneberg E, Kamphuisen PW. Bleeding risk and reversal strategies for old and new anticoagulants and antiplatelet agents. J Thromb Haemost 2011;9: 1705–12.
44. Schulman S, Bijsterveld NR. Anticoagulants and their reversal. Transfus Med Rev 2007;21(1):37–48.
45. Mayer S, Brun N, Begtrup K, et al. Efficacy and safety of recombinant activated factor VII for acute intracerebral hemorrhage. N Engl J Med 2008;258(20): 2127–37.
46. Lubetsky A, Yonath H, Olchovsky D, et al. Comparison of oral vs. intravenous phytonadione (vitamin K1) in patients with excessive anticoagulation: a prospective randomized controlled study. Arch Intern Med 2003;163(2):2469.
47. Wilson S, Watson H, Crowther M. Low-dose oral vitamin K therapy for the management of asymptomatic patients with elevated international normalized ratios: a brief review. CMAJ 2004;170(5):821.
48. Dezee K, Shimeall W, Douglas K, et al. Treatment of excessive anticoagulation with phytonadione (vitamin K): a meta-analysis. Arch Intern Med 2006; 166(4):391.
49. Crowther M, Julian J, McCarty D, et al. Treatment of warfarin-associated coagulopathy with oral vitamin K: a randomized controlled trial. Lancet 2000; 356(9241):1551.
50. Horlocker T, Wedel D, Rowlingson J, et al. Regional anesthesia in the patient receiving antithrombotic or thrombolytic therapy: American Society of Regional Anesthesia and Pain Medicine evidence-based guidelines (third edition). Reg Anesth Pain Med 2010;35(1):64–101.
51. Douketis J, Spyropoulos A, Spencer F, et al. Perioperative management of antithrombotic therapy: antithrombotic therapy and prevention of thrombosis, 9th edition: American College of Chest Physicians evidence-based clinical practice guidelines. Chest 2012;141(2):e326S–50S.
52. Crowther MA, Ginsberg JB, Kearon C, et al. A randomized trial comparing 5-mg and 10-mg warfarin loading doses. Arch Intern Med 1999;159:46–8.
53. Harrison L, Johnston M, Massiocotte MP, et al. Comparison of 5-mg and 10-mg loading doses in initiation of warfarin therapy. Ann Intern Med 1997;126(2):133.
54. Kovacs MJ, Rodger M, Anderson DR, et al. Comparison of 10-mg and 5-mg warfarin initiation nomograms together with low-molecular-weight heparin for

outpatient treatment of acute venous thromboembolism. A randomized, double-blind, controlled trial. Ann Intern Med 2003;189(9):714.

55. McKenna R, Cole ER, Vasan U. Is warfarin sodium contraindicated in the lactating mother? J Pediatr 1983;103:325–7.

56. Ginsburg JS, Kowalchuk G, Hirsh J, et al. Heparin therapy during pregnancy. Risks to the fetus and mother. Arch Intern Med 1989;149(10):2233–6.

57. Vetter A, Perera G, Leithner K, et al. Development and in vivo bioavailability study of an oral fondaparinux delivery system. Eur J Pharm Sci 2010;41:489–97.

58. Lindhoff-Last E, Willeke A, Thalhammer C, et al. Hirudin treatment in a breast-feeding women. Lancet 2000;335:467–8.

Anticoagulation in Pregnant Patients with Mechanical Heart Valves: Clinical Considerations

Molly J. Stout, MD*, Anthony O. Odibo, MD, MSCE

KEYWORDS

- Mechanical heart valves • Anticoagulation • Warfarin • Pregnancy

KEY POINTS

- Pregnancy in women with mechanical heart valves should be managed collaboratively with a cardiologist and a maternal fetal medicine specialist.
- Warfarin use may be associated with decreased valve thrombosis complications.
- Heparin compounds may be substituted during organogenesis for fetal benefit.
- Maternal and fetal benefits and risks must be discussed with the patient in the context of her specific situation to best choose an anticoagulation regimen.

IMPORTANT EPIDEMIOLOGY FACTS OF VALVULAR HEART DISEASE

Valvular heart disease can be congenital or acquired. In the United States most maternal heart disease in women of reproductive age is congenital, complicates 1% of all pregnancies, and accounts for 20% of nonobstetric maternal deaths.[1,2] Worldwide, cardiac valvular disease is predominantly rheumatic (acquired) in etiology. Because of improved survival of children with congenital cardiac anomalies, patients are living to reproductive years, and in developed countries congenital heart disease comprises 50% of maternal heart disease during pregnancy.[3,4]

Preconception counseling and collaborative management with an experienced cardiologist are important for discussion of pregnancy-specific risks in the context of the specific maternal lesion and preconception medication planning. With respect to mechanical heart valves in pregnancy, preconception discussion with maternal fetal medicine specialists and a cardiologist can address several of the pregnancy-specific issues associated with mechanical heart valves and anticoagulation that are addressed in this article.

Department of Obstetrics and Gynecology, Washington University in Saint Louis, 660 South Euclid Campus, Box 8064, St. Louis, MO 63110, USA
* Corresponding author.
E-mail address: stoutm@wudosis.wustl.edu

Clin Lab Med 33 (2013) 357–365
http://dx.doi.org/10.1016/j.cll.2013.03.021
0272-2712/13/$ – see front matter © 2013 Elsevier Inc. All rights reserved.

HEART VALVE TYPES, LOCATION, AND RISK OF THROMBOEMBOLISM

There are three general types of mechanical prosthetic valves: (1) bileaflet, (2) tilting disk, and (3) caged-ball. The St. Jude bileaflet valve is the most widely used mechanical prosthesis worldwide.[5] Mechanical valves in the mitral position are more thrombogenic than those in the aortic position. Even with appropriately dosed anticoagulation valve thromboembolism occurs in 0.6 to 3.3 per 100 patient years for patients with bileaflet mechanical valves.[5]

PHARMACOLOGIC CHARACTERISTICS OF COMMONLY USED ANTICOAGULANT DRUGS
Vitamin K Antagonists

Vitamin K antagonists, such as warfarin, interfere with the conversion between vitamin K and vitamin K epoxide, which ultimately alters the required carboxylation of vitamin K–dependent coagulation factors 2, 7, 9, and 10 to active proteins. Proteins C and S, which function to attenuate the coagulation pathway, are also inhibited by vitamin K antagonists. This inhibition of proteins C and S by vitamin K antagonists can produce a transient prothrombotic effect at the initiation of therapy before the more dominant inhibition of factors 2, 7, 9, and 10. Warfarin is water soluble and easily absorbed from the gastrointestinal tract with a half-life of 36 to 42 hours. There are many drug-drug interactions that can either decrease or potentiate the anticoagulant activity of warfarin:

- Amoxicillin (potentiation effect)
- Azithromycin (potentiation effect)
- Metronidazole (potentiation effect)
- Amiodarone (potentiation effect)
- Propranolol (potentiation effect)
- Omeprazole (potentiation effect)
- Citalopram (potentiation effect)
- Sertraline (potentiation effect)
- Nafcillin (inhibition effect)
- Mesalamine (inhibition effect)
- Sucralfate (inhibition effect)

Careful attention to polypharmacy in patients on vitamin K antagonist therapy minimizes the risk that the addition of a new medication will put the patient at risk for being either subtherapeutic or supratherapeutic.[6]

After administration of warfarin an effect in the international normalized ratio (INR) usually occurs within 2 to 3 days. Initiation doses of 5 mg can be started and then adjusted to the goal INR. If rapid anticoagulation is desired either unfractionated heparin (UFH) or low-molecular-weight heparin (LMWH) should be used with warfarin and continued until the goal INR has been reached for at least 2 consecutive days. Then, INR surveillance should be performed every 2 to 3 days until the desired dose response (**Table 1**) has been reached. Repeat testing can be monthly in patients on stable dosage.[6]

The primary adverse effect of vitamin K antagonists is the increased risk for bleeding. Complications, such as acute thrombosis, skin necrosis, and limb gangrene (caused by thrombosis of capillaries in the subcutaneous fat) occur rarely. Reversal of vitamin K antagonists is needed when an urgent procedure is required and the INR is therapeutically or supratherapeutically elevated. The risk for bleeding associated with the procedure compared with the risk for valve thrombosis needs to be considered. Phytonadione (vitamin K_1) can be used orally to reverse the warfarin effect; however, this strategy

Table 1
Summaries of American Heart Association and American College of Chest Physician recommendations for management of mechanical heart valves in pregnancy

American Heart Association[24]	American College of Chest Physicians[23]
All patients with mechanical heart valves require continuous therapeutic anticoagulation	In patients with a mechanical *aortic* valve, vitamin K antagonist therapy with a target INR of 2.5 (range 2–3) is recommended
Women requiring anticoagulation and attempting pregnancy should be monitored with pregnancy tests for prompt therapeutic decision making	In patients with a mechanical *mitral* valve vitamin K antagonist therapy with a target INR of 3 (range 2.5–3.5) over lower INR targets
Pregnant women who elect to stop warfarin between weeks 6 and 12 should receive intravenous UFH, dose-adjusted subcutaneous UFH, or dose-adjusted LMWH	For pregnant patients with mechanical values one of the following three regimens is recommended:
For pregnant women the risks and benefits of UFH, LMWH, or heparin should be discussed fully weighing maternal and fetal risks and benefits	1. Adjusted-dose BID LMWH throughout pregnancy (dose adjusted to manufacturers peak anti-Xa 4 h after injection)
Monitoring goals:	2. Adjusted-dose UFH throughout pregnancy administered subcutaneously every 12 h to keep aPPT two times control
LMWH: BID dosing with anti-Xa levels 0.7–1.2 U/mL 4 h after administration	3. UFH or LMWH until 13th wk with substitution by vitamin K antagonist until close to delivery when UFH or LMWH is resumed
UFH: aPTT two times control	If thought to be at very high risk for thromboembolism (older-generation prosthesis, mitral position, history of thromboembolism) vitamin K antagonists throughout pregnancy with replacement by UFH or LMWH close to delivery is recommended
Warfarin: INR goal = 3 (range 2.5–3.5)	
Warfarin should be discontinued and continuous intravenous UFH started 3–4 wk before planned delivery	
It is reasonable to avoid warfarin between weeks 6 and 12 of gestation because of the high risk of fetal defects	For pregnant women with prosthetic valves at high risk of thromboembolism the addition of 75–100 mg/d of aspirin is recommended
It is reasonable to resume UFH 4–6 h after delivery and begin oral warfarin in the absence of significant bleeding	
It is reasonable to give low-dose aspirin (75–100 mg/d) in the second and third trimesters	

Abbreviations: aPTT, activated partial thromboplastin time; INR, international normalized ratio; LMWH, low-molecular-weight heparin; UFH, unfractionated heparin.

requires 2 to 3 days for normalization. If more urgent reversal is required intravenous phytonadione or blood products, such as fresh frozen plasma, may be used.[6]

Unfractionated Heparin

Heparin produces its major anticoagulant effect by inactivating factor X and preventing the conversion of prothrombin to thrombin.[7] UFH is administered either intravenously or subcutaneously with dose adjustment to achieve a therapeutic activated partial thromboplastin time (aPTT) of two times the control for patients with mechanical heart valves. In patients with lupus anticoagulant the aPTT may be elevated because of the effect of lupus anticoagulant protein and thus these patients may need to be followed with anti–factor Xa level. Heparin binding proteins and the increased plasma volume and altered coagulation profile of pregnancy may require higher doses in pregnant women to maintain a therapeutic aPTT compared with a nonpregnant patient.[8] Approximately 3% of patients receiving UFH develop heparin-induced thrombocytopenia (HIT).[9] Pregnancy-related causes of thrombocytopenia should be considered (discussed elsewhere in this issue), but for patients who received heparin therapy HIT must also be considered in the differential diagnosis for new thrombocytopenia.[10] The management of patients with HIT is described elsewhere,[11] and in the article by Fuller and coworkers elsewhere in this issue. Long-term treatment (over years and dose related) with UFH is associated with osteoporosis but most commonly the maternal benefit of anticoagulation outweighs the small risk for osteoporosis. However, the adverse bone effect may need to be considered in patients requiring long-term UFH anticoagulation with comorbidities, which also may jeopardize bone health (eg, chronic steroids or immobilization). Heparin molecules (UFH and LMWH) are large and do not cross the placenta. UFH and LMWH are too large for placental transport and thus fetal anticoagulation effect is avoided. Maternal treatment does not cause fetal anticoagulation.

Low-Molecular-Weight Heparin

LMWH is used commonly in lieu of UFH because of several studies that have documented that LMWH is as safe and effective as UFH[12–17] and it is increasingly being used during pregnancy for anticoagulation because of easier dosing and improved side effect profile. Compared with UFH, LMWH has a decreased risk for HIT and osteoporosis. However, the LMWH package insert contains a manufacturer warning based on postmarketing reports of valve thrombosis in women with prosthetic heart valves receiving LMWH anticoagulation suggesting that although no causal relationship can be established, LMWH has been inadequately studied in women with prosthetic heart valves.[18] Surveillance of adequate anticoagulation with LMWH is followed with anti-Xa trough levels obtained 4 hours after dose is administered.

The decision to substitute LMWH (or UFH) for vitamin K antagonists during organogenesis must weigh the maternal risk for suboptimal anticoagulation and valve thrombosis; risk of fetal exposure to vitamin K antagonists; and fetal and maternal risks if an urgent procedure is required (eg, stroke, valve replacement, thrombolysis) in the case of valve thromboses. Patients must understand these risks and benefits and be involved in clinical decision making. Furthermore, joint decision making between maternal fetal medicine providers and cardiologists is optimal. For example, women with a particularly high-risk clinical situation (mitral position, first-generation caged-ball or dual mechanical valves, history of previous blood clot, or in atrial fibrillation) may be best managed with continuous warfarin, whereas women with lower risk for thrombosis may choose to switch to heparin medications during organogenesis.

WARFARIN EMBRYOPATHY

Vitamin K antagonists do cross the placenta and thus have the potential for fetal teratogenicity and anticoagulation. Warfarin exposure is associated with an increased risk for miscarriage and fetal warfarin embryopathy. Warfarin embryopathy (critical time period is 6–9 weeks gestation) characteristically includes nasal or midface hypoplasia with nasal alar grooves, and epiphyseal stippling. Epiphyseal stippling appears as multiple calcific foci in abnormally developing bone.[19] Because warfarin crosses the placenta the fetus becomes anticoagulated and thus can have fetal intracranial hemorrhage. Fetal intracranial hemorrhage can occur during labor and vaginal delivery, but can also occur antepartum and may be suspected with irregular echogenic patterns or distortion of normal brain anatomy.[20] Typically transitioning off of warfarin to either UFH or LMWH is performed close to delivery (at approximately 35–36 weeks or earlier if signs or symptoms of preterm delivery) to allow the fetal coagulation profile to return to normal and minimize the risk for intracranial hemorrhage secondary to labor and delivery.

In addition to warfarin embryopathy, an association with an increased risk for stillbirth has been reported. Chan and colleagues[21] reported 21% risk for stillbirth in pregnancies where warfarin was used throughout as compared with 15% risk when heparin was substituted between weeks 6 and 12. Vitale and colleagues[22] reported a possible dose-dependent effect of fetal complications with fewer miscarriages, stillbirths, and cases of warfarin embryopathy with doses of less than 5 mg. Extensive data to definitively document a dose-response relationship or a dose below which fetal risk is negligible do not exist. For warfarin treatment during pregnancy, as with any other medication, the clinical dogma of the "lowest therapeutic dose" should be used so as to avoid the dual risk of subtherapeutic treatment: thrombotic consequences in the maternal patient while still exposing the fetus to the potential for adverse outcomes.

BALANCE OF MATERNAL AND FETAL RISKS

Management of women with mechanical heart valves during pregnancy requires balancing maternal risk of valve thrombosis versus the fetal risk of anticoagulant exposure. Choice of mechanical versus bioprosthetic valves at the time of valve replacement is a trade off of durability versus thrombogenicity. In general, mechanical valves offer increased durability with the downside of requiring life-long full anticoagulation, whereas bioprosthetic valves do not require lifelong anticoagulation but may not be as durable as mechanical valves. In women of reproductive age, because of their long anticipated life span, a mechanical valve may be preferred. The anticoagulants of choice in patients with mechanical valves are vitamin K antagonists. Although vitamin K antagonists are not used commonly during pregnancy, the presence of a mechanical valve is one indication for vitamin K antagonist treatment even during pregnancy. The considerations for maximizing benefit and minimizing risk to maternal and fetal patients in cases of mechanical heart valves in pregnancy are addressed next.

The two most dreaded complications during pregnancy with maternal mechanical valves are fetal warfarin embryopathy and maternal valve thrombosis. No research trials have been performed to definitively answer whether one anticoagulation regimen is superior during organogenesis, during later pregnancy, or around the time of labor and delivery. The risk for valve thrombosis is related to valve position (mitral more than aortic); presence of multiple artificial valves; blood flow gradients across the valve; and other risk factors for coagulation (inherited thrombophilias, atrial fibrillation).

Pregnancy poses a specific risk because of the increased coagulable state consistent with normal pregnancy physiology. Thrombosis of a mechanical valve can be a life-threatening event. Symptoms may include heart failure, low cardiac output, altered valve closure sounds, new and pathologic murmurs, and evidence on transthoracic or transesophageal echocardiography of abnormal leaflets. Reoperation and fibrinolytic therapy in cases of valve thrombosis are associated with significant mortality (>15%)[5] and thus prevention of valve thrombosis is of utmost importance.

The most effective anticoagulant for use in patients with mechanical valves is vitamin K antagonists (eg, warfarin). Although these drugs are the preferred treatment of valve thrombus prophylaxis special consideration in women of reproductive age is needed because of the risk for warfarin embryopathy. Some experts have recommended substituting heparin during weeks 6 to 12 to minimize the risk for warfarin embryopathy.[10,23,24] The following retrospective studies show how different treatment regimens, outcome endpoints, and patient noncompliance make it difficult to determine the best management approach. In a systematic review by Chan and colleagues,[21] three anticoagulation regimens were compared: (1) oral anticoagulants (vitamin K antagonists) throughout pregnancy without interruption; (2) heparin weeks 6 to 12 followed by oral anticoagulation; and (3) heparin use throughout pregnancy. They report a 6% risk for warfarin embryopathy in the liveborn infants and a nearly 25% spontaneous abortion rate in women who received oral anticoagulation throughout pregnancy (regimen 1). When regimen 2 was used (substitution of heparin for weeks 6–12) fetal anomalies decreased to 3.4%. With regimen 3 (heparin throughout), there were no cases of congenital fetal anomalies but there was a 33% risk for thromboembolic complications and a 15% risk for maternal death.[21]

A retrospective evaluation of 356 women with artificial (combined mechanical or bioprosthetic) valves from Denmark reported no thromboembolisms in patients treated with warfarin throughout pregnancy, three thromboembolisms in patients treated with heparin throughout pregnancy, and one thromboembolism in patients treated with warfarin with heparin substituted weeks 6 to 12. There were two neonatal deaths in the warfarin-throughout group and no neonatal deaths in the heparin-throughout and warfarin plus heparin substitution groups.[25]

Another retrospective cohort of 31 women (47 pregnancies) compared complications of three anticoagulation regimens in patients with mechanical heart valves: (1) substitution of warfarin with therapeutic dose enoxaparin and aspirin before 6 weeks of gestation and continued throughout pregnancy; (2) substitution of warfarin with therapeutic dose enoxaparin from 6 to 12 weeks of gestation and again from 36 weeks until delivery (with aspirin throughout pregnancy); and (3) warfarin and aspirin throughout pregnancy switching to therapeutic enoxaparin plus aspirin at 36 weeks.[26] Seven thromboembolic complications occurred, five in the antenatal period and two postpartum. Five of the seven events were on enoxaparin, but in all five cases the authors report patient noncompliance or subtherapeutic anti–factor Xa levels as potential confounders for these events. There were no cases of thromboembolism in pregnancies treated predominantly with warfarin. One case of fetal hydrocephalus, two stillbirths with fetal intracerebral hemorrhage, and one case of warfarin embryopathy occurred in women taking warfarin.

Without definitive randomized control trials to guide decision-making, management of pregnancies in women with mechanical heart valves must be based on interpretation of observational data and extrapolation of known physiologic and pharmacologic phenomena.

PREGNANCY MANAGEMENT
Maternal Complications of Anticoagulant Therapy

Complications of anticoagulant therapy in pregnant patients is similar to that seen in nonpregnant patients including risk for supratherapeutic or subtherapeutic dosing, risk for bleeding, risk for HIT, osteoporosis, bruising, and pain at injection sites for heparin compounds. However, these complications must be weighed against the potentially catastrophic risk for thrombotic events especially during the prothrombotic state of pregnancy.

Early Pregnancy Considerations

In the absence of randomized trial data to suggest a superior anticoagulation strategy, the American College of Chest Physicians and the American Heart Association support multiple anticoagulation strategies during pregnancy as acceptable treatment plans (see **Table 1**). A careful assessment of maternal and fetal risks is required. For example, a patient who presents in the late first or early second trimester of pregnancy for prenatal care may have passed the gestational age for which transition to heparin provides any benefit and oral vitamin K antagonist therapy could be continued. Similarly, a patient with the highest risk thrombogenic profile (caged-ball valve, associated thrombophilia, cardiac arrhythmia, or thrombosis history) may accept the fetal risks to avoid the joint maternal and fetal risks of valve thrombosis and its associated therapy. However, a patient with a lower thrombosis risk profile may, in consultation with a maternal fetal medicine physician and cardiologist, choose to substitute heparin compounds during weeks 6 to 12. Multiple acceptable anticoagulation strategies according to the American College of Chest Physicians and the American Heart Association are summarized in **Table 1**.

Peridelivery and Postdelivery

Warfarin crosses the placenta and thus mother and fetus are therapeutically anticoagulated. The fetal liver is immature and likely takes a longer time to reverse the anticoagulation relative to the normalization of maternal INR. Labor and delivery with a therapeutic INR increases the risk for fetal bleeding events including intracerebral bleeds. Thus, typically around 35 to 36 weeks, or earlier in the case of symptoms of preterm labor, heparin therapy can be initiated while the effect of the vitamin K antagonist wanes in the mother and the fetus. Therapeutic anticoagulation with heparin precludes regional anesthesia during labor because of the risk for dural hematoma and may increase the risk for maternal blood loss. Joint decision making between cardiology and perinatology specialists should be performed to decide whether to allow a short peridelivery time frame during which no anticoagulation is used (thereby allowing for regional anesthesia) or whether to accept the risk for maternal bleeding complications and continue therapeutic heparin throughout labor and delivery. If spontaneous labor occurs while the mother is therapeutically anticoagulated on warfarin, one must assume that the fetus is also therapeutically anticoagulated, and cesarean section should be considered to avoid the risk for fetal intracranial hemorrhage sequelae from labor and delivery. After delivery, resumption of oral anticoagulation with vitamin K antagonists can be performed, often with the use of a heparin bridge until therapeutic. The American College of Chest Physicians suggests continuation of warfarin therapy during lactation. Warfarin is highly protein bound, is not readily detected in breast milk, and importantly does not cause anticoagulation in breastfeeding infants. Warfarin should be used postpartum in lactating women with mechanical heart valves without hesitation.[10]

SUMMARY

Pregnancy management with mechanical heart valves is best done collaboratively with experienced cardiologists and maternal fetal medicine specialists. All anticoagulation options are associated with risks and benefits. In light of the absence of definitive research to suggest a superior regimen, the risks, benefits, and limitations of each strategy should be discussed with the patient and specific attention given to her individual clinical situation.

REFERENCES

1. Kuklina E, Callaghan W. Chronic heart disease and severe obstetric morbidity among hospitalisations for pregnancy in the USA: 1995-2006. BJOG 2011; 118(3):345–52.
2. Burlingame J, Horiuchi B, Ohana P, et al. The contribution of heart disease to pregnancy-related mortality according to the pregnancy mortality surveillance system. J Perinatol 2012;32(3):163–9.

3. Merz WM, Keyver-Paik MD, Baumgarten G, et al. Spectrum of cardiovascular findings during pregnancy and parturition at a tertiary referral center. J Perinat Med 2011;39(3):251–6.

4. Simpson LL. Maternal cardiac disease: update for the clinician. Obstet Gynecol 2012;119(2 Pt 1):345–59.

5. Otto CM, Bonow RO. Valvular heart disease: a companion to Braunwald's heart disease. 3rd edition. Philadelphia, PA: Elsevier; 2009.

6. Ageno W, Gallus AS, Wittkowsky A, et al. Oral anticoagulant therapy: antithrombotic therapy and prevention of thrombosis, 9th ed: American College of Chest Physicians Evidence-Based Clinical Practice Guidelines. Chest 2012;141(Suppl 2):e44S–88S.

7. Gray E, Hogwood J, Mulloy B. The anticoagulant and antithrombotic mechanisms of heparin. Handb Exp Pharmacol 2012;(207):43–61.

8. Chunilal SD, Young E, Johnston MA, et al. The APTT response of pregnant plasma to unfractionated heparin. Thromb Haemost 2002;87(1):92–7.

9. Warkentin TE, Levine MN, Hirsh J, et al. Heparin-induced thrombocytopenia in patients treated with low-molecular-weight heparin or unfractionated heparin. N Engl J Med 1995;332(20):1330–5.

10. Bates SM, Greer IA, Middeldorp S, et al. VTE, thrombophilia, antithrombotic therapy, and pregnancy: antithrombotic therapy and prevention of thrombosis, 9th ed: American College of Chest Physicians Evidence-Based Clinical Practice Guidelines. Chest 2012;141(Suppl 2):e691S–736S.

11. Linkins LA, Dans AL, Moores LK, et al. Treatment and prevention of heparin-induced thrombocytopenia: antithrombotic therapy and prevention of thrombosis, 9th ed: American College of Chest Physicians Evidence-Based Clinical Practice Guidelines. Chest 2012;141(Suppl 2):e495S–530S.

12. Quinlan DJ, McQuillan A, Eikelboom JW. Low-molecular-weight heparin compared with intravenous unfractionated heparin for treatment of pulmonary embolism: a meta-analysis of randomized, controlled trials. Ann Intern Med 2004;140(3):175–83.

13. Eikelboom JW, Anand SS, Malmberg K, et al. Unfractionated heparin and low-molecular-weight heparin in acute coronary syndrome without ST elevation: a meta-analysis. Lancet 2000;355(9219):1936–42.

14. Weitz JI. Low-molecular-weight heparins. N Engl J Med 1997;337(10):688–98.

15. Lepercq J, Conard J, Borel-Derlon A, et al. Venous thromboembolism during pregnancy: a retrospective study of enoxaparin safety in 624 pregnancies. BJOG 2001;108(11):1134–40.

16. Sanson BJ, Lensing AW, Prins MH, et al. Safety of low-molecular-weight heparin in pregnancy: a systematic review. Thromb Haemost 1999;81(5):668–72.

17. Greer I, Hunt BJ. Low molecular weight heparin in pregnancy: current issues. Br J Haematol 2005;128(5):593–601.

18. Lovenox [package insert]. Saint Louis, MO: Sanofi-Aventis Pharmaceuticals; 2011.

19. Wainwright H, Beighton P. Warfarin embryopathy: fetal manifestations. Virchows Arch 2010;457(6):735–9.

20. Sherer DM, Anyaegbunam A, Onyeije C. Antepartum fetal intracranial hemorrhage, predisposing factors and prenatal sonography: a review. Am J Perinatol 1998;15(7):431–41.

21. Chan WS, Anand S, Ginsberg JS. Anticoagulation of pregnant women with mechanical heart valves: a systematic review. Arch Intern Med 2000;160(2):191–6.

22. Vitale N, De Feo M, De Santo LS, et al. Dose-dependent fetal complications of warfarin in pregnant women with mechanical heart valves. J Am Coll Cardiol 1999;33(6):1637–41.

23. Guyatt GH, Akl EA, Crowther M, et al. Introduction to the ninth edition: antithrombotic therapy and prevention of thrombosis, 9th ed: American College of Chest Physicians Evidence-Based Clinical Practice Guidelines. Chest 2012; 141(Suppl 2):48S–52S.

24. Bonow RO, Carabello BA, Kanu C, et al. ACC/AHA 2006 guidelines for the management of patients with valvular heart disease: a report of the American College of Cardiology/American Heart Association Task Force on Practice Guidelines (writing committee to revise the 1998 Guidelines for the Management of Patients With Valvular Heart Disease): developed in collaboration with the Society of Cardiovascular Anesthesiologists: endorsed by the Society for Cardiovascular Angiography and Interventions and the Society of Thoracic Surgeons. Circulation 2006;114(5):e84–231.

25. Sillesen M, Hjortdal V, Vejlstrup N, et al. Pregnancy with prosthetic heart valves: 30 years' nationwide experience in Denmark. Eur J Cardiothorac Surg 2011; 40(2):448–54.

26. McLintock C, McCowan LM, North RA. Maternal complications and pregnancy outcome in women with mechanical prosthetic heart valves treated with enoxaparin. BJOG 2009;116(12):1585–92.

Anticoagulation in Management of Antiphospholipid Antibody Syndrome in Pregnancy

Michael D. Lockshin, MD

KEYWORDS

- Antiphospholipid antibody • Lupus anticoagulant • Systemic lupus erythematosus
- Anticoagulation • Pregnancy

KEY POINTS

- Antiphospholipid antibodies (anticardiolipin, antibody to β_2 glycoprotein I, lupus anticoagulant) are associated with fetal death, prematurity, growth restriction, and preeclampsia.
- Among the antiphospholipid antibodies, lupus anticoagulant is the best predictor of adverse outcome.
- Coexisting systemic lupus erythematosus and/or history of prior thrombosis worsen pregnancy prognosis.
- Although heparin and aspirin are considered standard therapy, treatment trials have not been performed in risk-stratified populations; recommended therapies may therefore be less effective than thought.
- Low-dose heparin (in patients without a history of thrombosis) is as effective as full anticoagulant doses; low-molecular-weight heparin is likely as effective as unfractionated heparin.
- Many new therapy options are under investigation, but performing clinical trials in this population will be difficult.

HISTORY AND DEFINITION

In 1906 Wassermann and colleagues[1] described a complement fixation test for syphilis that is based on the binding of an IgG or IgM antibody from an infected person to cardiolipin, which is a negatively charged phospholipid derived from beef hearts. Because patients who could not have contracted syphilis sometimes had positive test results, a confirmation test was subsequently devised demonstrating the ability of patient serum to immobilize the spirochete *Treponema pallidum*,[2] leading to the

No conflicts of interest.
No unlabelled drug use discussion.
The Barbara Volcker Center for Women and Rheumatic Disease, Hospital for Special Surgery, Weill Cornell Medical College, 535 East 70th Street, New York, NY 10021, USA
E-mail address: LockshinM@hss.edu

label of biologic false-positive (BFP) reactors for persons whose serum reacted in the cardiolipin ("Wassermann") test but not in the immobilization test. Initially BFP was a medical curiosity of no known clinical significance, until, in 1952, Conley and Hartmann[3] described prolongation of an in vitro clotting test in patients who had systemic lupus erythematosus (SLE), many of whom were also BFP. Because these patients experienced hemorrhage, they named the factor *lupus anticoagulant* (LAC). Work thereafter by Rapaport and colleagues,[4] Bowie and colleagues,[5] and others demonstrated that LAC is an antibody to a phospholipid associated with thrombosis rather than with hemorrhage; it binds and thus sequesters the negatively charged phospholipids that initiate clotting in the in vitro assays.[6] Case reports in the 1970s and early 1980s from Sweden, France, England, and Holland suggested an association among LAC, BFP, and fetal death.[7–16]

From the first description until 1983, testing for LAC was tedious, difficult to perform, and unreliable in inexperienced hands. Demonstration of LAC required fresh whole blood specimens for in vitro clotting tests, which began with an abnormal screening test, most often a partial thromboplastin time (PTT) or kaolin clotting time (KCT), but not prothrombin time. Proof that it was an anticoagulant, an inhibitor of clotting, rather than a factor deficiency requires follow-up testing in which patient plasma prolongs the PTT or KCT of normal plasma; if the abnormality is caused by deficiency, normal plasma will correct the test.

In 1983 Hughes' group in England proposed a simple radioimmunoassay as a proxy for the LAC test.[17] The assay uses cardiolipin as the test antigen, can be performed in most clinical laboratories, and, most importantly, can be performed on stored serum. Within a year the radioimmunoassay was revised to an even simpler and less expensive enzyme-linked immunosorbent assay (ELISA). A positive result in this ELISA is now called the *anticardiolipin antibody* (aCL).

In 1990 several groups simultaneously discovered that what is called aCL does not bind cardiolipin directly but requires a cofactor, β_2 glycoprotein I (β_2GP-I), also known as apolipoprotein H; an assay for antibody to β_2GP-I was devised (aβ_2GP-I).[18,19] Today LAC, aCL, and aβ_2GP-I are collectively known as antiphospholipid antibodies (aPLs).

BIOLOGIC ACTIVITY OF APLS

All of the terms used to describe aPLs are misnomers. Except when directed against prothrombin, LAC is a procoagulant; it is an anticoagulant only in vitro. aCL does not directly bind cardiolipin (or other negatively charged phospholipids), but rather does so through its binding to β_2GP-I, which itself binds the phospholipid.

β_2GP-I is a complex molecule with 5 domains. The fifth domain, in combination with a membrane protein cofactor, most likely Toll-like receptor 2 or 4 (TLR2, TLR4),[20,21] binds to a negatively charged phospholipid, specifically the phosphatidylserine that is exteriorized when a cell is activated or dying. Pathogenic aPL binds to a peptide in the first domain of β_2GP-I.[22] aPL binding to β_2GP-I–TLR4 initiates both intracellular and extracellular processes that result in tissue damage (see later discussion).

Other antibodies are commonly associated with aPL, such as antibodies to prothrombin (which, in depleting prothrombin, may cause hemorrhage) or to the prothrombin-phospholipid complex.[23,24] The biologic importance of these associated antibodies is now being discovered. Animal models for both thrombosis and pregnancy loss, in which animals are either immunized to produce aPL or have it passively infused, strongly suggest that the aPL itself is directly pathogenic and is not a passive marker or bystander.[25]

aPL can be induced, usually transiently, by several infections, such as Epstein-Barr virus, Lyme, leprosy, and, of course, syphilis.[26] Some infection-induced aPLs, such as that induced by the syphilis spirochete, bind directly to membrane phospholipids, bypassing the β_2GP-I pathway, and differ from the pathogenic aPL found in patients with SLE.[27] aPLs induced by leprosy are likely β_2GP-I–dependent and pathogenic.

Today, the target for pathogenic aPL is thought to be conformationally altered β_2GP-I bound to TLR4. The pathophysiologic model proposes that the antibody may arise as a result of an (unidentified) infection in a genetically prepared host; it causes no harm until cell injury or perhaps virally induced endothelial cell activation, and exteriorizes the negatively charged phospholipid phosphatidylserine to the outer cell membrane. At that time, β_2GP-I binds to the cell membrane phosphatidylserine–TLR4 complex and undergoes a conformational change that activates complement in the extracellular space and/or triggers intracellular activation, which results in upregulation of adhesion and other molecules. These events lead to inflammation, thrombosis, and clinically recognized disease.[22] aPL may also interfere with trophoblast development, maturation, and invasion.[28] Under normal circumstances β_2GP-I is thought to be a molecule that protects endothelial integrity.[29]

CLINICAL ASSOCIATIONS

After the introduction of the anticardiolipin ELISA, several papers in the mid-1980s confirmed and strengthened the association between aPL and pregnancy complications, and also between aPL and recurrent venous or arterial thromboses. Initially restricted to fetal death, pregnancy morbidity associated with aPL now includes fetal growth restriction, prematurity, and early or severe preeclampsia.

Together with the definition of aPL, a clinical definition of what is now known as antiphospholipid syndrome (APS) evolved. International consensus conferences in 1999 (Sapporo, Japan)[30] and 2006 (Sydney, Australia)[31] provide the following criteria for APS:

- A patient must have both serologic and clinical findings.
- Serologic criteria must include LAC (positive) and/or high-titer ($\geq$40 units) IgG or IgM aCL and/or high-titer ($\geq$40 units) IgG or IgM aβ_2GP-I.
- Tests must be positive on 2 occasions at least 12 weeks apart.
- Clinical criteria include recurrent thromboses and/or recurrent pregnancy losses, defined as at least one loss of an apparently normal fetus after 12 weeks, or 3 consecutive losses of apparently normal fetuses at less than 12 weeks, without other causes, such as infection.

IgA antibody does not fulfill the definition for either aCL or aβ_2GP-1 because it is unreliably determined in commercial laboratories. Similarly, assays for antibodies to other phospholipids, such as phosphatidylserine and phosphatidylethanolamine, have not undergone rigorous standardization procedures nor clinical association studies, and therefore are not included. Low-titer antibody is insufficiently closely associated with clinical events, and may be transient after infection, and therefore does not fulfill the criteria for APS.

Many other clinical features occur in patients with APS but are not included in the criteria, including the following:

- Thrombocytopenia
- Livedo reticularis
- Cardiac valve vegetations
- Renal thrombotic microangiopathy

- Cognitive dysfunction
- Hyperintense nonenhancing white matter lesions on brain magnetic resonance imaging
- Catastrophic antiphospholipid syndrome in which multiple widespread thromboses occur over a short period[32]

Recent articles suggest that patients presenting with different manifestations, such as pregnancy loss or thrombosis, likely represent different subgroups, and that risks experienced by one group are not necessarily applicable to another.[33]

ANTICOAGULATION AS TREATMENT

Because historically the recognition of APS evolved from recognizing the relationship between aPL and thrombosis, and because the association between aPL and SLE was an early discovery, initial treatment recommendations focused on immunosuppressive therapy for both the thrombotic and the pregnancy morbidity forms of the disease. High-dose corticosteroid therapy failed.[34,35] Because early reports had sought and found placental thrombosis, and because of the association between aPL and peripheral thrombosis, anticoagulation with heparin was introduced, given that warfarin was disfavored in pregnancy because of teratogenicity. Early papers on pregnancy also emphasized the association between genetic hypercoagulable states (factor V Leiden, prothrombin 20210, antithrombin III) and recurrent pregnancy loss, and a putative increase in pregnancy failure in patients having both aPL and genetic hypercoagulability, supporting the hypothesis that placental thrombosis was the mechanism at fault.[36]

The first papers on fetal loss in patients with aCL or LAC did not address therapy.[13,37,38] The next generation of papers focused on the (generally negative) results of treatment with high-dose corticosteroids.[34,35] Thereafter a series of papers, including a few randomized controlled studies, found better fetal outcome in patients taking heparin and aspirin compared with untreated patients or those treated with aspirin alone,[39–41] but not all investigators agreed.[42] Studies in patients with genetic thrombopathies or in those likely to develop preeclampsia mostly failed to show efficacy of either aspirin or heparin.[43] Some articles emphasized a good prognosis in untreated patients with aPL or APS.[44,45] The available studies are small; as a rule, they do not stratify patients according to either serologic or clinical risk profile, nor do they examine different fetal outcomes, such as growth restriction or prematurity, as opposed to fetal death.

The studies that most clearly supported the use of heparin are those of Rai and colleagues[39] and of Kutteh and colleagues.[40,41] In the study by Rai and colleagues,[39] pregnant women who had aPL, mostly but not exclusively defined by LAC, and who had had 3 or more miscarriages were prospectively randomized to either aspirin or aspirin and heparin treatment. Treatment groups had similar numbers of prior miscarriages but were not otherwise described. The live birth rate among 45 women who received 75 mg of aspirin plus 5000 units of unfractionated heparin twice daily was 71% compared with 42% among 45 women who received aspirin alone. Women who received heparin had a median decrease in lumbar spine bone density of 5.4%. Kutteh and colleagues,[40,41] using a similar study design and entry criteria, found that 80% of 25 women treated with heparin plus low-dose aspirin had viable pregnancies (essentially all at term) compared with 44% of women treated with aspirin alone. They then compared 25 women treated with anticoagulant-dose heparin (80% survival) versus 25 women treated with low-dose heparin (76% survival), concluding, as in the animal experiments, that heparin's efficacy may not reside in its anticoagulant properties. Although less systematic, subsequent studies have argued that low-molecular-weight heparin is equivalent to unfractionated heparin in efficacy, as it is in the animal model.[46]

Animal models demonstrate that aCL has a direct, causative role in fetal loss and that heparin prevents fetal loss. A particularly informative set of experiments in mice further shows that heparin, but not fondaparinux or warfarin, prevents aCL-induced fetal resorption, and that complement deficiency or inactivation is equally protective.[47] The low-dose heparin trial (inactivating complement but not preventing thrombosis) by Kutteh and colleagues[40,41] would seem to confirm this, and Rai and colleagues[39] also used subanticoagulant doses. These data are consistent with the hypothesis that heparin's efficacy is from its anticomplement activity, and thus place complement activation and inflammation at the head of the pathogenetic line, with thrombosis being a downstream, terminal event. More recent human studies question whether genetic hypercoagulable states truly lead to pregnancy loss and whether these need be treated at all,[43,44] again diminishing the prothrombotic theory of recurrent pregnancy loss.

TREATMENT RECOMMENDATIONS

Standard treatment to prevent adverse pregnancy outcome, based mostly on consensus data rather than on clinical trials, continues to be

- Prophylactic doses, such as 0.5 mg/kg/d of low-molecular-weight heparin (enoxaparin) or 5000 u twice daily of unfractionated heparin plus low-dose (81 mg) aspirin for patients who have not had prior thrombosis. It is best to consider checking, once or twice during treatment, anti–factor Xa activity 4 hours after the last dose for a level of 0.2 to 0.6 U/mL.
- Full anticoagulant doses, such as 1 mg/kg every 12 hours of enoxaparin or 10,000 to 12,000 units unfractionated heparin every 12 hours in those who have had prior thrombosis. Treatment dose must be monitored by anti–factor Xa activity, because PTT is usually abnormal in patients with LAC. Target anti–factor Xa 4 hours after the last dose for a level of 0.5 to 1.1 U/mL if twice-daily dosing, or 1.0 to 2.0 U/mL if once-daily dosing.
- Treatment begins at conception and continues for 6 to 12 weeks postpartum if the patient has no history of thrombosis, and indefinitely if the patient has a history.
- Dosing will need to be reduced if renal impairment is present.

RISK STRATIFICATION

A difficulty in interpreting the available data is that recent work strongly suggests that not all patients with aPL are at equal risk for pregnancy loss, and that past studies that did not risk stratify may be invalid. Papers discussing aPLs have not clearly distinguished risks that might be differently distributed among the different antibodies, aCL, aβ₂GP-1, and LAC, nor have treatment studies attempted to risk stratify according to clinical diagnosis.

Only recently have studies begun to stratify patients according to prepregnancy risk profile. In its setting criteria for the classification of APS, an international consensus team emphasized that risk is increased only by sustained high titers aCL and aβ₂GP-1 and of IgG or IgM isotype, and as opposed to low titers of IgA aCL or transient high titers of IgG aCL or IgM aCL.[31] Concomitantly, clinical studies confirmed the increased risk attributable to coexisting SLE, prior thrombosis history, smoking, and trigger factors (eg, surgery, trauma, oral contraceptive therapy, sepsis).[48] Systematic risk stratification analyses for pregnancy treatment studies are unavailable.

A parallel article on aPL-associated thrombosis began to argue that risk could be graded by serologic profile, that, depending on investigator, high titer, triple (aCL, $a\beta_2$GP-1, and LAC) positivity, $a\beta_2$GP-1 alone, LAC alone, or antibody to a peptide found in domain 1 (of 5 domains) of β_2GP-1 more precisely predicted thrombotic risk.[49] Other investigators focused on clinical risk profile: occurrence of trauma, surgery, or delivery; smoking; preexisting atherosclerosis; and prior thrombi.[48]

Until recently, no study has been large enough, or has considered a sufficient number of variables, to allow determination of treatment efficacy in a risk-stratified patient group.

Ruffatti and colleagues,[50] emphasizing serology, retrospectively compared 57 women with APS who either lost pregnancies or delivered before 34 weeks ("unsuccessful") versus 57 women with APS who had successful pregnancies. To isolate predictive clinical features, this study matched successful and unsuccessful pregnancies according to treatment with heparin, aspirin, or both together. The investigators concluded that triple positivity was the best predictor of fetal loss. Concerns about this conclusion are that the patients were collected between 1986 and 2009 ($a\beta_2$GP-1 was not identified until 1990[18,19] and did not become a clinical assay until several years later); only 38 of the 57 (67%) women with unsuccessful pregnancies and 45 of the 57 (79%) with successful pregnancies in fact had all 3 tests performed; and those with unsuccessful pregnancies differed from those with successful pregnancies in having much more associated autoimmune disease (49% vs 12%), prior thrombosis (49% vs 21%), both pregnancy morbidity and prior thrombosis (32% vs 4%), and other APS-related manifestations (35% vs 12%).

The author's own studies[51] show similar outcomes but lead to different conclusions. Between 2003 and 2011, the author's group enrolled 144 pregnant patients with aPL into a prospective observational study; all were tested for aCL, $a\beta_2$GP-1, and LAC at core laboratories at enrollment, in each trimester, and at 3 months postpartum; LAC was determined using 3 separate methods (screening with PTT, dilute Russell's viper venom time, or dilute prothrombin time). The investigators did not analyze pregnancies lost before 12 weeks, nor did they alter therapy chosen by the treating physician. Of the 144 patients, 57 had SLE. Using multivariate analysis, the investigators concluded that the most powerful predictor of adverse pregnancy outcome (fetal death, prematurity, growth restriction, and/or preeclampsia) is lupus anticoagulant. Other adverse predictors include diagnosis of SLE, prior thrombosis, and young maternal age. Surprisingly, neither adverse prior pregnancy history nor high-titer aCL or $a\beta_2$GP-1 IgG or IgM isotypes (without concomitant LAC) added to the prediction model. Triple positivity was no more predictive than its dominant component, LAC. The study was not a treatment trial, and confounding bias by treatment indication cannot be excluded; however, when only patients who had positive test results for LAC are considered, heparin therapy was not associated with improved outcome, whereas aspirin was. Patients whose test results were negative for LAC had uniformly good outcomes despite whether heparin or aspirin was administered.

The author's review of available information suggests the following: aPL is associated with recurrent pregnancy loss; among aPLs, LAC is the most powerful predictor; other clinical features, especially coexisting SLE, contribute to pregnancy risk; and no study to date has sufficiently stratified patients to support an unequivocal recommendation of heparin treatment for prophylaxis against pregnancy loss, nor are clear guidelines for either dose or type of heparin available.

FUTURE TREATMENTS AND TRIAL DESIGN

The biology of aPL-associated tissue damage suggests alternatives to anticoagulation as treatment for APS.[29,52] If complement activation is truly a critical early step in the process that leads to fetal death, as it seems to be in animal models, products that prevent complement activation may be of benefit; eculizumab, a C5 inhibitor, successfully interrupted recurring catastrophic antiphospholipid syndrome in 1 patient.[53] Experimental animal models indicate that peptides that block the binding of antibody to β_2GP-1 are also effective.[54] It may be possible to remove or block aPL synthesis, or to prevent upregulation of the adhesion molecules that, presumably, are the final step in vascular insufficiency and placental failure. Other anecdotal treatments include plasmapheresis and intravenous immunoglobulin. These new treatment opportunities and others have been reviewed elsewhere.[29,55,56]

However, safe and ethical clinical trials will be difficult to design. Most clinics now achieve greater than 80% fetal survival in women who do not have SLE and who have had 2 or more consecutive fetal losses, implying that, if positive aPL results, history of recurrent fetal loss, and no underlying illness are the only entry criteria, very large numbers of patients will have to be treated to demonstrate success, and the safety of an intervention will have to be guaranteed at a very high level. If studies are restricted to women stratified to be at very high risk (history of prior losses, coexisting SLE, positive LAC results, history of prior thrombosis), very few study subjects will be available, but few will be needed to prove efficacy. Because modern neonatology enables survival of very premature or ill infants, outcome criteria for clinical trials will have to include prematurity, growth restriction, preeclampsia, and death, which will add variables to the analysis; similarly, analysis will not truly be complete until the infants have reached at least school age and possibly teen years to determine long-term outcomes of the intervention. These rigorous criteria will be difficult to fulfill, but couples experiencing repeated pregnancy loss continue to plead for the challenges to be met.

REFERENCES

1. Wassermann A, Neisser A, Bruck C. Eine serodiagnostische Reaktion bei Syphilis. Deutsche medicinische Wochenschrift, Berlin 1906;32:745–6.
2. Nielsen HA, Reyn A. The Treponema pallidum immobilization test. Bull World Health Organ 1956;14:263–88.
3. Conley CL, Hartmann RC. A hemorrhagic disorder caused by circulating anticoagulants in patients with disseminated lupus erythematosus. J Lab Clin Invest 1952;31:621–2.
4. Mueh JR, Herbst KD, Rapaport SI. Thrombosis in patients with the lupus anticoagulant. Ann Intern Med 1980;92:156–9.
5. Bowie EJ, Thompson JH, Pascuzzi CA, et al. Thrombosis in systemic lupus erythematosus despite circulating anticoagulants. J Lab Clin Med 1963;62:416–30.
6. Thiagarajan P, Shapiro SS, De Marco L. Monoclonal immunoglobulin M lambda coagulation inhibitor with phospholipid specificity. Mechanism of a lupus anticoagulant. J Clin Invest 1980;66:397–405.
7. Nilsson IM, Åstedt B, Hedner U, et al. Intrauterine death and circulating anticoagulant ("antithromboplastin"). Acta Med Scand 1975;197:153–9.
8. Soulier JP, Boffa MC. Avortements á répétition, thromboses et anticoagulant circulant anti-thromboplastine: trois observations. Nouv Presse Med 1980;9:859–64.
9. Firkin BG, Howard MA, Radford N. Possible relationship between lupus inhibitor and recurrent abortion in young women. Lancet 1980;2:366.

10. Abramowsky CR, Vegas ME, Swinehart G, et al. Decidual vasculopathy of the placenta in lupus erythematosus. N Engl J Med 1980;303:668–72.

11. Carreras LO, Defreyn G, Machin SJ, et al. Arterial thrombosis, intrauterine death and "lupus" anticoagulant: detection of immunoglobulin interfering with prostacyclin formation. Lancet 1981;1:244–6.

12. De Wolf F, Carreras LO, Moerman P, et al. Decidual vasculopathy and extensive placental infarction in a patient with repeated thromboembolic accidents, recurrent fetal loss and a lupus anticoagulant. Am J Obstet Gynecol 1982;142:829–34.

13. Hughes GR. Thrombosis, abortion, cerebral disease, and the lupus anticoagulant. Br Med J (Clin Res Ed) 1983;287(6399):1088–9.

14. Lubbe WF, Palmer SJ, Butler WS, et al. Fetal survival after prednisone suppression of maternal lupus-anticoagulant. Lancet 1983;1:1361–3.

15. Reece EA, Romero R, Clyne LP, et al. Lupus-like anticoagulant in pregnancy. Lancet 1984;1:344–5.

16. Gårdlund B. The lupus inhibitor in thromboembolic disease and intrauterine death in the absence of systemic lupus. Acta Med Scand 1984;215:293–8.

17. Harris EN, Gharavi AE, Boey ML, et al. Anticardiolipin antibodies: detection by radioimmunoassay and association with thrombosis in systemic lupus erythematosus. Lancet 1983;2:1211–4.

18. Galli M, Comfurius P, Maassen C, et al. Anticardiolipin antibodies (ACA) directed not to cardiolipin but to a plasma cofactor. Lancet 1990;335:1544–7.

19. McNeil HP, Simpson RJ, Chesterman CN, et al. Antiphospholipid antibodies are directed against a complex antigen that includes a lipid binding inhibitor of coagulation: b2 Glycoprotein I (apolipoprotein H). Proc Natl Acad Sci U S A 1990;87:4120–4.

20. Allen KL, Fonseca FV, Betapudi V, et al. A novel pathway for human endothelial cell activation by antiphospholipid/anti-β2 glycoprotein I antibodies. Blood 2011;119:884–93.

21. Mulla MJ, Brosens JJ, Chamley LW, et al. Antiphospholipid antibodies induce a pro-inflammatory response in first trimester trophoblast via the TLR4/MyD88 pathway. Am J Reprod Immunol 2009;62:96–111.

22. Salmon JE, Girardi G, Lockshin MD. The antiphospholipid syndrome as a disorder initiated by inflammation: implications for the therapy of pregnant patients. Nat Clin Pract Rheumatol 2007;3:140–7.

23. Erkan D, Bateman H, Lockshin MD. Lupus anticoagulant-hypoprothrombinemia syndrome associated with systemic lupus erythematosus: report of 2 cases and review of literature. Lupus 1999;8:560–4.

24. Amengual O, Atsumi T, Koike T. Pathophysiology of thrombosis and potential targeted therapies in antiphospholipid syndrome. Curr Vasc Pharmacol 2011;9:606–18.

25. Girardi G, Redecha P, Salmon JE. Heparin prevents antiphospholipid antibody-induced fetal loss by inhibiting complement activation. Nat Med 2004;10:1222–6.

26. Ribeiro SL, Pereira HL, Silva NP, et al. Anti-β2-glycoprotein I antibodies are highly prevalent in a large number of Brazilian leprosy patients. Acta Reumatol Port 2011;36:30–7.

27. Levy RA, de Meis E, Pierangeli S. An adapted ELISA method for differentiating pathogenic from nonpathogenic aPL by a beta 2 glycoprotein I dependency anticardiolipin assay. Thromb Res 2004;114:573–7.

28. Han CS, Mulla MJ, Brosens JJ, et al. Aspirin and heparin effect on basal and antiphospholipid antibody modulation of trophoblast function. Obstet Gynecol 2011;118:1021–8.

29. Meroni PL, Borghi MO, Raschi E, et al. Pathogenesis of antiphospholipid syndrome: understanding the antibodies. Nat Rev Rheumatol 2011;7:330–9.
30. Wilson WA, Gharavi AE, Koike T, et al. International consensus statement on preliminary classification criteria for definite antiphospholipid syndrome. Arthritis Rheum 1999;42:1309–11.
31. Miyakis S, Lockshin MD, Atsumi T, et al. International consensus statement on an update of the classification criteria for definite antiphospholipid syndrome (APS). J Thromb Haemost 2006;4:295–306.
32. Erkan D, Lockshin MD. Non-criteria manifestations of antiphospholipid syndrome. Lupus 2010;19:424–7.
33. Meroni PL, Raschi E, Grossi C, et al. Obstetric and vascular APS: same autoantibodies but different diseases? Lupus 2012;21:708–10.
34. Lockshin MD, Druzin ML, Qamar T. Prednisone does not prevent recurrent fetal death in women with antiphospholipid antibody. Am J Obstet Gynecol 1989; 160:439–44.
35. Cowchock ES, Reece EA, Balababan D, et al. Repeated fetal losses associated with antiphospholipid antibodies: a collaborative randomized trial comparing prednisone with low dose heparin treatment. Am J Obstet Gynecol 1992;166: 1313–23.
36. Bradley LA, Palomaki GE, Bienstock J, et al. Can Factor V Leiden and prothrombin G20210A testing in women with recurrent pregnancy loss result in improved pregnancy outcomes?: results from a targeted evidence-based review. Genet Med 2012;14:39–50.
37. Lockshin MD, Druzin ML, Goei S, et al. Antibody to cardiolipin predicts fetal distress or death in pregnant patients with systemic lupus erythematosus. N Engl J Med 1985;313:152–6.
38. Branch DW, Scott JR, Kochenour NK, et al. Obstetric complications associated with the lupus anticoagulant. N Engl J Med 1985;313:1322–6.
39. Rai R, Cohen H, Dave M, et al. Randomised controlled trial of aspirin and aspirin plus heparin in pregnant women with recurrent miscarriage associated with phospholipid antibodies (or antiphospholipid antibodies). BMJ 1997;314:253–7.
40. Kutteh WH. Antiphospholipid antibody-associated recurrent pregnancy loss: treatment with heparin and low-dose aspirin is superior to low-dose aspirin alone. Am J Obstet Gynecol 1996;174:1584–9.
41. Kutteh WH, Ermel LD. A clinical trial for the treatment of antiphospholipid antibody-associated recurrent pregnancy loss with lower dose heparin and aspirin. Am J Reprod Immunol 1996;35:402–7.
42. Farquharson RG, Quenby S, Greaves M. Antiphospholipid syndrome in pregnancy: a randomized, controlled trial of treatment. Obstet Gynecol 2002;100: 408–13.
43. Manuck T, Branch DW, Lai Y, et al. Antiphospholipid antibodies and pregnancy outcomes in women heterozygous for factor V Leiden. J Reprod Immunol 2010; 85:180–5.
44. Cohn DM, Goddijn M, Middeldorp S, et al. Recurrent miscarriage and antiphospholipid antibodies: prognosis of subsequent pregnancy. J Thromb Haemost 2010;8:2208–13.
45. Laskin CA, Spitzer KA, Clark CA, et al. Low molecular weight heparin and aspirin for recurrent pregnancy loss: results from the randomized, controlled HepASA Trial. J Rheumatol 2009;36:279–87.
46. Check JH. The use of heparin for preventing miscarriage. Am J Reprod Immunol 2012;67:326–33.

47. Salmon JE, Girardi G. Antiphospholipid antibodies and pregnancy loss: a disorder of inflammation. J Reprod Immunol 2008;77:51–6.
48. Erkan D, Yazici Y, Peterson MG, et al. A cross-sectional study of clinical thrombotic risk factors and preventive treatments in antiphospholipid syndrome. Rheumatology (Oxford) 2002;41:924–9.
49. Ioannou Y, Rahman A. Domain I of beta2-glycoprotein I: its role as an epitope and the potential to be developed as a specific target for the treatment of the antiphospholipid syndrome. Lupus 2010;19:400–5.
50. Ruffatti A, Tonello M, Visentin MS, et al. Risk factors for pregnancy failure in patients with anti-phospholipid syndrome treated with conventional therapies: a multicentre, case-control study. Rheumatology (Oxford) 2011;50:1684–9.
51. Lockshin MD, Kim M, Laskin CA, et al. Prediction of adverse pregnancy outcome by the presence of lupus anticoagulant, but not anticardiolipin antibody, in patients with antiphospholipid antibodies. Arthritis Rheum 2012;64:2311–8.
52. Gelber SE, Salmon JE. Autoimmunity: effectiveness of treatments for pregnant women with APS. Nat Rev Rheumatol 2010;6:187–9.
53. Shapira I, Andrade D, Allen SL, et al. Brief report: induction of sustained remission in recurrent catastrophic antiphospholipid syndrome via inhibition of terminal complement with eculizumab. Arthritis Rheum 2012;64:2719–23.
54. de la Torre YM, Pregnolato F, D'Amelio F, et al. Anti-phospholipid induced murine fetal loss: novel protective effect of a peptide targeting the β2 glycoprotein I phospholipid-binding site. Implications for human fetal loss. J Autoimmun 2012;38:J209–15.
55. Erkan D, Lockshin MD. New approaches for managing antiphospholipid syndrome. Nat Clin Pract Rheumatol 2009;5:160–70.
56. Pierangeli SS, Erkan D. Antiphospholipid syndrome treatment beyond anticoagulation: are we there yet? Lupus 2010;19:475–85.

Inherited Thrombophilia
Diagnosis and Anticoagulation Treatment in Pregnancy

Nazli Hossain, MBBS, FCPS[a],*, Michael J. Paidas, MD[b]

KEYWORDS

- Inherited thrombophilia • Heparin • Adverse pregnancy outcome

KEY POINTS

- Screening for inherited thrombophilia includes factor V Leiden (FVL), prothrombin gene mutation 20210A (PGM), and natural anticoagulants antithrombin III, protein C and protein S.
- Screening for less common thrombophilia, methyltetrahydrofolate reductase and plasminogen activator inhibitor antigen is not recommended for adverse pregnancy outcomes.
- Screening for inherited thrombophilia in recurrent pregnancy losses at less than 10 weeks of gestation is not recommended.
- Screening for inherited thrombophilia for adverse pregnancy outcome is not justified.
- Anticoagulant therapy for adverse pregnancy outcome should be considered investigational.
- Large, well-designed, multicenter trials are required to determine whether anticoagulation is beneficial in a range of adverse pregnancy outcomes.
- Heparin and/or aspirin therapy is not indicated to prevent the recurrence of unexplained early pregnancy loss, or losses associated with FVL or PGM.

INTRODUCTION

The association between inherited thrombophilia and deep vein thrombosis is well established. However, gaps in knowledge exist in the association of inherited thrombophilia and adverse pregnancy outcome. Adverse pregnancy outcome, sometimes called placenta-mediated complications, including preeclampsia, preterm labor,

[a] Department of Obstetrics & Gynecology, Dow University of Health Sciences, Karachi 74200, Pakistan; [b] Baxter Clinical Fellowship Program, Yale Division of Maternal Fetal Medicine, Department of Obstetrics, Gynecology and Reproductive Sciences, National Hemophilia Foundation, Yale Women and Children's Center for Blood Disorders, Yale University School of Medicine, 333 Cedar Street, FMB 339B, New Haven, CT 06520-8063, USA
* Corresponding author.
E-mail address: Nazli.hossain@duhs.edu.pk

Clin Lab Med 33 (2013) 377–390
http://dx.doi.org/10.1016/j.cll.2013.03.025
0272-2712/13/$ – see front matter

intrauterine growth restriction, and small for gestational age, have been attributed to excessive thrombosis and inflammation at the uteroplacental interface.[1] This linkage resulted in widespread screening for thrombophilia in women with adverse pregnancy outcome. Anticoagulant therapy was initially liberally administered for prevention of adverse pregnancy outcome, based on case-control studies, coincident with widespread screening for inherited thrombophilic conditions in the setting of adverse pregnancy outcomes. However, well-designed randomized trials were initiated and some have been completed in the past few years. Results of these randomized trials have provided critical evidence-based data to serve as a guide for clinicians faced with managing patients with one or more of the common obstetric complications (**Table 1**).

This article focuses on the prevalence of different inherited thrombophilias, their association with adverse pregnancy outcome, and possible beneficial effects of anticoagulant therapy.

Factor V Leiden and Adverse Pregnancy Outcome

Factor V Leiden (FVL) is the most common inheritable thrombophilia, and is also the most common causal factor for venous thromboembolic disease. Among Europeans, FVL heterozygosity is found among 5.3% of the population.[2] Sweden has the highest prevalence of all the European countries. The prevalence of FVL heterozygosity in the United States varies between 3% and 8%.[3] Prevalence is uncommon in the Asian and African races. Factor V, in activated form FVa, causes the conversion of prothrombin to thrombin. It is subsequently acted on by activated protein C (APC), to cause inactivation of VIIIa. FVL mutation refers to specific mutation of the amino acid guanine with adenine substitution in the FV gene, which predicts substitution of amino acid glutamine at the cleavage site of APC. The result is increased procoagulant activity, reflected as increased levels of D-dimer and prothrombin fragments F1+2. Diagnosis is based on screening for APC resistance using a second-generation coagulation assay, and can be followed by DNA analysis of the FV gene. The second-generation assay has shown 100% sensitivity and specificity for FVL.[4] The FVL mutation is inherited as an autosomal dominant disorder. The lifetime risk of venous thromboembolism (VTE) in heterozygous individuals is 5% to 8%, whereas, in homozygous individuals, this risk is increased more than 25-fold. FVL has been implicated in pregnancy complications such as:

- Early pregnancy loss
- Late pregnancy loss

Table 1	
Recent trials of anticoagulant use in prevention of adverse pregnancy outcome (APO)	
Study	**ClinicalTrial.gov**
TIPPS	ISRC TN87441504
FRUIT	ISRC TN 87325378
ALIFE	ISRC TN 58496168
SPIN	ISRC TN 06774126
HAPPY	Eudra CT 2006-004205-26

Abbreviations: ALIFE, Anticoagulant for Living Fetuses; FRUIT; Fragmin in Pregnant Women with a History of Uteroplacental Insufficiency and Thrombophilia; HAPPY, Heparin in Pregnant Women with Previous Placenta-mediated Pregnancy Complications; SPIN, Scottish Pregnancy Intervention Study; TIPPS, Thrombophilia in Pregnancy Prophylaxis Study.

- Preeclampsia
- Abruptio placentae
- Intrauterine growth restriction

FVL AND PREGNANCY LOSS

FVL has been extensively studied for associations with early and late pregnancy loss. In a cohort of more than 400 patients with adverse pregnancy outcome, we showed that inherited thrombophilia was not associated with pregnancy loss before 10 weeks, but was associated with loss at greater than 14 weeks' gestation.[5] In this high-risk cohort, the presence of 1 or more maternal thrombophilias protected against recurrent losses at less than 10 weeks (1 thrombophilia, odds ratio [OR] 0.55, 95% confidence interval [CI] 0.33–0.92; >1 thrombophilia, OR 0.48, 95% CI 0.29–0.78). In contrast, the presence of maternal thrombophilia(s) was modestly associated with an increased risk of losses at more than 10 weeks (1 thrombophilia, OR 1.76, 95% CI 1.05–2.94; >1 thrombophilia, OR 1.66, 95% CI 1.03–2.68). This association was greater with euploid losses compared with aneuploid losses. In a population-based study including more than 32,700 women, FVL was associated with pregnancy loss between 10 and 39 weeks of gestation (OR 3.46, 95% CI 2.53–4.72).[6] In an incident case–control study of women with recurrent pregnancy losses, screening of couples was carried out for the FV allele. The investigators concluded that FVL was not associated with early recurrent loss.[7] In Asian people, recurrent pregnancy loss was not associated with inherited thrombophilia.[8]

FVL AND PREECLAMPSIA

The association between FVL and preeclampsia is controversial.

In early literature, an association was seen between preeclampsia and FVL. Kupfer-minc,[9] in a study of 110 women with adverse pregnancy outcome, showed an association between preeclampsia and FVL (OR 5.3; 95% CI 2.0–4.3). This association was also seen with recurrent preeclampsia. In a prospective study, women with recurrent preeclampsia were screened for inherited thrombophilia. Screening was positive in 34% (OR 2.5, 95% CI 1.2–5.1).[10] In a meta-analysis of pregnancy complications with inherited thrombophilia, no association was seen between FVL and preeclampsia (OR 1.23, 95% CI 0.89–1.70).[11] Similar results were seen in other prospective studies. In a prospective case-cohort study from Germany, 491 FVL carriers and 1055 controls were observed for pregnancy complications like preeclampsia, stillbirth, and intrauterine growth restriction. The investigators concluded that being an FVL carrier was not associated with the pregnancy complications discussed earlier.[12]

FVL AND ABRUPTIO PLACENTAE

Compared with preeclampsia, studies exploring the association between abruptio placentae and FVL are few. In a retrospective case-control study, Procházka and colleagues[13] compared 180 cases of abruptio placentae with 196 controls. FVL was found in 14% compared with 5.1% among controls (OR 3.0, 95% CI 1.4–6.7). In another case-control study, 50 cases with abruption, requiring immediate delivery were compared with 100 controls. Women heterozygous for FVL showed an association with abruptio placentae (OR 9.12, 95% CI 2.18–31.7, $P = .0005$)[14] In a recently published study from an Australian population, exploring adverse pregnancy outcome with inherited thrombophilia, FVL was a risk factor for stillbirth and abruptio placentae, but not for other adverse pregnancy outcomes.[15] However, the number of women with abruptio placentae was only 16, so caution should be exercised in interpreting the results of this study.

Prothrombin Gene Mutation 20210A and Adverse Pregnancy Outcome

Prothrombin gene mutation 20210A (PGM) is less commonly seen than FVL; its prevalence is estimated to be around 2% to 3% in Europeans.[2] It is the second most common inherited thrombophilia seen in women with pregnancy-associated venous thromboembolism.

Earlier studies have shown a positive association between PGM and adverse pregnancy outcome. In a meta-analysis (The Thrombosis: Risk and Economic Assessment of Thrombophilia Screening [TREATS] study), Robertson colleagues[16] showed ORs and 95% CIs for women who were carriers of PGM:

- Preeclampsia: 2.54 (1.52–4.23)
- Small for gestational age neonates: 2.92 (0.62–13.70)
- Abruption: 7.71 (3.01–19.76)

Most of the studies included in this meta-analysis were small retrospective studies.

In a secondary analysis of an FVL study, 157 pregnant women identified with PGM were compared with women who were noncarriers of PGM for adverse pregnancy outcome. The investigators did not find any association between PGM carriers and preeclampsia, placental abruption, and fetal loss.[17] In an earlier case-control study the same group of investigators showed an association of PGM with early onset of severe preeclampsia.[17] In a multicenter case-control cohort study of 113 women with preeclampsia, no association was found between FVL and PGM mutation and risk for preeclampsia.[18] A recent meta-analysis also did not show an association of FVL and PGM with preeclampsia and small for gestational age.[11] PGM has been associated with VTE during pregnancy. A study of 119 women with VTE during pregnancy and the puerperium, versus 233 normal healthy women, showed that those with PGM had greater chances of VTE, 16.9% versus 1.3% without PGM (relative risk 15.2, 95% CI 4.2–52.6). The risk was further increased in women who had combined PGM and FVL.[19]

In a prospective study, women with pregnancy losses in either trimester, either recurrent or isolated, were screened for FVL and PGM. The frequency of PGM was not significant in any of these groups.[20] Kupferminc and colleagues,[21] in a matched-control study of women with midtrimester fetal growth restriction (birth weight less than third centile), showed an association with inherited thrombophilia. Sixty-nine percent of women had thrombophilia, compared with 14% in the control population. In a large hospital-based study of 496 women with intrauterine growth restriction (birth weight less than the 10th percentile), the OR for PGM was 0.92 (95% CI 0.36–2.35), which was not significant for any association. Similar results were shown for other thrombophilias, and investigators concluded that there were no associations between maternal or newborn polymorphisms associated with thrombophilia and an increased risk of intrauterine growth restriction.[22]

PROTEIN S DEFICIENCY AND ADVERSE PREGNANCY OUTCOME

Protein S (PS), along with antithrombin and protein C (PC), is a natural anticoagulant. It is synthesized in the endothelium, and circulates in both free and bound forms (complement protein). Free PS acts as cofactor with PC, and causes inactivation of factor Va and VIIIa. PS antigen shows a physiologic decrease during pregnancy. The decrease in levels has been observed from as early as the first trimester, to a mean level of 46%.[23] Significant interassay and intra-assay variations have been noted because of this physiologic change in circulating levels. Congenital PS deficiency is a recognized risk factor for venous thromboembolism and adverse pregnancy outcome. The prevalence of PS deficiency is higher in Asian people than in white people.[24] Regarding obstetric complications and PS deficiency, data are available for fetal demise and intrauterine growth restriction. In an earlier meta-analysis, PS deficiency was associated with recurrent fetal loss (14.72, 0.99–218.01) and late nonrecurrent fetal loss (7.39, 1.28–42.63).[25] In a retrospective case-control study, women with intrauterine growth restriction had significantly lower levels of functional and free PS compared with the control group: functional PS 54.07% ± 24.72% versus 65.20% ± 17.95% (P<.005), and free PS 42.88% ± 11.01% versus 56.64% ± 13.30% (P<.0001), respectively.[26] In a larger study, women with identified anticoagulant deficiency had an improved live birth rate with anticoagulant therapy.[27] Fewer recent data are available with other obstetric complications and PS deficiency.

ANTITHROMBIN III DEFICIENCY AND ADVERSE PREGNANCY
Outcome

Antithrombin III (AT) deficiency is an uncommon thrombophilia, but it has the greatest lifetime risk for thromboembolic events. Its prevalence in the general population is estimated to be between 0.5 and 5 per 1000.[28] In a cohort of 9669 healthy blood donors, AT deficiency was identified in 16 persons.[29] There are 2 types of AT deficiency. Type 1 AT deficiency is quantitative, and is seen in 80% of symptomatic cases. Type 2 AT deficiency is qualitative, and is more prevalent than type 1 (1.45 per 1000, compared with 0.21 per 1000).[29] The risk of thrombosis in AT-deficient individuals has been estimated to be around 51%.[30] AT deficiency has been associated with recurrent miscarriage, preeclampsia, and fetal growth restriction.[31]

AT levels have been found to be decreased in women with PIH. In a recent study, levels of natural anticoagulants AT, PS, and PC were compared between preeclamptic, healthy pregnant, and nonpregnant women. Levels of AT were significantly decreased in women with preeclampsia (P<.001).[32] Larciprete and colleagues[33] screened women with adverse pregnancy outcome (preeclampsia, abruptio placentae, intrauterine growth restriction, and the syndrome of hemolysis, elevated liver enzymes, and low platelet count [HELLP]) for individual thrombophilias. AT deficiency was significantly associated with preeclampsia, but FVL and PGM were not associated with preeclampsia. In a retrospective study of 1493 women, 114 women were identified with PIH or pregnancy-induced AT deficiency (PIATD). AT deficiency was identified in women with PIH, as well as in women without PIH. These investigators found that coagulation-fibrinolysis was significantly more enhanced and the postpartum reduction in the hematocrit value was significantly larger in women with PIATD, irrespective of the presence or absence of hypertension, than in women without PIATD.[34] There are reports studying the association of PIATD and excessive weight gain in the last weeks of pregnancy with eclampsia.[35] However, this observation has been made in only a small number of patients and needs to be investigated in a larger cohort.

Hyperhomocysteinemia and Adverse Pregnancy Outcome

Increased serum levels of circulating homocysteine have been linked to thrombosis. Thrombosis results from mutations in the methionine metabolic pathway, including cytoplasmic enzyme methyltetrahydrofolate reductase (MTHFR). This enzyme causes conversion of 5,10-methylenetetrahydrofolate to 5-methylenetetrahydrofolate, which converts circulating homocysteine to methionine. Recent data have shown weak evidence of hyperhomocysteinemia with VTE.[36] Associations have been shown between increased levels and preeclampsia, fetal loss, and abruptio placentae. The Hordaland study (a community-based study conducted in Norway) was designed to assess serum levels of homocysteine with various common diseases. Within the study, serum values and pregnancy outcome were assessed for 5883 pregnant women. The investigators found increased levels of homocysteine with stillbirth (OR 2.03, 95% CI 0.98–4.21).[37] Association with increased total homocysteine levels was also seen with small-for-gestational-age in a meta-analysis, although the difference in birth weight was small (31 g: 95% CI −13, −51 g).[38] The American College of Obstetricians and Gynecologists (ACOG) does not recommend testing for MTHFR or fasting homocysteine levels in evaluation of thrombophilia.[39] ACOG also recommends against testing for uncommon thrombophilia like PAI-1 gene, protein Z deficiency.

SCREENING FOR THROMBOPHILIA

It is important to identify a group of women who should be offered screening for acquired (antiphospolipid antibody syndrome [APS]) and inherited thrombophilia (eg, FVL, ATIII). Screening for thrombophilia is a controversial issue. The ACOG guideline does not recommend screening for inherited thrombophilia and treatment with anticoagulant in women with a previous history of adverse pregnancy outcome (severe preeclampsia, abruptio placentae, fetal loss), because there is insufficient evidence.[39] The ACOG guideline does recommend that screening for acquired thrombophilia (APS) may be appropriate in women with a history of fetal loss. It is also recommended that women with preterm birth before 34 weeks of gestation caused by severe preeclampsia, eclampsia, or intrauterine growth restriction should be screened for acquired thrombophilia.[40] There is strong evidence that those with positive values for LA, anticardiolipin antibodies, and anti-β2-glycoptrotein I antibodies are more at risk for thrombosis and pregnancy morbidity than those with only a single positive test.[41] This topic is discussed in the article by Lockshin elsewhere in this issue. **Table 2** lists the screening methods for inherited thrombophilias.

There are clinical situations in which screening for inherited thrombophilia is recommended.

- Women with personal history of VTE with nonrecurrent cause (fracture, prolonged immobilization, surgery), when pregnant and untreated, and with thrombophilia have a recurrence risk of 16% (OR 6.5, 95% CI 0.8–56.3).
- Women with a first-degree relative or sibling, having VTE at age less than 50 years, should be screened for thrombophilia.
- Venous thromboembolism in a child requires screening for siblings and first-degree relatives. The risk of venous thromboembolism in first-degree relative is greater for deficiencies of natural anticoagulants (PS, PC, and AT).[42]

ROLE OF ANTICOAGULANT THERAPY IN PREVENTION OF ADVERSE PREGNANCY OUTCOME

Anticoagulant therapy has been used to prevent pregnancy complications in women with and without known thrombophilia (**Table 3**). The mechanism of heparin action is still uncertain. Heparin in vivo increases circulating levels of maternal sFlt-1, but this may be an epiphenomenon.[43] Kuperminc and colleagues[44] used low-molecular-weight heparin (LMWH) in a dose of 1 mg/kg body weight in women with recognized thrombophilia and adverse pregnancy outcome. In this retrospective cohort, the stillbirth rate was significantly decreased in women in whom LMWH was used (0% compared with 7%, $P = .06$). In the recently published Fragmin in Pregnant Women

Table 2		
Inherited thrombophilia screening methods		
Thrombophilia	**Laboratory Test**	**Comments**
FVL mutation	Screening by second-generation assay Confirmation by DNA analysis	—
PG20210A mutation	DNA analysis	—
Protein S	Functional assay	Confirmation of deficiency is required outside of pregnancy and postpartum period
Protein C	Functional assay	—
ATIII deficiency	Functional assay	—
Lupus anticoagulant	Functional assay	Needs to be repeated after 12 wk
Anticardiolipin antibodies IgG and IgM	ELISA	Needs to be repeated after 12 wk
Beta 2 glycoproteins, IgM, IgG	ELISA	Needs to be repeated after 12 wk

Abbreviations: ATIII, antithrombin III; ELISA, enzyme-linked immunosorbent assay; IgG, immunoglobulin G; IgM, immunoglobulin M.

with a History of Uteroplacental Insufficiency and Thrombophilia (FRUIT) study, conducted in women with inherited thrombophilia and history of early preeclampsia at less than 34 weeks, women were randomized to receive either aspirin 80 mg alone or aspirin with LMWH. Investigators showed a decrease in the risk of recurrent preeclampsia (risk difference [RD] 8.7%, CI of RD 1.9%–15.5%, $P = .012$).[45] In a nonrandomized, observational study, women carriers for FVL or PGM, with a history of venous thrombosis or obstetric complications were prescribed LMWH with or without ASA. The risk of VTE in women on LMWH was significantly reduced (OR 0.05, 95% CI 0.01–0.21). The risk of fetal loss was also decreased (OR 0.52, 95% CI 0.29–0.94). These results were not seen in women on ASA therapy alone. The investigators

Table 3				
Studies of anticoagulant therapy in women with inherited thrombophilia				
Author (Year), Reference	**Inherited Thrombophilia**	**Type of Study**	**Intervention**	**Live Birth Rate (%)**
Kupferminc et al,[44] 2011	FVL, PGM, PS, PC	Retrospective	LMWH	—
Grandone et al,[60] 2008	PS, PC, ATIII	Retrospective	LMWH	87.5
Marinov et al,[61] 2011	FVL, PGM, PAI	Prospective	Aspirin + LMWH	70
de Vries et al,[45] 2012	FVL, PGM, PS, PC	Prospective	Aspirin + LMWH or aspirin alone	NR
Gris et al,[47] 2011	FVL, PGM	Prospective, randomized	LMWH/no LMWH	NR
Tormene et al,[46] 2012	FVL, PGM	Observational	LMWH ± aspirin	73
Leduc et al,[62] 2007	PC, PS, ATIII, FVL,	Retrospective	LMWH + ASA/ASA	NR
Kovac et al,[63] 2013	PC, PS, ATIII, FVL,	Prospective	LMWH	93
De Sancho et al,[64] 2012	—	Retrospective	LMWH	NR

Abbreviations: LMWH, low-molecular-weight heparin; NR, not reported.

concluded that LMWH improved live birth rate in women with FVL or PGM.[46] In a follow-up of the NOHA study, women with FVL or PGM and preeclampsia in their first pregnancy were randomized to LMWH (enoxaparin) or no LMWH after positive pregnancy test in 112 women. The primary outcome was composite of adverse pregnancy outcome (preeclampsia, abruptio placentae, and fetal loss). Enoxaparin was associated with a lower frequency of primary outcome: 8.9% (n = 10/112 vs 25% [28/112], $P = .004$, hazard ratio = 0.32, 95% CI 0.16–0.66, $P = .002$).[47] Studies have also been conducted in women without any known thrombophilia, but who had adverse pregnancy outcome in antecedent pregnancy. The aim of these studies was to show whether adverse pregnancy outcome can be prevented by the use of anticoagulant therapy. One such large, multicenter study was completed recently. In this study, 135 women with adverse pregnancy outcome in antecedent pregnancy were randomized to receive LMWH or were kept on medical surveillance alone. Primary outcomes were a composite of adverse pregnancy outcome. The investigators did not find any significant difference in primary end points between the 2 groups and concluded that the absolute event risk difference between treatment arms (2.2; −1.6 to 16.0) was not statistically significant ($P = .76$).[48] The trial was registered at http://ricerca-clinica.agenziafarmaco.it as EudraCT 2006-004205-26.

Several other studies have been conducted in women with placenta-mediated complications without any thrombophilia screening (**Table 4**). The primary aim of these

Table 4
Studies of anticoagulant therapy in women without inherited thrombophilia

Author (Year), Reference	Previous APO	Type of Study	Intervention	Outcome
Kupferminc et al,[49] 2011	Preeclampsia, AP, FGR	Prospective	LMWH	Overall adverse outcome 9.4% vs 60% (treated vs untreated), $P = .001$
Urban et al,[65] 2007	Preeclampsia, IUGR	Retrospective	LDA, LDA + LMWH	IUGR (OR = 0.16; 95% CI 0.03–0.98) Spe (OR = 0.08; CI 0.01–0.96)
Sergio et al,[66] 2006	Preeclampsia	Prospective	LDA + LMWH	Improved: GA at delivery, ($P = .05$); BW ($P<.01$); preeclampsia ($P<.01$)
Yu et al,[67] 2010	IUGR	Prospective	LMWH/Danshen + dextrose water	Increased birth weight ($P = .0000$) and greater GA at delivery ($P = .0003$)
Rey et al,[68] 2009	Preeclampsia, IUFD, AP	Prospective, randomized	LMWH/no LMWH	Improved primary outcome (OR 0.15; CI 0.03–0.70)
Gris et al,[47] 2011	Preeclampsia	NOH-PE	LMWH/no LMWH	Improved primary outcome, $P<.004$

Abbreviations: BW, birth weight; GA, gestational age; IUFD, intrauterine fetal distress; IUGR, intrauterine growth restriction; NOH-PE, The Nimes Obstetricians and Haematologist-Pre eclampsia; Spe, Severe Pre eclampsia.

studies was to determine whether heparin therapy can play any role in prevention of adverse pregnancy outcome. Kupferminc and colleagues[49] reported on a group of women with history of preeclampsia, fetal growth restriction, and abruptio placentae in antecedent pregnancy, without known thrombophilia. They were divided in 2 groups, one received LMWH, whereas the control group did not receive LMWH. There was decrease in incidences of severe preeclampsia and placental abruption in the study group in the index pregnancy (3.13% vs 20%, $P = .03$; and 0% vs 15%, $P = .03$, respectively). The respective incidence of fetal growth restriction was 6.25% versus 22.5%, and overall adverse outcome was 9.4% versus 60% ($P = .001$).[49] A Cochrane Review identified 14 studies in which heparin therapy was used as prophylaxis for prevention of placenta-mediated complications (preeclampsia, intrauterine growth restriction, birth weight, preterm birth, and perinatal mortality). Positive effects were seen for prevention of recurrent preeclampsia, eclampsia, and birth weight.[50] The use of anticoagulant in women with adverse pregnancy outcome with/without thrombophilia should still be considered investigational. There are studies in which investigators did not find any significant influence on maternal and perinatal outcome in asymptomatic women with thrombophilia. In a retrospective cohort study, the live birth rate was the same in asymptomatic women with diagnosed thrombophilia, with or without anticoagulant therapy.[51] Similar results were reported by investigators of the low molecular weight heparin/aspirin (HepASA) trial. Women with recurrent pregnancy losses with acquired or inherited thrombophilia or antinuclear antibodies were randomized to receive either LMWH/ASA or ASA alone. The live birth rate was 77% (LMWH/ASA) versus 79% in ASA-alone group.[52] LMWH did not confer any significant advantage on live birth rate. A consensus opinion on the use of anticoagulant therapy for prevention of adverse pregnancy outcome identified inherited thrombophilia, as one of the risk factors that may influence pregnancy outcome and concluded that heparin should be considered to be an investigational drug until robust evidence from large, well-conducted trials is available.[53]

ADVERSE EFFECTS OF ANTICOAGULATION DURING PREGNANCY

Common indications for use of anticoagulation during pregnancy include prevention of adverse pregnancy outcome in women with or without thrombophilia, and prevention or treatment of thromboembolism, including the very high-risk population of women with mechanical heart valves, whose management is beyond the scope of this article. Adverse effects associated with the use of heparin include risk of antenatal bleeding, thrombocytopenia, allergic skin reactions, and loss of bone mineral density (**Box 1**). See the article by Fuller and colleagues elsewhere in this issue.

In a retrospective cohort study of more than 600 women who were prescribed LMWH during pregnancy, there was no evidence of increased blood loss during cesarean deliveries, thrombocytopenia, or symptomatic osteoporotic fractures. The risk of allergic skin reactions was 0.03%. Investigators concluded that LMWH was safe in pregnancy.[54] Thrombocytopenia, known as heparin-induced thrombocytopenia (HIT), is a rare phenomenon, and may be early or delayed. It refers to an adverse reaction presenting as a prothrombotic disorder, secondary to antibody-mediated platelet activation and consumption. The relative risk ratio of HIT was less with LMWH than with unfractionated heparin (UFH), (risk ratio 0.24, 95% CI 0.07–0.82).[55] Heparin-induced allergic skin reactions are also reported in the literature. These reactions may be a manifestation of allergic reaction or of HIT phenomena. Allergic reaction is caused by delayed hypersensitivity, with skin biopsy showing lymphoid

Box 1
Adverse effects of heparin therapy

- Bleeding
- Heparin-induced thrombocytopenia
- Heparin-induced skin lesions
- Allergic, anaphylactoid reactions
- Osteoporosis
- Increase of liver enzymes
- Alopecia
- Hyperkalemia
- Impaired fracture healing

infiltration. All forms of LMWH used have shown association with allergic skin reactions.[56] The LIVE-Enoxapairin (LIVE-Enox) study showed a prevalence of skin lesions of around 3%. The nonbleeding complications of heparin therapy are caused by binding of heparin with molecules other than antithrombin.

The risk of osteoporosis is seen with long-term use of heparin. The risk is greater with UFH than with LMWH. In more than 2777 pregnancies, only 1 case of symptomatic osteoporotic fracture has been reported, with the use of LMWH.[57] In a prospective study of more than 100 pregnant women receiving anticoagulation, prevalence of bone loss as measured by densitometry was between 2% and 2.5%, irrespective of the type of heparin used.[58] Investigators in the Thrombophilia in Pregnancy Prophylaxis Study (TIPPS) trial did not identify decreased bone mineral density in women prescribed prophylactic doses of heparin in the antepartum and postpartum periods.[59]

REFERENCES

1. Hossain N, Paidas MJ. Adverse pregnancy outcome, the uteroplacental interface, and preventive strategies. Semin Perinatol 2007;31(4):208–12.
2. Michael J, Paidas CS, Hossain N, et al. Hemostasis and thrombosis in obstetrics & gynecology. Chichester, West Sussex, UK: John Wiley & Sons Ltd; 2011.
3. Kujovich JL. Factor V Leiden thrombophilia. Genet Med 2011;13(1):1–16.
4. Kapiotis S, Quehenberger P, Jilma B, et al. Improved characteristics of aPC-resistance assay: coatest aPC resistance by predilution of samples with factor V deficient plasma. Am J Clin Pathol 1996;106(5):588–93.
5. Roque H, Paidas MJ, Funai EF, et al. Maternal thrombophilias are not associated with early pregnancy loss. Thromb Haemost 2004;91(2):290–5.
6. Lissalde-Lavigne G, Cochery-Nouvellon E, Mercier E, et al. The association between hereditary thrombophilias and pregnancy loss. Haematologica 2005; 90(9):1223–30.
7. Pasquier E, Bohec C, Mottier D, et al. Inherited thrombophilias and unexplained pregnancy loss: an incident case-control study. J Thromb Haemost 2009;7(2): 306–11.
8. Hossain N, Shamsi T, Khan N, et al. Thrombophilia investigation in Pakistani women with recurrent pregnancy loss. J Obstet Gynaecol Res 2012;39:121–5.

9. Kupferminc MJ. Thrombophilia and preeclampsia: the evidence so far. Clin Obstet Gynecol 2005;48(2):406–15.

10. Facchinetti F, Marozio L, Frusca T, et al. Maternal thrombophilia and the risk of recurrence of preeclampsia. Am J Obstet Gynecol 2009;200(1): 46.e1–5.

11. Rodger MA, Betancourt MT, Clark P, et al. The association of factor V Leiden and prothrombin gene mutation and placenta-mediated pregnancy complications: a systematic review and meta-analysis of prospective cohort studies. PLoS Med 2010;7(6):e1000292.

12. Kjellberg U, van Rooijen M, Bremme K, et al. Leiden mutation and pregnancy-related complications. Am J Obstet Gynecol 2010;203(5):469.e1–8.

13. Prochazka M, Lubusky M, Slavik L, et al. Frequency of selected thrombophilias in women with placental abruption. Aust N Z J Obstet Gynaecol 2007;47(4): 297–301.

14. Facchinetti F, Marozio L, Grandone E, et al. Thrombophilic mutations are a main risk factor for placental abruption. Haematologica 2003;88(7):785–8.

15. Said JM, Higgins JR, Moses EK, et al. Inherited thrombophilias and adverse pregnancy outcomes: a case-control study in an Australian population. Acta Obstet Gynecol Scand 2012;91(2):250–5.

16. Robertson L, Wu O, Langhorne P, et al. Thrombophilia in pregnancy: a systematic review. Br J Haematol 2006;132(2):171–96.

17. Gerhardt A, Goecke TW, Beckmann MW, et al. The G20210A prothrombin-gene mutation and the plasminogen activator inhibitor (PAI-1) 5G/5G genotype are associated with early onset of severe preeclampsia. J Thromb Haemost 2005; 3(4):686–91.

18. Kahn SR, Platt R, McNamara H, et al. Inherited thrombophilia and preeclampsia within a multicenter cohort: the Montreal Preeclampsia Study. Am J Obstet Gynecol 2009;200(2):151.e1–9 [discussion: e1–5].

19. Gerhardt A, Scharf RE, Beckmann MW, et al. Prothrombin and factor V mutations in women with a history of thrombosis during pregnancy and the puerperium. N Engl J Med 2000;342(6):374–80.

20. Skrzypczak J, Rajewski M, Wirstlein P, et al. Incidence of hereditary thrombophilia in women with pregnancy loss in multi-center studies in Poland. Ginekol Pol 2012;83(5):330–6 [in Polish].

21. Kupferminc MJ, Many A, Bar-Am A, et al. Mid-trimester severe intrauterine growth restriction is associated with a high prevalence of thrombophilia. BJOG 2002;109(12):1373–6.

22. Infante-Rivard C, Rivard GE, Yotov WV, et al. Absence of association of thrombophilia polymorphisms with intrauterine growth restriction. N Engl J Med 2002;347(1):19–25.

23. Said JM, Ignjatovic V, Monagle PT, et al. Altered reference ranges for protein C and protein S during early pregnancy: implications for the diagnosis of protein C and protein S deficiency during pregnancy. Thromb Haemost 2010;103(5): 984–8.

24. Adachi T. Protein S and congenital protein S deficiency: the most frequent congenital thrombophilia in Japanese. Curr Drug Targets 2005;6(5):585–92.

25. Rey E, Kahn SR, David M, et al. Thrombophilic disorders and fetal loss: a meta-analysis. Lancet 2003;361(9361):901–8.

26. De Bonis M, Sabatini L, Galeazzi LR, et al. Maternal serum protein S forms in pregnancies complicated by intrauterine growth restriction. Eur J Obstet Gynecol Reprod Biol 2012;160(2):142–6.

27. Folkeringa N, Brouwer JL, Korteweg FJ, et al. Reduction of high fetal loss rate by anticoagulant treatment during pregnancy in antithrombin, protein C or protein S deficient women. Br J Haematol 2007;136(4):656–61.

28. Wells PS, Blajchman MA, Henderson P, et al. Prevalence of antithrombin deficiency in healthy blood donors: a cross-sectional study. Am J Hematol 1994; 45(4):321–4.

29. Tait RC, Walker ID, Perry DJ, et al. Prevalence of antithrombin deficiency in the healthy population. Br J Haematol 1994;87(1):106–12.

30. Demers C, Ginsberg JS, Hirsh J, et al. Thrombosis in antithrombin-III-deficient persons. Report of a large kindred and literature review. Ann Intern Med 1992;116(9):754–61.

31. Szilagyi A, Nagy A, Tamas P, et al. Two successful pregnancies following eight miscarriages in a patient with antithrombin deficiency. Gynecol Obstet Invest 2006;61(2):111–4.

32. Demir C, Dilek I. Natural coagulation inhibitors and active protein c resistance in preeclampsia. Clinics (Sao Paulo) 2010;65(11):1119–22.

33. Larciprete G, Gioia S, Angelucci PA, et al. Single inherited thrombophilias and adverse pregnancy outcomes. J Obstet Gynaecol Res 2007;33(4): 423–30.

34. Morikawa M, Yamada T, Yamada T, et al. Pregnancy-induced antithrombin deficiency. J Perinat Med 2010;38(4):379–85.

35. Yamada T, Kuwata T, Matsuda H, et al. Risk factors of eclampsia other than hypertension: pregnancy-induced antithrombin deficiency and extraordinary weight gain. Hypertens Pregnancy 2012;31(2):268–77.

36. Den Heijer M, Lewington S, Clarke R. Homocysteine, MTHFR and risk of venous thrombosis: a meta-analysis of published epidemiological studies. J Thromb Haemost 2005;3(2):292–9.

37. Refsum H, Nurk E, Smith AD, et al. The Hordaland Homocysteine Study: a community-based study of homocysteine, its determinants, and associations with disease. J Nutr 2006;136(Suppl 6):1731S–40S.

38. Hogeveen M, Blom HJ, den Heijer M. Maternal homocysteine and small-for-gestational-age offspring: systematic review and meta-analysis. Am J Clin Nutr 2012;95(1):130–6.

39. Lockwood C, Wendel G. Practice bulletin no. 124: inherited thrombophilias in pregnancy. Obstet Gynecol 2011;118(3):730–40.

40. Gonzalez-Nieto JA, Martin-Suarez I. Screening for antiphospholipid antibodies in women with pregnancy complications. Chest 2012;142(2):545 [author reply: 545–6].

41. Pengo V, Banzato A, Denas G, et al. Correct laboratory approach to APS diagnosis and monitoring. Autoimmun Rev 2012. [Epub ahead of print].

42. Bruce A, Massicotte MP. Thrombophilia screening: whom to test? Blood 2012; 120(7):1353–5.

43. Rosenberg VA, Buhimschi IA, Lockwood CJ, et al. Heparin elevates circulating soluble fms-like tyrosine kinase-1 immunoreactivity in pregnant women receiving anticoagulation therapy. Circulation 2011;124(23):2543–53.

44. Kupferminc MJ, Rimon E, Many A, et al. Low molecular weight heparin treatment during subsequent pregnancies of women with inherited thrombophilia and previous severe pregnancy complications. J Matern Fetal Neonatal Med 2011; 24(8):1042–5.

45. de Vries JI, van Pampus MG, Hague WM, et al. Low-molecular-weight heparin added to aspirin in the prevention of recurrent early-onset pre-eclampsia in

women with inheritable thrombophilia: the FRUIT-RCT. J Thromb Haemost 2012; 10(1):64–72.

46. Tormene D, Grandone E, De Stefano V, et al. Obstetric complications and pregnancy-related venous thromboembolism: the effect of low-molecular-weight heparin on their prevention in carriers of factor V Leiden or prothrombin G20210A mutation. Thromb Haemost 2012;107(3):477–84.

47. Gris JC, Chauleur C, Molinari N, et al. Addition of enoxaparin to aspirin for the secondary prevention of placental vascular complications in women with severe pre-eclampsia. The pilot randomised controlled NOH-PE trial. Thromb Haemost 2011;106(6):1053–61.

48. Martinelli I, Ruggenenti P, Cetin I, et al. Heparin in pregnant women with previous placenta-mediated pregnancy complications: a prospective, randomized, multicenter, controlled clinical trial. Blood 2012;119(14):3269–75.

49. Kupferminc M, Rimon E, Many A, et al. Low molecular weight heparin versus no treatment in women with previous severe pregnancy complications and placental findings without thrombophilia. Blood Coagul Fibrinolysis 2011; 22(2):123–6.

50. Dodd JM, McLeod A, Windrim RC, et al. Antithrombotic therapy for improving maternal or infant health outcomes in women considered at risk of placental dysfunction. Cochrane Database Syst Rev 2010;(6):CD006780.

51. Warren JE, Simonsen SE, Branch DW, et al. Thromboprophylaxis and pregnancy outcomes in asymptomatic women with inherited thrombophilias. Am J Obstet Gynecol 2009;200(3):281.e1–5.

52. Laskin CA, Spitzer KA, Clark CA, et al. Low molecular weight heparin and aspirin for recurrent pregnancy loss: results from the randomized, controlled HepASA Trial. J Rheumatol 2009;36(2):279–87.

53. Rodger MA, Paidas M, McLintock C, et al. Inherited thrombophilia and pregnancy complications revisited. Obstet Gynecol 2008;112(2 Pt 1):320–4.

54. Galambosi PJ, Kaaja RJ, Stefanovic V, et al. Safety of low-molecular-weight heparin during pregnancy: a retrospective controlled cohort study. Eur J Obstet Gynecol Reprod Biol 2012;163(2):154–9.

55. Junqueira DR, Perini E, Penholati RR, et al. Unfractionated heparin versus low molecular weight heparin for avoiding heparin-induced thrombocytopenia in postoperative patients. Cochrane Database Syst Rev 2012;(9):CD007557.

56. Schindewolf M, Lindhoff-Last E, Ludwig RJ, et al. Heparin-induced skin lesions. Lancet 2012;380(9856):1867–79.

57. Alban S. Adverse effects of heparin. Handb Exp Pharmacol 2012;207:211–63.

58. Casele H, Haney EI, James A, et al. Bone density changes in women who receive thromboprophylaxis in pregnancy. Am J Obstet Gynecol 2006;195(4):1109–13.

59. Rodger MA, Kahn SR, Cranney A, et al. Long-term dalteparin in pregnancy not associated with a decrease in bone mineral density: substudy of a randomized controlled trial. J Thromb Haemost 2007;5(8):1600–6.

60. Grandone E, De Stefano V, Rossi E, et al. Antithrombotic prophylaxis during pregnancy in women with deficiency of natural anticoagulants. Blood Coagul Fibrinolysis 2008;19(3):226–30.

61. Marinov B, Pramatarova T, Andreeva A, et al. Our experience with management of inherited thrombophilia during pregnancy: preliminary report. Akush Ginekol (Sofiia) 2011;50(Suppl 2):28–31 [in Bulgarian].

62. Leduc L, Dubois E, Takser L, et al. Dalteparin and low-dose aspirin in the prevention of adverse obstetric outcomes in women with inherited thrombophilia. J Obstet Gynaecol Can 2007;29(10):787–93.

63. Kovac M, Mikovic Z, Mitic G, et al. Does anticoagulant therapy improve pregnancy outcome equally, regardless of specific thrombophilia type? Clin Appl Thromb Hemost 2013. [Epub ahead of print].

64. De Sancho MT, Khalid S, Christos PJ. Outcomes in women receiving low-molecular-weight heparin during pregnancy. Blood Coagul Fibrinolysis 2012; 23(8):751–5.

65. Urban G, Vergani P, Tironi R, et al. Antithrombotic prophylaxis in multiparous women with preeclampsia or intrauterine growth retardation in an antecedent pregnancy. Int J Fertil Womens Med 2007;52(2–3):59–67.

66. Sergio F, Maria Clara D, Gabriella F, et al. Prophylaxis of recurrent preeclampsia: low-molecular-weight heparin plus low-dose aspirin versus low-dose aspirin alone. Hypertens Pregnancy 2006;25(2):115–27.

67. Yu YH, Shen LY, Zou H, et al. Heparin for patients with growth restricted fetus: a prospective randomized controlled trial. J Matern Fetal Neonatal Med 2010; 23(9):980–7.

68. Rey E, Garneau P, David M, et al. Dalteparin for the prevention of recurrence of placental-mediated complications of pregnancy in women without thrombophilia: a pilot randomized controlled trial. J Thromb Haemost 2009;7(1):58–64.

Catastrophic Antiphospholipid Syndrome

Diagnosis and Management in Pregnancy

Jose A. Gómez-Puerta, MD, PhD[a,b], Gerard Espinosa, MD, PhD[a],
Ricard Cervera, MD, PhD, FRCP[a,*]

KEYWORDS

- Antiphospholipid syndrome • Antiphospholipid antibodies
- Catastrophic antiphospholipid syndrome • Pregnancy • Puerperium • Thrombosis

KEY POINTS

- Pregnancy and puerperium periods are transient hypercoagulable states that predispose for the development of thrombosis, especially in those patients with an underlying susceptibility such as antiphospholipid syndrome (APS).
- The catastrophic APS (CAPS) syndrome is an unusual (<1%) but often life-threatening variant of the APS, characterized by the rapid appearance of multiple thromboses (mainly small vessel thromboses) that lead to multiorgan failure.
- In approximately 4% to 6% of cases, CAPS can appear during pregnancy or puerperium. A part of classical APS features, CAPS during the obstetric period may have some particular manifestations, such as HELLP syndrome, placental thrombosis, or myometrium thrombosis, among others.
- Because CAPS is not frequent in pregnancy, management is expert-based (not evidence-based) opinion. The management of CAPS during pregnancy and puerperium depends on fetal maturation and the presence of microangiopathic features. The recommended combined treatment includes anticoagulation, corticosteroids, plasma exchange, and/or intravenous immunoglobulins. Fibrinolytic therapy is another potentially useful therapy.

INTRODUCTION

The association between antiphospholipid antibodies (aPL) and pregnancy adverse outcome has been recognized for decades. Complications in pregnancy have been described in both early and late pregnancy, as well as postpartum. The most

Disclosure: The authors have nothing to disclose.
[a] Department of Autoimmune Diseases, Hospital Clinic, Villarroel 170, Barcelona 08036, Catalonia, Spain; [b] Section of Clinical Sciences, Division of Rheumatology, Immunology, and Allergy, Brigham and Women's Hospital, 221 Longwood Avenue, Boston, MA 02115, USA
* Corresponding author.
E-mail address: rcervera@clinic.cat

characteristic feature of the obstetric antiphospholipid syndrome (APS) is pregnancy loss. Pregnancy losses in patients with APS frequently occur after 10 weeks, compared with spontaneous abortions not associated with aPL, which most often occur earlier. Currently, recurrent pregnancy loss is a potentially treatable condition when it is associated with aPL.[1,2]

A wide number of other serious obstetric complications have been related to APS, including preeclampsia and related complications, such as HELLP (hemolysis, liver enzymes elevation, and low platelets) syndrome, fetal growth restriction, uteroplacental insufficiency, fetal distress, and medically induced preterm delivery.[3] Preterm delivery is reported in approximately 20% of patients with APS. In most cases, premature delivery is medically induced because of severe preeclampsia or placental insufficiency manifested by impaired fetal growth.[3] Other infrequently reported maternal APS complications include postpartum cardiopulmonary syndrome, chorea gravidum, and postpartum cerebral infarct, among others.[3]

Our group recently reported that those patients with a history of recurrent spontaneous abortions (<10 weeks) associated with aPL had a high risk of subsequent thrombosis after a long-term follow-up (7 years) (25.6 thrombotic events per 1000 patient-years). The risk was even higher than the risk of thrombosis in patients with recurrent spontaneous abortions associated with other thrombophilias. The odds ratio of thrombosis in relation to the presence or absence of aPL in patients with recurrent spontaneous abortions was 15.6 (95% confidence interval [CI] 3.2–70.5).[4]

PREGNANCY AS A HYPERCOAGULABLE STATE

Pregnancy is a hypercoagulable state that encompasses a period of 10 to 11 months (including puerperium). The puerperium is the time of greatest risk for thrombosis. Approximately, 80% of thrombotic events occur in the first 3 to 4 weeks after delivery and is explained not only by the immobility but also by the trauma of pelvic vessels in the course of delivery leading to endothelial damage.[5]

Hypercoagulability during the obstetric period is explained by many factors, including abnormalities in coagulation proteins (increased levels of factors II, V, VII, VIII, X, and XII, as well as von Willebrand factor, and decreased levels of protein S and activated protein C) and abnormalities in the fibrinolytic system (low plasma fibrinolytic activity during pregnancy, labor, and delivery) with decreased activity of tissue plasminogen activator. The most important changes occur in the levels of factor VIII and fibrinogen, each of which increase twofold to threefold.[6,7]

Risk factors for thrombosis during pregnancy are listed in **Table 1**. Preexisting risk factors for thrombosis during pregnancy include age older than 35 years, obesity (body mass index >30), smoking, multiparity, and a personal or family history of deep vein thrombosis (DVT) or thrombophilia. Acquired or transient risk factors include bed rest, immobility for 4 days or longer, weight gain of more than 21 kg during pregnancy, previous use of assisted reproductive techniques, twin pregnancy, hyperemesis, dehydration, medical-related problems (ie, infections), preeclampsia, severe varicose veins, or blood transfusions.[8,9]

DEFINITION OF CATASTROPHIC APS

The life-threatening variant of the APS, known as catastrophic APS (CAPS), was described for the first time more than 20 years ago.[10] CAPS is characterized by an aggressive form of the disorder in which clotting occurs at several sites in the vasculature (mainly, small vessel thromboses) over a short period of time that most often

Table 1
Risk factors for thrombosis during pregnancy

Thrombophilic Disorders	Causes Related to Pregnancy	Other Risk Factors for Thrombosis
Antithrombin deficiency	Immobility	Previous history of deep vein thrombosis
Factor V Leiden	Multiparity	Obesity (body mass index >30)
Antiphospholipid antibodies	Weight gain >21 kg	Age >35 y
Hyperhomocysteinemia	Assisted reproductive techniques	Smoking
Homozygous MTHFR C677T	Twin pregnancy	Blood transfusions
Protein C deficiency	Preeclampsia	Dehydration
Protein S deficiency	Antepartum hemorrhage	Infections
Prothrombin gene mutation	Hyperemesis	Severe varicose veins
Plasminogen activator inhibitor-1 (PAI-1) 4G/5G	Cesarean section	Systemic lupus erythematosus

leads to multiorgan failure.[10] Since the first description, several large series have been published.[11–13]

Because of the rarity of this syndrome, the European Forum on Antiphospholipid Antibodies created in 2000 an international registry of patients with CAPS (CAPS Registry, http://infmed.fcrb.es/es/web/caps). The registry documents the clinical, laboratory, and therapeutic data of the published cases with this condition, as well as of many additional patients whose data have been submitted for registration. Currently, approximately 400 patients have been collected in the international Web-based registry for CAPS.

CLINICAL FEATURES AND LABORATORY FINDINGS OF CAPS

The detailed analysis of the first 280 patients included in the CAPS Registry[13] shows that 72% are female, with a mean age of 37 years (range, 11–60). Forty-six percent suffered from primary APS, 40% from systemic lupus erythematosus (SLE), 5% from lupuslike disease, and 9% from other autoimmune diseases. Patients may develop CAPS de novo, without any previous history of a thrombosis (46%); however, the database also shows that a prior history of DVT, fetal loss, or thrombocytopenia are the most frequently encountered aPL-associated previous manifestations. A precipitating factor for the episode of CAPS was reported in 53% of patients. The most common precipitating factors were infections (22%) and surgical procedures (10%). Other less common triggers included anticoagulation withdrawal, malignancies, lupus "flares," or, infrequently, appearance during pregnancy or puerperium (ie, after a cesarean section or fetal loss).[13,14]

The manifestations of CAPS are diverse and include multiorgan involvement (ie, lung, heart, kidney, skin, and central nervous system disease, among other manifestations). There is a high prevalence of lung involvement in CAPS, mainly in the form of acute respiratory distress syndrome (ARDS) and pulmonary hemorrhage. Abdominal pain is a common symptom as a feature of multiple intra-abdominal complications. Additionally, other less-common manifestations in the classical form of APS may be present, including bone marrow necrosis, digital ulcers, genital organ involvement (ovary, uterus, testes), or osteonecrosis, among others. The main clinical manifestations from a series of 280 patients with CAPS are listed in **Table 2**.

The most common laboratory findings of CAPS include thrombocytopenia (46% of cases), hemolytic anemia (35%), in many occasions accompanied by schistocytes (thrombotic microangiopathic hemolytic anemia [MHA]) (16%), and disseminated intravascular coagulation (15%). Recently, we reported that those patients with MHA had a higher rate of CAPS relapses than those patients without MHA. The presence of MHA features in patients with CAPS who relapsed was 72% and in those who did not relapse was 7% (*P*<.0001).[15] Regarding the autoantibody profile, the immunoglobulin G (IgG) isotype of anticardiolipin antibodies (aCL) was detected in 83% of the patients, IgM aCL in 38%, and lupus anticoagulant in 82%.[13]

Among the 280 patients, 56% recovered from the CAPS event. Considering the presence or absence of a single treatment, recovery occurred more frequently in those patients treated with anticoagulants (63%); however, most patients received a combination of medical therapies. The highest recovery rate (69%) was achieved by the combination of anticoagulants plus corticosteroids plus plasma exchange and/or intravenous immunoglobulins. Not all treatments are successful. Some cases of

Table 2
Clinical manifestations of catastrophic antiphospholipid syndrome

First Clinical Manifestation of the Catastrophic Episode	No.	%
Pulmonary involvement	67	24
Neurologic involvement	50	18
Renal involvement	49	18
Cutaneous involvement	28	10
Cardiac involvement	27	10
Adrenal involvement	3	1
Organ involvement during the episode		
Kidney	180	71
Lung	163	64
Brain	158	62
Heart	131	51
Skin	128	50
Liver	85	33
Gastrointestinal	60	25
Peripheral venous thrombosis	59	23
Spleen	48	19
Adrenal glands	33	13
Peripheral artery thrombosis	27	11
Pancreas	19	8
Retina	17	7
Peripheral nerve	12	5
Bone marrow	10	4

Data from Cervera R, Bucciarelli S, Plasin MA, et al. Catastrophic antiphospholipid syndrome (CAPS): descriptive analysis of a series of 280 patients from the "CAPS Registry". J Autoimmun 2009;32(3–4):240–5.

CAPS are refractory, meaning some patients die despite the use of these therapies or patients suffer recurrent episodes of CAPS.[16]

CAPS DURING PREGNANCY AND PUERPERIUM

We previously reported the maternal and fetal characteristics of 15 cases with CAPS presenting during pregnancy and the puerperium.[17] Apart from typical CAPS manifestations, we found some particular features in this group: HELLP syndrome was seen in 53%, placental infarctions in 27%, and pelvic vein thrombosis and myometrium thrombotic microangiopathy in 7% of cases.

For this current review article, we have analyzed and reported on the data collected in the CAPS Registry until January 2013 (Cervera, 2013, unpublished data). Nineteen (4.6%) of 409 catastrophic events were presented during pregnancy or puerperium. In all, 10 (53%) patients had primary APS, and 9 (47%) had SLE. The mean (SD) age at the time of the catastrophic APS event was 27.9 (6.2) years. Previous APS manifestations were present in 74% of cases. Ten (53%) patients had previous abortions or fetal losses, 32% had previous DVT, and 16% previous arterial thrombosis.

The main clinical manifestations were renal, central nervous system, liver, and skin involvement (58% each). Other manifestations included pulmonary involvement in 9 (47%) patients (ARDS in 6 patients), adrenal involvement in 3 (15%) patients, and bone marrow necrosis in 2 (10%) patients. We also compared the clinical features of those patients with CAPS related to pregnancy and puerperium with those with CAPS not related to pregnancy and puerperium (**Table 3**). Briefly, a previous history of abortions and liver involvement were more common in CAPS occurring during the obstetric period, whereas previous thrombotic APS manifestations were more frequent in patients with CAPS outside the obstetric period.

Among the laboratory features, thrombocytopenia was found in 73% of patients and hemolytic anemia in 58%. IgG aCL was positive in 89% of patients, IgM aCL in 42%, lupus anticoagulant in 63%, schistocytes were present in 31%, and positive Coombs test in 5% of patients. Approximately one-third of patients with CAPS developed serologic or hematologic evidence of disseminated intravascular coagulation (DIC) during the course of their multiorgan illness.[18] The serologic features of DIC found in these patients may be explained on the basis of extensive small vessel endothelial damage, as it is also seen accompanying ARDS and systemic inflammatory response syndrome.

Regarding treatment, 84% of patients received anticoagulation treatment, 84% corticosteroids, 32% plasma exchange, 32% intravenous immunoglobulins, 21% cyclophosphamide, 16% dialysis, and 5% fibrinolytics.

DIAGNOSIS OF CAPS

For the diagnosis of CAPS, it is important to have a high clinical suspicion and identify factors that may be useful in the differential diagnosis of other thrombotic microangiopathic disorders presenting during pregnancy. These factors include a history of recurrent spontaneous abortions, previous history of thrombosis (arterial and/or venous) or manifestations of an associated autoimmune disease, including livedo reticularis, Raynaud phenomenon, and others.[19] In the absence of these factors before the acute event, the diagnosis is often a challenge for clinicians and sometimes is not possible to confirm until days or weeks later. Importantly, sometimes aPL may be transiently negative at the time of thrombosis.[20]

During the 10th International Congress on aPL in Taormina, Sicily, Italy, in 2002, the proposed preliminary classification criteria for CAPS were accepted (**Box 1**).[21] These

Table 3
Comparison between clinical manifestations in CAPS related and not related to pregnancy and puerperium[a]

	CAPS Related to Pregnancy and Puerperium n = 19	CAPS Not Related to Pregnancy and Puerperium n = 390	P Value
Mean age	27.7 ± 6.2	39.9 ± 35	.214
Previous APS manifestations, %	51.8	73.7	.04
Previous DVT, %	31.6	27.4	.820
Previous peripheral arterial thrombosis, %	15.8	22.8	.640
Previous abortions, %	52.6	15.6	<.0001
CAPS manifestations, %			
Deep vein thrombosis	21.1	24.4	.851
Peripheral arterial thrombosis	0	14.4	.180
Cardiac involvement	52.6	50.3	.981
Pulmonary involvement	47.4	58.5	.609
Renal embolism	52.6	72.8	.140
Central nervous system involvement	57.9	57.4	.976
Skin involvement	57.9	47.4	.373
Livedo reticularis	5.3	21.3	.09
Liver involvement	57.9	36.4	.05
Bone marrow necrosis	10.5	3.1	.081
Thrombocytopenia	73.7	59.7	.501

Abbreviations: APS, antiphospholipid syndrome; CAPS, catastrophic antiphospholipid syndrome; DVT, deep vein thrombosis.
[a] CAPS Registry Data, 2013, unpublished.

criteria were subsequently validated in clinical settings demonstrating that they are useful for epidemiologic studies.[22] More recently, during the 13th International Congress on aPL in Galveston, Texas, in 2010, a "Catastrophic APS Task Force" was developed by the meeting organization committee. The aim of that Task Force was to design a step-by-step approach for clinicians with diagnostic algorithms based on the 3 anchoring diagnostic points, namely the previous history of APS or aPL, the involvement of 3 or more organs, and the histologic confirmation of microthrombosis. A detailed explanation of the different algorithms is outside the scope of the current review, but is accessible for interested readers.[23]

DIFFERENTIAL DIAGNOSIS

Careful differential diagnosis is mandatory in the presence of a patient with multiorgan thromboses and failures during pregnancy or puerperium. This should include CAPS as well as other microangiopathic syndromes that may have overlapping features of (1) thrombotic microangiopathy, (2) hemolytic anemia, (3) thrombocytopenia, and (4) involvement of central nervous and renal systems.[24]

CAPS must be distinguished from other thrombotic microangiopathies during the obstetric period (**Table 4**). These conditions include preeclampsia, HELLP, thrombotic thrombocytopenic purpura, hemolytic–uremic syndrome, and acute fatty liver of pregnancy, among others. Because the diagnosis is not always simple owing to overlap of

---

Box 1
Preliminary criteria for the classification of CAPS

1. Evidence of involvement of 3 or more organs, systems, and/or tissues[a]

2. Development of manifestations simultaneously or in less than a week

3. Confirmation by histopathology of small-vessel occlusion in at least 1 organ or tissue[b]

4. Laboratory confirmation of the presence of antiphospholipid antibodies (lupus anticoagulant and/or anticardiolipin antibodies[c]

Definite catastrophic APS

- All 4 criteria

Probable CAPS

- All 4 criteria, except for only 2 organs, systems, and/or tissues involved

or

- All 4 criteria, except for the absence of laboratory confirmation at least 6 weeks apart because of the early death of a patient never previously tested for aPL before the CAPS event

or

- Criteria 1, 2, and 4

or

- Criteria 1, 3, and 4 and the development of a third event in more than a week but less than a month, despite anticoagulation

[a] Usually, clinical evidence of vessel occlusions, confirmed by imaging techniques when appropriate. Renal involvement is defined by a 50% rise in serum creatinine, severe systemic hypertension (>180/100 mm Hg), and/or proteinuria (>500 mg/24 h).
[b] For histopathological confirmation, significant evidence of thrombosis must be present, although vasculitis may coexist occasionally.
[c] If the patient had not been previously diagnosed as having an APS, the laboratory confirmation requires that the presence of antiphospholipid antibodies must be detected on 2 or more occasions at least 6 weeks apart (not necessarily at the time of the event), according to the proposed preliminary criteria for the classification of definite APS.

---

clinical and laboratory features between the different syndromes, it is important to identify some particular clues, including the time of onset for each one. These conditions are discussed in more detail in the article by Adams and colleagues elsewhere in this issue.

TREATMENT

A more detailed approach for the treatment of APS during pregnancy is discussed in the article by Lockshin elsewhere in this issue. A meta-analysis about the use of anticoagulant therapies during the obstetric period was published recently.[25] The investigators reported that anticoagulant therapy was associated with a mean incidence of major bleeding during the antenatal period of 1.41% (95% CI: 0.60%–2.41%) and of 1.90% (95% CI: 0.80%–3.60%) during the first 24 hours after delivery. The estimated mean incidence of recurrent venous thromboembolism during pregnancy was 1.97% (95% CI: 0.88%–3.49%).

Because the prevalence of CAPS is very low, randomized clinical trials on treatment have not been feasible. Recommendations for the management of CAPS during pregnancy or puerperium come from a small series of patients and previous expert-based

Table 4
Differential diagnosis of thrombotic microangiopathies during pregnancy

Syndrome	MAHA	Thrombocytopenia	Coagulopathy	Hypertension	Renal Disease	CNS Disease	ADAMTS13 Activity	Time of Onset
Preeclampsia	+	+	±	+++	+	+	Low	3rd trimester
HELLP	++	+++	+	±	+	±	Mild to moderate decreased	3rd trimester, occasionally during puerperium
HUS	+	++	±	±	+++	±	Low or absent	Puerperium
TTP	+++	+++	±	±	±	+++	Low (usually <5%) or absent	2nd trimester
AFLP	+	+	+++	±	±	+	NA	3rd trimester
CAPS	++	+++	++	+	++	+	NA	2nd and 3rd trimester and puerperium

Abbreviations: ADAMTS-13, von Willebrand factor-cleaving protease; AFLP, acute fatty liver of pregnancy; CAPS, catastrophic antiphospholipid syndrome; CNS, central nervous system; HELLP, hemolysis, liver enzymes elevation, and low platelets; HUS, hemolytic–uremic syndrome; MAHA, microangiopathic hemolytic anemia; NA, not available; TTP, thrombotic thrombocytopenic purpura.

(not evidence-based) recommendations for the management of CAPS. First, evaluate fetal maturation; once pulmonary maturation is present, a prompt caesarean intervention is recommended. Full anticoagulation should be started as soon as CAPS is suspected and reversed for the surgery, but it should be started again as soon as possible at the puerperium (depending on the surgical procedures and complications). Low-molecular-weight heparin could be the drug of choice for preventing obstetric complications and CAPS, because of its anticoagulant and anti-inflammatory properties. However, if thrombosis occurs close to labor, unfractionated heparin use is recommended because of its short duration and because it can be relatively easily reversed using protamine sulfate. Combined treatment with steroids, plasma exchange sessions, and/or intravenous immunoglobulins, as in other CAPS events, are also recommended. Because streptokinase and, probably, other thrombolytic agents do not cross the placenta, thrombolysis is another reasonable option for some particular scenarios, such as massive pulmonary embolism.[9]

Several additional treatments have been used in patients with refractory CAPS, including rituximab, defibrotide, and eculizumab[16]; however, none of them have been used during pregnancy or puerperium. Eculizumab, a humanized monoclonal antibody against complement protein C5, is currently approved for the treatment of paroxysmal nocturnal hemoglobinuria and is a promising therapy in CAPS.

It is important to bear in mind that preterm delivery is the strongest risk factor for an adverse neonatal outcome, but it can be life saving for the mother and the fetus.

After the resolution of a CAPS episode, the patient must continue long-term anticoagulation as secondary thromboprophylaxis, but steroids should be tapered and plasma exchange sessions and intravenous immunoglobulins stopped.

Patients with a previous history of CAPS should be advised on the risks of pregnancy as trigger of a new CAPS episode. If the general clinical situation does not contraindicate pregnancy, full anticoagulation with heparin and aspirin should be prescribed during pregnancy and puerperium. Regarding delivery management, these patients can undergo an attempt at vaginal delivery with cesarean birth done for usual obstetric indications or if a new CAPS episode is suspected.

ACKNOWLEDGMENTS

The authors thank Dr Ignasi Rodríguez for his work in the management of the CAPS Registry.

REFERENCES

1. Branch DW, Khamashta MA. Antiphospholipid syndrome: obstetric diagnosis, management, and controversies. Obstet Gynecol 2003;101(6):1333–44.
2. Cervera R, Balasch J. The management of pregnant patients with antiphospholipid syndrome. Lupus 2004;13(9):683–7.
3. Carmona F, Balasch J. Obstetric complications of antiphospholipid syndrome. In: Asherson RA, Cervera R, editors. The antiphospholipid syndrome II: autoimmune thrombosis. Amsterdam: Elsevier; 2000. p. 205–11.
4. Martinez-Zamora MA, Peralta S, Creus M, et al. Risk of thromboembolic events after recurrent spontaneous abortion in antiphospholipid syndrome: a case-control study. Ann Rheum Dis 2012;71(1):61–6.
5. Jacobsen AF, Skjeldestad FE, Sandset PM. Incidence and risk patterns of venous thromboembolism in pregnancy and puerperium—a register-based case-control study. Am J Obstet Gynecol 2008;198(2):233.e1–7.

6. Brenner B. Haemostatic changes in pregnancy. Thromb Res 2004;114(5–6): 409–14.

7. Toglia MR, Weg JG. Venous thromboembolism during pregnancy. N Engl J Med 1996;335(2):108–14.

8. Gomez-Puerta JA, Sanin-Blair J, Galarza-Maldonado C. Pregnancy and catastrophic antiphospholipid syndrome. Clin Rev Allergy Immunol 2009;36(2–3): 85–90.

9. Greer IA. Thrombosis in pregnancy: updates in diagnosis and management. Hematology Am Soc Hematol Educ Program 2012;2012:203–7.

10. Asherson RA. The catastrophic antiphospholipid syndrome. J Rheumatol 1992; 19(4):508–12.

11. Asherson RA, Cervera R, Piette JC, et al. Catastrophic antiphospholipid syndrome. Clinical and laboratory features of 50 patients. Medicine (Baltimore) 1998;77(3):195–207.

12. Asherson RA, Cervera R, Piette JC, et al. Catastrophic antiphospholipid syndrome: clues to the pathogenesis from a series of 80 patients. Medicine (Baltimore) 2001;80(6):355–77.

13. Cervera R, Bucciarelli S, Plasin MA, et al. Catastrophic antiphospholipid syndrome (CAPS): descriptive analysis of a series of 280 patients from the "CAPS Registry". J Autoimmun 2009;32(3–4):240–5.

14. Gomez-Puerta JA, Cervera R, Espinosa G, et al. Pregnancy and puerperium are high susceptibility periods for the development of catastrophic antiphospholipid syndrome. Autoimmun Rev 2006;6(2):85–8.

15. Espinosa G, Rodriguez-Pinto I, Gomez-Puerta JA, et al. Relapsing catastrophic antiphospholipid syndrome: potential role of microangiopathic hemolytic anemia in disease relapses(1). Semin Arthritis Rheum 2012. [Epub ahead of print].

16. Espinosa G, Berman H, Cervera R. Management of refractory cases of catastrophic antiphospholipid syndrome. Autoimmun Rev 2011;10(11):664–8.

17. Gomez-Puerta JA, Cervera R, Espinosa G, et al. Catastrophic antiphospholipid syndrome during pregnancy and puerperium: maternal and fetal characteristics of 15 cases. Ann Rheum Dis 2007;66(6):740–6.

18. Asherson RA, Espinosa G, Cervera R, et al. Disseminated intravascular coagulation in catastrophic antiphospholipid syndrome: clinical and haematological characteristics of 23 patients. Ann Rheum Dis 2005;64(6):943–6.

19. Cervera R, Espinosa G, Bucciarelli S, et al. Lessons from the catastrophic antiphospholipid syndrome (CAPS) registry. Autoimmun Rev 2006;6(2):81–4.

20. Hughes GR, Khamashta MA. Seronegative antiphospholipid syndrome. Ann Rheum Dis 2003;62(12):1127.

21. Asherson RA, Cervera R, de Groot PG, et al. Catastrophic antiphospholipid syndrome: international consensus statement on classification criteria and treatment guidelines. Lupus 2003;12(7):530–4.

22. Cervera R, Font J, Gomez-Puerta JA, et al. Validation of the preliminary criteria for the classification of catastrophic antiphospholipid syndrome. Ann Rheum Dis 2005;64(8):1205–9.

23. Erkan D, Espinosa G, Cervera R. Catastrophic antiphospholipid syndrome: updated diagnostic algorithms. Autoimmun Rev 2010;10(2):74–9.

24. Espinosa G, Bucciarelli S, Cervera R, et al. Thrombotic microangiopathic haemolytic anaemia and antiphospholipid antibodies. Ann Rheum Dis 2004;63(6):730–6.

25. Romualdi E, Dentali F, Rancan E, et al. Anticoagulant therapy for venous thromboembolism during pregnancy: a systematic review and a meta-analysis of the literature. J Thromb Haemost 2013;11(2):270–81.

Index

Note: Page numbers of article titles are in **boldface** type.

A

Abruptio placentae, in factor V Leiden, 379–380
Acute fatty liver of pregnancy, 336
Acute myocardial infarction, 246–247, 250–251
ADAMTS13 deficiency, thrombocytopenia in, 333–335
Allograft monitoring, in pregnant, diabetic, renal transplant patients, 261
Alpha-fetoprotein, in aneuploidy screening, 272, 274–275
American Diabetes Association classification, of diabetic
    complications, 244
Anemia, **281–291**
    aplastic, 288–289
    autoimmune hemolytic, 287
    classification of, 283–284
    clinical presentation of, 283
    hemolytic. *See* Hemolytic anemia.
    hereditary spherocytosis and elliptocytosis, 286–287
    in glucose-6-phosphate dehydrogenase deficiency, 287–288
    iron deficiency, 285
    macrocytic, 284–285
    megaloblastic, 284–286
    microcytic, 284
    normocytic, 284
    paroxysmal nocturnal hemoglobinuria, 289–290
    pathogenesis of, 283
    physiologic, 281–283
    red cell morphology classification of, 283–285
    sickle cell, **293–310**
    sideroblastic, 284, 286
Anencephaly, in diabetic embryopathy, 210
Anesthesia, regional
    anticoagulant use and, 351
    in thrombocytopenia, 332
Aneuploidy screening, in diabetes mellitus, **271–280**
    cell-free fetal DNA in, 277
    factors affecting, 273–274
    false-positive rates in, 277
    first-trimester, 275–277
    history of, **272**
    overview of, 273
    second-trimester, 274–275
    serum methods for, 274–277

Clin Lab Med 33 (2013) 401–411
http://dx.doi.org/10.1016/S0272-2712(13)00043-7
0272-2712/13/$ – see front matter © 2013 Elsevier Inc. All rights reserved.

labmed.theclinics.com

Moving?

Make sure your subscription moves with you!

To notify us of your new address, find your **Clinics Account Number** (located on your mailing label above your name), and contact customer service at:

Email: journalscustomerservice-usa@elsevier.com

800-654-2452 (subscribers in the U.S. & Canada)
314-447-8871 (subscribers outside of the U.S. & Canada)

Fax number: 314-447-8029

Elsevier Health Sciences Division
Subscription Customer Service
3251 Riverport Lane
Maryland Heights, MO 63043

ELSEVIER

Printed and bound by CPI Group (UK) Ltd, Croydon, CR0 4YY

22/10/2024

01777749-0001